Medical Child Abuse

Beyond Munchausen Syndrome by Proxy

Thomas A. Roesler, MD
Carole Jenny, MD, MBA, FAAP

Editor: Diane E. Beausoleil
Copy Editor: Kate Larson
Marketing Manager: Linda Smessaert
Production Manager: Theresa Wiener
Design: Linda Diamond
Production: Mary Williamson

Library of Congress Control Number: 2008935843
ISBN: 978-1-58110-136-2
MA0280

The recommendations in this publication do not indicate an exclusive course of treatment or serve as a standard of care. Variations, taking into account individual circumstances, may be appropriate.

Copyright © 2009 American Academy of Pediatrics. All Rights Reserved. No part of this publication may be reproduced or transmitted in any form or by any means, electronic or mechanical, including photocopying, recording, or any information retrieval system without written permission form the publisher (fax permissions editor at 847/434-8780).

The Licensed Material is being used for illustrative purposes only and any person depicted in the Licensed Material is a model.

Printed in the United States of America.

9-203/0908

Last digit is the print number: 9 8 7 6 5 4 3 2 1

TO BILL, BETTY, VANCE, AND ALICE

Contents

	Acknowledgments	vii
	Introduction	1
Chapter 1	The Case for a New Paradigm	17
Chapter 2	Medical Child Abuse	43
Chapter 3	How Did We Get Here?	61
Chapter 4	Uncommon Manifestations of Battered Child Syndrome	77
Chapter 5	Why Has It Taken So Long?	93
Chapter 6	So, Why *Do* They Do It?	111
Chapter 7	Description of 115 Cases Referred for Possible Munchausen Syndrome by Proxy	131
Chapter 8	Introduction to Treatment	155
Chapter 9	Identifying Medical Child Abuse	165
Chapter 10	Stopping the Abuse	199
Chapter 11	Providing for Ongoing Safety	219
Chapter 12	Treating the Physical Consequences	239
Chapter 13	Treating the Psychological Consequences	259
Chapter 14	Physicians as Part of the Problem	279
Chapter 15	Lawyers as Part of the Solution	293
Chapter 16	Where Do We Go From Here?	309
	Index	327

Acknowledgments

Our friends, family, and colleagues know that the ideas presented in this book have been evolving over a number of years. They have seen us through seemingly endless visions and revisions. As a result we feel honored and obligated to acknowledge many people who have helped advised, supported, tolerated, disagreed with, and encouraged us.

We have exposed the concepts in this book to many audiences over the past few years by deciding early on to talk about medical child abuse to any group that expressed interest. Sometimes the response was warm and inviting. Other times we met skepticism and disbelief. The result was a continuous, rolling process of peer review that we think has resulted in a much better book.

Having said this, we also realize that it continues to be a work in progress. We go to press thinking of new contradictions, new issues, and new examples that seem to prove or disprove a point. We hope the book promotes interest in the ideas expressed but also stimulates people to engage in a fierce but friendly debate.

It is appropriate to begin acknowledgments by thanking our family, especially our children, siblings, nephews, and nieces, for letting us borrow their names (without their knowledge) to identify our case examples.

Staff of our respective programs have been constantly involved not only in the evaluation and treatment of children suspected of having been medically abused but also in helping us give birth to the concepts included here. Michelle Rickerby, Pamela High, Jack Nassau, Robyn Mehlenbeck, Kristin Bruning, Patricia Flam, Francesca Pingitori, Mary-Ellen Mullin, Mary Anne Costello, Kerry Burke, Lynn Pascale, Ana Santos, Donna Silva, Christine Haddad, Diane DerMarderosian, Heather Chapman, Ann Boland, John Peterson, Tracy Bergeron, Lauren Minotis, Ayana Bass, and Linda Vieira all held things together at the Hasbro Children's Partial Hospital Program while Tom took a sabbatical to work on this project.

Staff from the ChildSafe program, including Christine Barron, Amy Goldberg, Kathy Fitzgerald, Jane Ferguson, Laurie Sawyer, Maryellen Ouellette, and a number of current and prior Fellows in Child Protection have protected Carole from herself on too many occasions.

In addition to her role as best friend and confidant Michelle Rickerby read and commented on several drafts of the book. Other readers include Gregory Fritz, Pamela High, Suzanne Starling, Tom Dwyer, Kim Oats, Mary Sawicki, and John Stirling. Reena Isaac and Debra Ersenio-Jenssen have been on the forefront of applying medical child abuse concepts in the legal arena.

Our greatest thanks go to Tim David and Alex Levin, who both did critical reviews of the manuscript.

We also want to acknowledge colleagues who have made so many contributions to understanding child abuse in the medical setting. Some of these people are friends, others are acquaintances, and others we know only through their writings.

Roy Meadow, Donna Rosenberg, Randell Alexander, David Southall, Alex Levin, Mary Sheridan, Herbert Schrier, Judith Libow, and Marc Feldman are only some of the pioneers in this field. No one can begin to understand this kind of child abuse without reading their work and appreciating their insights.

So many others have made major contributions. Terence Donald and Jon Jureidini wrote papers over a decade ago that we could have used as an outline for this book. Mary Eminson, Robert Postlethwaite, Christian Bools, Robert McClure, David Jones, Kenneth Feldman, Tona McGuire, James Griffith, and Catherine Ayoub are all names you will see often in the following pages.

Colin Morley, Mary Bryk, Stephen Boros, Geoffrey Fisher, Ian Mitchell, Jenny Gray, Arnon Bentovim, Teresa Parnell, Kathryn Artingstall, David Hall, Paul Hyman, Birgit Berg, Martin Samuels, Thomas Truman, David Beck, Beatrice Yorker, Gwen Adshead, and David Waller have all made major contributions. These are only a few of the people whose ideas have nurtured our thoughts.

Mary Sanders came to National Jewish Hospital 15 years ago and helped us see things differently. With Brenda Bursch she wrote the best guide to understanding complex cases and coming to thoughtful and fair conclusions.

We certainly must also thank Diane Beausoleil, our editor; Kate Larson, our copy editor; and Mark Grimes and others at the American Academy of Pediatrics for their help in making this book a reality.

Most of all we want to acknowledge C. Henry Kempe, Carole's first mentor who was also instrumental in promoting Tom and Carole's long collaboration.

Thomas A. Roesler
Carole Jenny

Decatur Island, WA

Introduction

The protective obligation of parents, particularly mothers, toward their children may be one of the few universally accepted obligations in society. —Levin and Sheridan, 1995[1]

Medical child abuse occurs when a child receives unnecessary and harmful or potentially harmful medical care at the instigation of a caretaker. In this book we describe how to identify and treat medical child abuse. But before we do this we must clear away some confusing thinking that has caused problems for the medical and child protection communities for decades. We have subtitled this book *Beyond Munchausen Syndrome by Proxy*. We think, and many of our colleagues agree, that it is time to stop using, once and for all, the term *Munchausen syndrome by proxy (MSBP)*. Munchausen syndrome by proxy and its other names, including *factitious disorder by proxy* and *pediatric condition falsification,* have outlived their usefulness. In this book we make the case that what we have been calling MSBP is simply a form of child abuse, having much more in common with other types of child abuse than it has characteristics that set it apart.

True, it has always been assumed that MSBP is child abuse. However, when MSBP was first described our understanding of child abuse was still in its infancy. We have in the intervening years come to learn a great deal about the ways children can be harmed by caretakers. There have been significant advances in our ability to diagnose and treat many types of child abuse. But during this time the term *MSBP* and the understanding of what it meant seemed to set it apart from other forms of child maltreatment. It came to be assumed, or so it seems, that there was child abuse and then there was also MSBP. Somehow the violation of the rules of parenting seen in this type of child abuse was of a different nature than when children were physically, sexually, or emotionally abused by their parents. We feel looking back from the perspective of 3 decades that the child protection community, and in particular physicians and other medical personnel responsible for identifying child abuse, took a wrong turn in 1977 and it has taken this long to get back on track.

An incident occurred approximately 15 years ago that marked a major turning point in our thinking. We were discussing with a prosecuting attorney the case of a child who had experienced 22 life-threatening events in the hospital while in the presence of his mother. The mother had devised a way to make her child aspirate liquids. He would be perfectly well one minute, begin coughing, turn blue, and then begin a several-day process of recovery from aspiration pneumonia. At one point he ended up on a respirator for 5 days and we feared that he had experienced severe hypoxic brain damage. Although no one ever observed her in the act, we concluded that she gave her child a drink from her ever-present can of soda, held his nose, and in doing so caused him to inhale the liquid. The result ranged from vigorous coughing that resolved in a few minutes to pneumonia requiring intubation.

We helped make the decision that security personnel escort the mother from the hospital while keeping the child safe on the ward. Next we petitioned the court on behalf of the boy for a no-contact order to ensure the mother would not be allowed to visit. When we told the prosecuting attorney the child had experienced near fatal child abuse, he responded, "Oh really? I thought this was a Munchausen by proxy case." The bright, inquisitive attorney had been doing his homework and had read that the problem in cases like this was that mothers had their own needs met by having their children be sick. He had never prosecuted a "Munchausen by proxy case" before and was anxiously preparing himself. We wanted his help in ensuring the mother not have a chance to kill her child. He wanted to talk about the mother's fascinating and strange behavior. We went away thinking that somehow we all had our priorities backward. Our response to this event was to begin a period of questioning ourselves, researching what others had to say about MSBP and, eventually, to write this book.

It has been more than 30 years since Roy Meadow, a pediatric nephrologist from Great Britain, published the first paper describing what he called

Munchausen syndrome by proxy.[2] In that paper he documented 2 children whose illnesses had long gone undiagnosed. In one instance a 6-year-old girl underwent multiple evaluations over many years for recurrent urinary tract infections and hematuria, or bloody urine. Once he came to the realization that the mother might be the source of the problem, Meadow was able, by some careful detective work, to determine that the child's mother had handled the only urine samples that contained blood. By contaminating the child's urine with her own bloody urine the mother had created a situation where her child required multiple diagnostic tests, many of which were intrusive and potentially dangerous. The second child was a toddler who died of salt poisoning. His confusing symptoms made sense if one concluded that the child might be receiving a lethal dose of salt from his diet. The only person who could have given him the salt was his own mother.

The subtitle of Meadow's original paper was "The Hinterland of Child Abuse." In the intervening decades, MSBP has moved from "the hinterland" to the mainstream of public awareness. American television newsmagazine programs such as *20/20* have featured stories about MSBP. Munchausen syndrome by proxy has entered popular culture. A Hollywood movie, *The Sixth Sense,* had as part of its plot a child who "saw" through his special powers a dead child showing him where she hid a video she made of her mother poisoning her. Jonathan Kellerman[3] made MSBP a central theme of his novel, *The Devils Waltz.* The popular singer Eminem wrote and performed a song about his own experience as a victim of MSBP at the hands of his mother. The autobiography of Julie Gregory,[4] *Sickened,* is subtitled, *The Memoir of a Munchausen by Proxy Childhood.* In it she detailed what it was like to grow up in an abusive environment where, among other things, she and her mother tried to deceive doctors into giving her medical care, including heart surgery she did not need. In Great Britain, news stories regarding MSBP have been a staple both in the popular press and for special programs broadcast by the BBC.

In this country there has been a series of widely publicized cases such as that of Kathy Bush in Florida[5] or Laurie Williamson in Texas.[6] Kathy Bush's daughter, Jennifer, had more than 200 hospitalizations, more than 40 surgeries, multiple bouts of polymicrobial sepsis (bloodstream infections with several different bacteria at the same time), and numerous other illnesses that went away soon after she was removed from her mother's care. Her mother took Jennifer to meet Hillary Clinton at the White House during the debate regarding access to health care. Newspaper articles about Jennifer and her mother appeared in the Florida press for many years.

A simple computer search today yields more than 400 articles regarding MSBP in the medical literature. The medical community has documented innumerable ways in which children can be hurt through receiving harmful and unnecessary medical care. A Google search using the term *Munchausen syndrome by proxy* generated 195,000 citations, with the first reference being a Web site sponsored by MAMA (Mothers Against Munchausen syndrome by proxy Allegations). This group provides a rallying point for parents who feel they have been unjustly accused. Clearly, the concept of MSBP is no longer obscure, no longer lurking in the hinterlands.

Yet, while MSBP has assumed a presence in the public consciousness, by no means is the concept well understood. Not only the public but also the medical community continues to have difficulty understanding just what MSBP might be. Typically people respond to a mention of MSBP by saying, "Isn't that where the mother makes her child sick?" Invariably someone will raise the question, "How could a mother ever do such a thing?" Or, conversely, "How could the doctor keep doing all those tests when he thought nothing was really wrong?" Physicians, when confronted with MSBP, for reasons we are just now beginning to comprehend, react as if they are discovering something entirely new—not something we have been discussing for nearly 30 years.

One manifestation of this confusion is a backlash phenomenon currently underway in Great Britain. There is a movement to retry a large number of cases where children were removed from their parents after MSBP was diagnosed.[7] Prominent physicians, including Roy Meadow himself, and David Southall, who has documented, using covert video surveillance, dozens of children being smothered by their parents, have come under considerable scrutiny because of their testimony in MSBP cases. Southall has had an extremely difficult road. He had his privileges restricted and then reinstated after a 2-year investigation of his work. The investigation cost more than 750,000 British pounds.[8] Subsequently he was accused again of serious professional misconduct and was struck from the medical register (lost his license to practice medicine.)[9]

Roy Meadow has been writing and lecturing about MSBP ever since he submitted the first paper in 1977. His research has been widely admired and even led to his being knighted for his work on behalf of children. He was elected the first president of the Royal College of Paediatrics and Child Health in Great Britain. Recently, an inquiry into his testimony given in a high-profile case led to his being stricken from the register of physicians in Great Britain. He was accused of misusing statistics in a way that resulted in a mother being found guilty of smothering her child. The mother was subsequently acquitted when it was determined that evidence was withheld in the original trial. Fortunately, Meadow appealed the decision by the General Medical Council and was eventually reinstated.[9]

We feel that MSBP is no longer a useful concept, and that Meadow, by inventing it, helped to create an environment that has been counterproductive, and in his own case, disastrous. Yet, the reader will surely appreciate from our many references to his work in the coming pages how much we respect his contributions. He has always shown the greatest empathy for mothers and has been most thoughtful in his observations. He has been the voice of reason, bringing people back from extreme positions. We agree wholeheartedly with the editorial in *Lancet*[10] that censuring Meadow was wrong. We also agree that decisions by the General Medical Council could have the effect of significantly undermining efforts to protect an entire generation of children.[11]

Let us be clear. In saying that it is time to stop using the term *Munchausen syndrome by proxy,* in no way are we suggesting that children are not the victims of child abuse. The boy we wanted to protect from his mother almost died because of what she did to him. Furthermore, because she lied about what she was doing, he was subjected to many dangerous medical procedures. Meadow was unable to save the life of the little boy he described in his original paper. Decades later he learned that the mother of the boy, who had training as a nurse, confessed to using a tube she inserted in his nose to give him the salt solution that killed him.[12]

In writing this book we intend to give no specific comfort to parents who have subjected their children to unnecessary and harmful or potentially harmful medical care. Indeed, our primary concern has to do with their children. Our object is to turn the focus of concern away from what parents might be thinking or feeling toward what their children are experiencing.

The purpose of this book is to reintegrate the evaluation and treatment of this particular kind of child abuse into the general field of child maltreatment. We do offer parents who previously abused their children medically and who truly want their children to be healthy and happy an opportunity to reestablish a collaborative partnership with the medical care community and to participate in the *appropriate* medical treatment of their children. And we hope to offer our medical colleagues a conceptual framework that allows them to enter into this collaborative partnership whenever possible.

To do this we have written essentially 2 different books. The first book makes the case for bringing what has been called MSBP back into the mainstream as medical child abuse. The second starts with the premise that we are evaluating and treating child abuse and details our experience over the last 15 years with more than a hundred children referred for possible medical child abuse.

In the first book we begin with the state of things as they are today. Even though almost 3 decades have passed, the field has more questions than answers. Is MSBP really an illness? If it is, what should we call it? If it is an illness and we have a name for it, how serious is it, how prevalent is it, and can it be treated? If it is not an illness, what have we been talking about all this time? These questions and more, and evidence for both sides of the controversy, make up Chapter 1. This discussion provides a justification for undergoing a thorough reevaluation of the concept as we attempt to move beyond MSBP.

By now, Kuhn's [13] concept of paradigm shift as it pertains to the development of scientific thought has become well accepted. He advanced the idea that the progress of scientific thinking is a balance between organizing concepts, "paradigms," and facts to support them. As we make more observations, we gather more facts. Sometimes we continue to preserve an organizing concept long after it fails to incorporate all the facts successfully. At a certain point, however, the edifice comes tumbling down. Facts no longer fit. The balance between theory and observation has been lost. We need to apply a new paradigm. We are at that point now with MSBP. Chapter 1 documents how unwieldy the concept has become.

Chapter 2 describes the new conceptual framework, medical child abuse. The test of any new paradigm is whether it can make clear what previously was confusing. Usually a new paradigm will seem straightforward, almost simple, compared with the one it is replacing. Such is the case with medical child abuse. In Chapter 2 we define medical child abuse as a child receiving unnecessary and harmful, or potentially harmful, medical care at the instigation of a caretaker. A child who has been purposefully suffocated is the victim of a physical assault. If that child undergoes an intrusive and potentially harmful medical procedure, bronchoscopy for example, because a parent deceived the doctor, the child is the victim of medical child abuse perpetrated by the parent. The doctor is the implement the parent uses to carry out the abuse.

We document the many ways medical child abuse is similar to physical child abuse, sexual child abuse, or psychological child abuse. Of course, there are ways in which medical child abuse is distinct from other forms of abuse, but they are few. We also make the case that medical child abuse is totally distinct from malpractice. In malpractice doctors provide bad medical care, care that does not meet the standards of treatment usually offered by other physicians in the community. With medical child abuse, the physician administers usual and customary, appropriate, well-intentioned treatment based on the information available to him or her provided by the caretaker.

Once having described the new concept, we find it necessary to go back and explore how, over 3 decades, we arrived at this point. A number of competent and thoughtful clinicians and researchers have been engaged in this debate. Why do we not have more to show for our efforts? The history of MSBP as a concept is covered in the next 2 chapters. That history is part of the larger picture of the medical community's awareness regarding child abuse.

Many people mark the beginning of child abuse as a pediatric concern to a groundbreaking paper by C. Henry Kempe and colleagues[14] in 1962 titled "The Battered Child Syndrome." In 1975 Kempe followed with "Unusual Manifestations of the Battered Child Syndrome," in which he invited his pediatric colleagues to be aware of unusual ways in which children might be maltreated.[15] Among the 20 or so published accounts by pediatricians that appeared over the next few years in response to his request for descriptions of unique forms of child abuse was the paper by Meadow published in 1977.

Chapter 3 describes the early years. We document the level of interest in these forms of child abuse prior to 1977 and the publication of "Munchausen

Syndrome by Proxy: The Hinterland of Child Abuse." Over the 5-year period between 1977 and 1982 pediatricians began mentioning more and more frequently, in their descriptions of unusual cases, *Munchausen syndrome by proxy*. For many people, the term seemed to crystallize their thoughts and concerns regarding this form of child abuse.

But the literature continued to be anecdotal. We were treated to carefully described case histories, one more fascinating than the next, elaborating the numerous ways in which parents could harm their children in a medical setting. Missing from this discussion were the "everyday cases." Almost in passing authors made mention of how common it was to see a parent who exaggerated their child's symptoms even to the point of putting the child in harm's way, or described a parent who refused to follow prescribed treatment, or who overused prescribed medications. For the most part, the cases we read about in medical journals involved children being poisoned many times. What about the child who might have been poisoned only once?

There is a term, *availability heuristic*,[16,17] that describes the difficulty of trying to make generalizations from a series of extreme cases. If one looks down from an airplane at the tops of mountains sticking up through the clouds and never sees the valleys between them, it is difficult to describe the terrain in a meaningful way. This has been one of our problems in trying to understand this particular type of abusive health-seeking behavior. Chapter 3 ends with the publication, in 1987, of a paper by Rosenberg titled "Web of Deceit: A Literature Review of Munchausen Syndrome by Proxy."[18] In it she summarized information from 117 cases. Her view of the mountaintops has had a significant impact on thinking regarding MSBP.

In Chapter 4 we discuss developments in characterizing specific illnesses, the "uncommon manifestations of the battered child syndrome" referred to by Kempe. In a way, this chapter describes how the field might have developed had the term *MSBP* never been introduced. It documents how much we have learned about many ways parents can abuse their children in a medical setting. We discuss specific symptom presentations, such as polymicrobial sepsis and recurrent apnea, which are associated with children experiencing unnecessary and harmful medical care.

In the next 2 chapters we conclude our effort to reintegrate medical child abuse into the larger framework of child maltreatment by addressing 2 important questions. The first, discussed in Chapter 5, involves why it took so long for the medical and child abuse communities to realize that MSBP as a concept was not working and that a simple solution was readily at hand. We show that many thoughtful participants in the debate had questions along the way and gave answers similar to what we are proposing today. We offer our answer to the question by describing how the medical profession has responded to discovering its own involvement in the abuse.

As physicians become involved in the investigation of most forms of child abuse the first question is, "What happened to the child?" and then, "What has to happen to make it stop?" Once these questions have been addressed one can examine, "Why did it happen?" In medical child abuse the tendency is to reverse the order of concern and jump prematurely to "why." We think this is the result of the medical profession's profound sense of guilt and shame about having been induced to do something harmful to a child.

In Chapter 6 we ask and answer the question, "What about motivation?" Because there has been so much attention focused on the motivation of perpetrators of this kind of child maltreatment, experts have advanced many hypotheses. We review psychological and sociological theories. We look at how and why patients lie to their physicians and how some families have a tradition of expressing feelings through physical symptoms.

We conclude that the reasons for perpetrating this type of abuse do not differ much from other forms of child maltreatment and that in the end the most important question is, "What does one need to know to protect the child?"

With the discussion of these 2 topics, "Why did it take so long?" and, "What about motivation?" we bring to a close the theoretical discussion. We hope we have convinced the reader to reconceptualize MSBP as a specific type of child abuse, one that can respond to evaluation and treatment strategies used in other forms of child maltreatment. But we have a lot of work left to do.

Book 2 (Chapter 7) begins with a summary of our involvement in 115 cases over the past 12 years. We present the data from a retrospective chart review involving evaluation and treatment of children who, at some point, were considered to be suffering from MSBP. These children and their families have in common only the fact that someone suspected MSBP.

Many of them meet our criteria for medical child abuse. Others do not. Some have died from assault at the hands of their parents. In other cases we found ourselves dealing with an anxious parent, a manipulative child, or a frustrated referring physician. Because of this range of presentations, we feel our experience with these children and families represents the situation one is more likely to face in the real world. This is our attempt to look at both the peaks and valleys to understand the terrain.

We looked at the diagnoses treated, the medical treatment the children received, and whether objective medical signs and symptoms could justify the care. We examined the behaviors of caretakers that precipitated care and documented evidence of illness exaggeration, illness fabrication, and illness induction. We determined the extent of involvement with the child protection system. In this chapter we include clinical vignettes of youngsters who then get discussed in detail in subsequent chapters as part of the description of the management of medical child abuse.

Continuing with the theme that medical child abuse is a subset of child maltreatment, we begin the discussion of the evaluation and treatment of medical abuse with some general principles regarding treatment of all types of child abuse. There are 5 basic steps in child protection. The first is to identify the child who is being harmed or is at risk of being harmed. The second is to stop the harm. The third step is to ensure that the harm will not resume (ie, that one can maintain ongoing safety of the child). The fourth step is to treat the physical and psychological consequences of the abuse. Finally, we want to accomplish these 4 steps while maintaining, as best we can, the integrity of the family unit. All of these principles apply in the treatment of medical child abuse.

Chapter 8 introduces 2 early cases that exemplify these principles but also call attention to some special features of medical child abuse. We wish to make the point that successful evaluation and treatment of medical child abuse must build on the strategies we have developed for dealing with other forms of child maltreatment. If we were to invent an entirely new system to treat medical abuse the task would be overwhelming. Fortunately, a well-established system to protect children exists in most developed countries, and the use of this system is the key to proceeding successfully.

The next chapter is the first of 5 addressing aspects of evaluation and treatment of child abuse. Chapter 9 deals with identifying abuse. Everything follows from this step. Treatment cannot proceed if the child being abused is not recognized. We emphasize the necessity of practicing good medicine, and in doing so keeping in mind the possibility that one might not be receiving accurate medical information from caretakers. We discuss the varying perspectives of primary care and specialty care physicians engaged in the evaluation of medical abuse.

In many cases it is the physician providing care who must determine that the medical care being offered is harmful. At a certain point the treatment relationship changes from working with the family to feeling a need to protect the child. We discuss treatment strategies that serve as diagnostic indicators. In addition, in this chapter we discuss specific issues in identifying medical abuse such as the use of covert video surveillance.

In Chapter 10 we discuss stopping the abuse. Because there is a continuum of presentations of medical abuse from mild to severe, as with other types of child maltreatment, steps required to stop the abuse differ depending on the severity. With medical child abuse, however, there is the special situation that medical care previously given must be stopped, and a new, revised treatment program established. Central to this process is the need to develop a consensus of the medical professionals before beginning a new treatment protocol. A specific technique that has come to be called *the informing session* is presented in detail. We also discuss how to involve the child protection community, and in particular the multidisciplinary, hospital-based, child protection team.

The child protection team is the cornerstone of an effective child protection network. Our team meets weekly and involves pediatricians specializing in child abuse, child psychiatrists, and pediatric specialists from our tertiary care children's hospital. Representatives of the local child protection agency, police, prosecutors, and other community resources interested in child protection attend regularly.

It is widely recognized that attempting to evaluate and treat child abuse without the use of a multidisciplinary team is almost impossible. Medical child abuse is still an unusual presentation for our team. The weekly meeting is typically taken up dealing with children with bad physical injuries, allegations of sexual abuse, and issues regarding neglect. Because medical child abuse comes up less frequently, it is all the more incumbent on the medical team to help other multidisciplinary team members understand the complex medical and psychological issues. In this chapter we detail the process of bringing the community into focus to enable it to deal with this more unusual type of child abuse.

Chapter 11 takes up the next principle of child abuse treatment, ensuring that the abuse does not reoccur. Consistent with treatment for other types of abuse we follow the guideline that one should provide the minimum intervention necessary to guarantee the ongoing safety of the child. We discuss the pros and cons of hospitalization and other out of home placements, medical foster care, and termination of parental rights.

While treatment of medical child abuse clearly involves identification and interruption of the maltreatment, it also includes dealing with the consequences of the abuse. In chapters 12 and 13 we take up treatment of the psychological and physical damage experienced by the child. As noted earlier, all phases of child abuse treatment need to take into consideration the protection of the child in the least restrictive environment. This usually means working with the strengths of the family unit to reconstitute the family as completely as possible while maintaining the safety of the child.

Many of the children in our series were evaluated and treated in a specialized pediatric/child psychiatric treatment environment that is particularly well suited to dealing with issues that span medical and emotional concerns. In Chapter 12 we describe this treatment program, with particular emphasis on the formation of a therapeutic environment capable of dealing with the types of family dysfunction represented by the perpetrators and victims of medical abuse. In our treatment program we address issues of many types of patients, including teenagers with diabetes and behavioral issues, grade school–aged children with long-standing failure to thrive, and a host of other medical/psychiatric problems. Within this environment a child with an unexplained medical condition who lives in a family with intense emotional needs feels welcome and appreciated. We share our experience and discuss some of the difficulties in duplicating our treatment model.

Chapter 13 deals with the treatment of psychological sequelae of medical child abuse. Children abused by receiving harmful medical care respond in the same way as other maltreated children. They experience the abuse as a betrayal by caretakers that affects their ability to make ongoing relationships. They exhibit symptoms of post-traumatic stress disorder (PTSD) and the depression and anxiety symptoms that often accompany PTSD. And they develop cognitive distortions, adaptations to a life situation that result in making choices such as participating in the unnecessary medical treatment–seeking behavior introduced by their caretaker. We give examples of these consequences of medical child abuse and outline treatment strategies.

In discussing our treatment model we make significant use of the cases reviewed in our case series. Obviously, a child who needs to be removed from his home with parental rights terminated is going to represent a different treatment challenge than a youngster in a family where we are actively engaged in helping family members become functional enough to decrease their use of medical care to an appropriate level.

Chapter 14 we titled "Doctors as Part of the Problem." The feature of medical child abuse that distinguishes it most clearly from other forms of child maltreatment is the involvement of the medical community as the instrument of abuse. As a correlate, the medical community is essential in stopping medical abuse and ensuring that it does not reoccur. As befits their central role, doctors can be extremely helpful or somewhat obstructive. We have several illustrative examples of the strategies one sometimes finds necessary to generate a therapeutic network around the child needing protection from medical abuse.

When we were in medical school we were taught that incest was an extremely rare phenomenon. In fact, the child psychiatry text we used cited prevalence rates of one in a million. Since then we have come to understand that sexual abuse, including incest, is relatively common. Communicating this to other professionals including physicians and judicial personnel has been a long, slow process. That process, however, is far ahead of where we currently stand with regard to medical abuse. It may take another 10 years for us to educate our colleagues to the variety of presentations of medical child abuse and the degree of harm children can experience. In this chapter we share our experiences, including some prominent successes and some ignominious failures.

The companion chapter (Chapter 15) to our discussion of physician involvement is a description of "Lawyers as Part of the Solution." The point at which members of the medical profession move to advocate for a child needing protection from close family members often entails involving colleagues from the legal world, prosecuting attorneys or attorneys functioning as "guardians ad litem." They can be an asset or, in some situations, can make things worse for the children and families we are trying to help. In this chapter we will see how the use of "medical child abuse" in various jurisdictions around the country has simplified the judicial process and has begun to rewrite criminal code and child protection procedures.

In the final chapter, "Where Do We Go From Here," we offer some conclusions and discuss how the child protection community can incorporate medical abuse into their ongoing work. We make suggestions for research criteria and outline the areas where we think research is needed.

We want to take a minute to discuss the use of case material in writing this book. Events from the lives of literally hundreds of children and families have been published over the past 30 years in an attempt to understand the medical abuse phenomenon. In citing many of these cases we are republishing personal facts, descriptions of illnesses, and accounts of doctor-patient relationships. It is difficult to imagine writing a book of this nature without trying to understand the lives of real people, without attempting to make sense of sometimes painful truths. In addition to the case material that has been published previously, we have added numerous accounts from our personal experience with patients and their families.

In describing aggregate data, we have followed established research methodology including obtaining institutional review approval for chart review. However, when we use anecdotal information to illustrate a point, we have chosen to err on the side of protecting the identity of patients. To this end we have chosen to leave out specific identifying details, or we have purposefully changed information that might be used to recognize a child or family. We have taken care not to change details in a way that would affect the usefulness or meaning of the anecdote. We understand this stance leaves us open to charges of having fictionalized accounts. This is a risk we are willing to take for the sake of our patients. We ask the reader to keep faith with us.

What we have learned in working with these children, their families, and the medical community is that things are never as they seem. Despite all our efforts, the children perceived to be victims of medical abuse do not fit in one box. The children are as diverse as any other population of children seen in doctors' offices. The families they live in share no single set of identifying criteria. It is not easy to identify or categorize the motivations of the people who inflicted harm on their children. There do not seem to be any shortcuts. Each situation is like a ball of string. Once you begin pulling at one piece you become committed to untangling the entire ball.

References

1. Levin AV, Sheridan MS, eds. *Munchausen Syndrome by Proxy: Issues in Diagnosis and Treatment*. New York, NY: Lexington Books; 1995
2. Meadow R. Munchausen syndrome by proxy. The hinterland of child abuse. *Lancet.* 1977;2(8033):343-345
3. Kellerman J. *The Devil's Waltz*. New York, NY: Random House; 2003
4. Gregory J. *Sickened: The Memoir of a Munchausen by Proxy Childhood*. New York, NY: Bantam Books; 2003
5. Schreier H. On the importance of motivation in Munchausen by proxy: the case of Kathy Bush. *Child Abuse Negl.* 2002;26(5):537-549
6. Spring mother found guilty in child-injury trial. *Houston Chronicle*. April 25, 2008
7. Doward J. Ministers told child harm theory was flawed. *Observer.* January 25, 2004
8. White C. Leading UK paediatrician reinstated. *BMJ.* 2001;323(7318):885
9. Rose D. New guidance says doctors 'must be alert to signs of child abuse'. *The Times*. March 19, 2008
10. Horton R. A dismal and dangerous verdict against Roy Meadow. *Lancet.* 2005;366:277-278
11. Jenny C. The intimidation of British pediatricians. *Pediatrics.* 2007;119(4):797-799
12. Meadow SR. Who's to blame—mothers, Munchausen or medicine? *J R Coll Physicians Lond.* 1994;28(4):332-337
13. Kuhn TS. *The Structure of Scientific Revolutions*. Chicago, IL: University of Chicago Press; 1962
14. Kempe CH, Silverman FW, Steele BF, Droegemueller W, Silver H. The battered child syndrome. *JAMA.* 1962;181:17-24
15. Kempe CH. Uncommon manifestations of the battered child syndrome. *Am J Dis Child.* 1975;129:126-128
16. Rogers R. Diagnostic, explanatory, and detection models of Munchausen by proxy: extrapolations from malingering, and deception. *Child Abuse Negl.* 2004;28:225-238

17. Tversky A, Kahneman D. Availability: a heuristic for judging frequency and probability. In: Kahneman D, Slovic P, Teversky A, eds. *Judgement and Uncertainty: Heuristics and Biases.* Cambridge, UK: Cambridge University Press; 1982:163-178
18. Rosenberg DA. Web of deceit: a literature review of Munchausen syndrome by proxy. *Child Abuse Negl.* 1987;11(4):547-563

Chapter 1

The Case for a New Paradigm

Contrary to popular beliefs, this behavior is not rare and is not a syndrome of any known psychopathology. It is simply another, very dangerous, form of child abuse. —Boros et al, 1995[1]

Introduction

The term *Munchausen syndrome by proxy* (MSBP) was introduced early in the history of child abuse as a pediatric entity. It came into use when most child abuse was still referred to as *battered child syndrome*. While most of the field of child maltreatment has undergone continuous development toward conceptual clarification, the term *MSBP* has only become more problematic in its usage.

Roughly 10 years after C. Henry Kempe published about the battered child syndrome he recognized sexual abuse as another major subcategory of child maltreatment.[2] Physical and sexual abuse were soon joined in the literature by emotional or psychological abuse. The term *battered child syndrome* began to fade into the background. Subsequently, physical abuse underwent its own evolution as professionals recognized the importance of shaking infants in causing severe neurologic disease. The resulting illness presentation, *shaken baby syndrome*, is now more frequently referred to as a type of physical abuse, *abusive head trauma*.[3]

As we shall see, MSBP has had a number of synonyms. Yet, the concept the term represents has not evolved, as have other forms of child maltreatment. In this chapter we will discuss questions that remain unanswered regarding *MSBP*.

Is This Really a Syndrome?

For the general public denoting something as a syndrome is the same thing as calling it a disease. Meadow borrowed the "syndrome" part of his designation from Asher[4] who coined *Munchausen syndrome* as a tongue-in-cheek description of patients he felt had "hoodwinked" the medical profession. Meadow made no specific attempt in his initial paper to describe sentinel features of the new syndrome. Rosenberg,[5] however, in her review article was quite specific in her desire to describe a formal syndrome. She began by first explaining what constitutes a syndrome. She stated that a syndrome, in contrast to a disease, represents a "…cluster of symptoms and/or signs which are circumstantially related."

For her, the cluster of symptoms that define MSBP included[5]

"(1) Illness in a child which is simulated (faked) and/or produced by a parent or someone who is *in loco parentis;* and

(2) Presentation of the child for medical assessment and care, usually persistently, often resulting in multiple medical procedures; and

(3) Denial of knowledge by the perpetrator as to the etiology of the child's illness; and

(4) Acute symptoms and signs of the child abate when the child is separated from perpetrator."

Note that her initial cluster of symptoms *did not* include the motivation of the perpetrator, and *did* include a condition where the child must improve in the absence of the perpetrator. Child abuse professionals have long used clinical improvement in the absence of a potential perpetrator as confirmatory evidence that the condition was caused by that person. For example, a child with failure to thrive who begins gaining weight rapidly in the hospital while being fed by nurses is felt to require little other medical evaluation. The cause of the failure to thrive is assumed to be a product of the caretaker's difficulties with feeding. Rosenberg's criteria for MSBP as a syndrome have been used by many other authors.[6–17] More recently Rosenberg[18] has attempted to outline diagnostic criteria based on finding clear evidence of fabricated symptoms or induced symptoms. She has continued to pay little attention to motivation of the perpetrator. Meadow came to use Rosenberg's criteria, but he eventually added another condition involving the motivation of the perpetrator.[19]

Psychiatric diagnoses are codified in the diagnostic and statistical manual published by the American Psychiatric Association.[20] This manual is modified periodically. Munchausen syndrome by proxy was not mentioned in versions of the manual prior to 1994 when a determination was made to include what are referred to as "research criteria" for a possible designation as a diagnosis in future editions. *Diagnostic and Statistical Manual of Mental Disorders, Fourth Edition (DSM-IV)* included research criteria for *factitious disorder by proxy (FDP)*. These criteria are different from those of Rosenberg and make the motivation of the perpetrator a central feature.

They include

A. Intentional production or feigning of physical or psychological signs or symptoms in another person who is under the individual's care.

B. The motivation for the perpetrator's behavior is to assume the sick role by proxy.

C. External incentives for the behavior (such as economic gain) are absent.

D. The behavior is not better accounted for by another mental disorder.

The propriety of calling MSBP a syndrome has been challenged for many years. For example, Fisher and Mitchell[21] reiterated that a syndrome must include a grouping of specific symptoms that occur together in a number of patients. They observed that, instead of similar symptoms occurring in a number of patients, children said to have MSBP have a myriad of presenting symptoms. "The victims present with a wide variety of symptoms and signs indicating the possible presence of varied medical illnesses and the perpetrators demonstrate an extensive assortment of psychopathologic dysfunctions, syndromes, and illnesses."[21]

Fisher and Mitchell concluded that MSBP does not meet criteria for being considered a discrete medical syndrome. Rather, they describe it as a set of circumstances or "…'situations' of fabrication observed and described by pediatricians on the basis of history, examination, and investigation." In other words, what physicians have been calling MSBP can more accurately be described as a series of events in the life of the child, something happening to the child, observed by a physician and not a discrete medical illness or syndrome. They offer as a comparable example the way that we look at child neglect. "In child neglect there are various parental psychological problems that interfere with the parent's awareness of the child's physical and emotional needs and in such cases it is not asserted that the neglecting parent has a syndrome known as 'child neglect.' "

More recently an entire book has been written about the question. Titled *Disordered Mother or Disordered Diagnosis*? the volume by Allison and Roberts[22] reviews the MSBP literature with a specific eye toward dismantling MSBP as a diagnostic category. The rhetorical aim of the work is made clear by the dedication. The authors, both professors of philosophy, write, "This book is dedicated to those mothers who have been wrongly accused of criminal abuse and neglect because they suffered from a nonexistent disorder." Throughout the book the authors imply that children have not experienced criminal abuse and neglect due to the efforts of parents who dissimulate, fabricate symptoms, or induce symptoms in their children. The book is written from the perspective of the adult accused of suffering from MSBP. Nowhere does it mention the authors have ever been involved in the diagnosis and treatment of children who have been victimized. They do make a reasonable argument that to find a child has been abused, it is not logically necessary to diagnose a parent with MSBP. Concomitantly, child abuse can exist whether the parent has been diagnosed with MSBP, depression, substance abuse, a personality disorder, or with no diagnosis at all. Mart,[23] a forensic psychologist, makes a similar case that calling MSBP a syndrome makes little logical sense.

While many people accept the designation of this particular type of behavior as a syndrome, others agree with Fisher and Mitchell[21] that the jury is still out. Rogers[24] makes what he describes as a first attempt to decide if MSBP can withstand rigorous scientific criteria that would establish it as a syndrome. He notes that the criteria to define a syndrome need to exclude cases that would represent other possible disease entities, include all possible cases for the described syndrome, and make allowance for researchers to begin describing outcome. He comments that Rosenberg's criteria are not adequate in this regard.

In summary, when comparing Rosenberg's criteria for MSPB with the *DSM-IV* criteria, we have 2 distinct descriptions of a medical condition, with 2 different sets of criteria, and adherents for both. In addition, there is another school of thought that denies the existence of MSBP as a syndrome or psychiatric diagnosis altogether. And, finally, as Rogers maintains, there might be a syndrome but we have not yet sufficiently described it.

What Should We Call It?

Meadow [6,13,25] has commented several times regarding his use of the term *Munchausen syndrome by proxy*. He admitted freely that he used journalistic license to come up with the term.[6] In a commentary published in 1991[25] he stated, "The term, and particularly its overuse, has led to problems (at times I have regretted coining it). Many lawyers, social workers, and sometimes doctors, seem to regard Munchausen syndrome by proxy as an identifiable disorder that afflicts certain women; it is common for the perpetrator to announce proudly 'I've got Munchausen syndrome by proxy, and the judge says I needn't go to prison providing I see the specialist and have treatment.'"

The origins of the terms *Munchausen syndrome* and *Munchausen syndrome by proxy* have been oft repeated. Briefly, Asher[4] named *Munchausen's syndrome* in 1951 in a paper about 3 patients who lied on numerous occasions in order to get admitted to the hospital. The Baron von Munchausen's name was synonymous for wildly exaggerated tales attributed to him in a popular book first written by Raspe[26] and subsequently by multiple authors in what became books of children's stories.

Shortly after MSBP was first used by Meadow in 1977, Burman and Stevens[27] published a case of nonaccidental poisoning and suggested the syndrome name should refer to Polle, a child of the Baron von Munchausen, who they said died under suspicious circumstances. The term *Polle syndrome* was used by various authors for the next few years.[28–34] However, Meadow and Lennert,[35] after a trip to Germany to visit the Baron's birthplace, clarified that the Baron von Munchausen did not have children but did marry, late in life, a 17-year-old woman who gave birth to a child presumably fathered by someone who was not the Baron. This child's name was not Polle but Maria. She died in infancy but not under suspicious circumstances. Polle is actually the name of the town where Maria was born.

Confusing the situation further, the term *Munchausen's syndrome by proxy* had actually been used, 1 year before Meadow published his landmark paper, by Money and Werlwas[36] to describe certain cases of psychosocial dwarfism. The 2 authors used the term to describe a condition involving severe child abuse resulting in lack of physical, psychological, and emotional development. Money eventually changed his designation to the *Kaspar Hauser syndrome*.[37]

Also in 1976, Sneed and Bell[38] published a paper titled "The Dauphin of Munchausen: Factitious Passage of Renal Stones in a Child." In their case report the authors note that a 10-year-old boy who was truant from school and getting in trouble with the authorities produced pebbles that he and his mother stated were passed from his urinary tract. The authors imply that it was the child who falsified his own illness but admitted that they could not separate out the contribution of his mother.

Another early candidate as a name for MSBP was the term *Meadow's syndrome*. Several authors felt that the syndrome he described should bear Meadow's name.[39–41] Other names included *doctor shopping*[42] and *the persistent parent*.[43]

Many writers continue to use the term *Munchausen syndrome by proxy*, the designation first used by Meadow in 1977.[15,44,45] Schreier and Libow[46] came to prefer *Munchausen by proxy syndrome*. This is the term they employ in their book *Hurting for Love*. They explained their reasoning by saying that *Munchausen syndrome by proxy* carries the implication that it is a variant of Munchausen syndrome differing only in the proxy use of a child. They feel that reversing the words makes it clear that we are talking about something quite distinct from Munchausen syndrome. Others have adopted this usage.[22,47,48]

Morris[49] first used the term *FDP*. Numerous authors have followed this usage.[21,50–53] As referred to earlier, when the committee of the American Psychiatric Association formulated research criteria for MSBP they used the term *FDP*. Bools[54] wrote a paper in 1996 describing 10 different types of FDP.

Gray and Bentovim[55] wrote about a group of children that others would classify as meeting criteria for MSBP. They disagreed, and thought that the condition from which these 41 children were suffering should be called *illness induction syndrome*. They argued that the term *MSBP* is esoteric and that *illness induction syndrome* represents an improvement over *FDP*. The 4 categories that made up their series included a group of children whose parents withheld food, a group with false allegations of allergies or food intolerance, a group of children whose parents alleged nonexistent symptoms or illnesses, and finally a group where parents induced symptoms. Many of the children in this last group were poisoned.

A significant effort to rename the condition came from a special task force of the American Professional Society on the Abuse of Children (APSAC) reported in the journal *Child Maltreatment*.[51] The task force, responding to the controversy regarding who should carry the diagnosis, decided to divide the entity and name one part *factitious disorder by proxy*, while designating the other part *pediatric condition falsification*. For this group FDP represents a psychiatric diagnosis given to the adult, the person who fabricates or induces illness. It corresponds closely to the research criteria in *DSM-IV*. Pediatric condition falsification is a diagnosis given to the child, or victim of abuse. The term designates a specific type of child abuse. The authors of the report indicate that one condition can exist without the other.[56] As Schreier [57] explains, "MBP [Munchausen by proxy] is then retained as the name applied to the disorder that contains these 2 elements, a diagnosis in the child and a diagnosis in the caretaker."

In his recent writings Meadow[19,58] refers to MSBP as *Munchausen syndrome by proxy abuse*. This usage is quite purposeful and has been adapted by others including Eminson and Jureidini.[59] Recently in Great Britain we have seen the term *Munchausen syndrome by proxy/fabricated and induced illness*.[60] This usage has been further modified into *fabricated or induced illness in a child by a carer*.[61]

With regard to this question we must conclude that there are numerous names for the condition with no single designation currently winning out.

If MSBP Is an Illness, to Whom Is the Diagnosis Assigned?

Meadow[6] wrote, "In the past I have resented being asked in court whether someone is 'suffering from Munchausen syndrome by proxy': it has seemed no more appropriate than being asked if a man who has buggered his stepson is 'suffering from sex abuse.'"

Meadow identified MSBP as a type of child abuse and assigned the diagnosis to the child as the victim of abuse. However, he has remained focused over a particular quality of mothers involved in MSBP, and has repeated his concern that the diagnosis be made only when the mother seeks a certain type of relationship with a medical care environment.[19] Rosenberg has also consistently designated the child as the recipient of the diagnosis.[44,62,63] "MBP is a pediatric, not a psychiatric, diagnosis."[62]

Factitious disorder, not otherwise specified (NOS), as described in the *DSM-IV*, is specifically a diagnosis assigned to an adult. It is a psychiatric diagnosis, a mental illness. Not everyone has been happy with this inclusion of MSBP behavior as a psychiatric diagnosis. Ford[64] was adamant on the subject: "… in the opinion of this author, the diagnosis of factitious disorder, not otherwise specified, when referring to FDP, should be reserved for the victim, not the perpetrator. Providing a formal psychiatric diagnosis for the perpetrator may allow for a defense on the basis of diminished responsibility because the behavior is related to a psychiatric disorder." Others have echoed his opinion.[6,59,65–67]

On the other side of this debate clinicians have been quite comfortable making a psychiatric diagnosis in the perpetrator of MSBP. Perhaps the most vocal early proponents of this last view is the team of Schreier and Libow.[46,68] Their book *Hurting for Love* is an extended discussion of the motivation of a caretaker to use her child in a "fetishistic manner."

As noted previously, the APSAC special task force on definitional issues concluded by assigning 2 diagnoses, one for the child, and one for the adult. Thus *pediatric condition falsification* is a description of a type of child abuse and is assigned to the child. *Factitious disorder by proxy* is a diagnosis given to the parent.

In summary, the question, "Who gets the diagnosis?" has been answered several ways. Some say the child gets the diagnosis, others say the caretaker gets the diagnosis, and some say both child and perpetrator get the diagnosis.

How Far Does the MSBP Concept Extend?

Soon after Meadow's original paper was published, case reports began accumulating in the literature of situations various authors felt were consistent with the new MSBP concept. As the number of published cases of a new syndrome grows, one would expect a consensus to develop regarding what is and what is not defined by the diagnostic entity. Here a consensus has never been reached. Instead, uses of the term *MSBP* seem to be multiplying.[69]

A concept originally restricted to children being abused by their parents fairly quickly was extended to any person being subjected to abuse by someone in a caretaker role.[70] For example, under the *DSM-IV* definition of factitious disorder, NOS, elderly people could be victims of FDP at the hands of their sons or daughters.[71] Serial killings of patients in hospitals by nurses and other health professionals have been described as a type of FDP.[72,73]

More recently, household pets have been described as victims of FDP.[74] Feldman[75] wrote about a 45-year-old woman who did not feed her dog, and called her veterinarian numerous times with complaints that the dog was suffering from gastrointestinal ailments. When the dog was placed in a kennel he ate ravenously and gained weight. The kennel operator refused to return the dog to his owner. The woman eventually acknowledged that she had starved the animal and was further characterized as someone who fabricated or exaggerated symptoms in her own personal life.

In 1998 a paper describing parents exhorting their children to excel in sports defined this activity as parental *achievement by proxy*.[76] Rosenberg[62] and Meadow[77] have both gone on record saying that children receiving multiple sexual abuse evaluations can be considered as having MSBP in some cases. Rand[78] asserted that that multiple sexual abuse evaluations represent a contemporary form of MSBP as opposed to the classical type. Fabricating stories about illness over the Internet has been described as *virtual factitious disorder by proxy*.[79] Children with behavior problems attributed to food intolerance seen in a clinic to evaluate allergies were felt to be victims of MSBP.[40]

More troublesome has been the description in the literature of case reports that seem to have little relationship to the original concepts of MSBP or FDP. In 1986 Ernst and Philp[80] wrote about a child with severe iron deficiency anemia. Over the first 13 months of the child's life she was brought to medical attention several times for ordinary childhood illnesses and was consistently found to be anemic. The child's mother was counseled to add iron to the diet on different occasions and consistently told to the doctors that she was doing so. When the child was finally hospitalized and begun on iron supplements she responded normally with rapid improvement in her serum hemoglobin levels. The authors concluded, reasonably, that the mother had been lying regarding giving iron to the baby. They went on to say that the mother was purposefully withholding iron from the baby's diet. This mother frequently missed scheduled appointments, and was described as having domestic turmoil at home. In the paper the authors offer no evidence of the mother desiring a special relationship with medical care providers.

The child did improve once removed from her caretaker. Her anemia was caused by her parent neglecting to feed her iron-fortified formula. But she was not persistently brought to medical attention for this illness. It would appear that simply because the mother lied to her physicians, she was felt to warrant a diagnosis of MSBP.

The iron deficiency case was reported relatively early in the history of MSBP. In 1995, 3 physicians from Turkey[81] writing in the *Journal of Pediatric Surgery* reported a case of a 2-year-old boy with recurrent stones in his urethra, calling it MSBP. The authors recount that this youngster had had a number of stones removed from his urethra over the 6 months prior to their evaluation. On analysis the stones were found to be silica based, such as one might find in the backyard. The story that emerged was that the boy's father, unable to get his first wife pregnant, took a second, illegal spouse who was the mother of the child brought for treatment. The first wife, angry with her husband, eventually admitted to inserting the stones as a means of getting back at him. The authors acknowledged that seeking a relationship to the medical care establishment had nothing to do with this presentation. Nor did anyone try to mislead the investigating physicians. While the wife was deceiving her husband, the father bringing his child for treatment was truly at a loss to explain why his son was having difficulty.

In 1998 Somani[82] reported a case of MSBP in the *International Journal of Dermatology*. A man presented with an unexplained burn on his cheek. His wife had caused it by putting acid on his face after he passed out from drinking alcohol. For several years she had been complaining about his excessive alcohol intake. She felt that if she burned him with acid each time he passed out he might be motivated to stop drinking.

Another case report[83] was described as "…a previously unreported case of an unusual dermatologic manifestation of MBP." The 1-year-old child had skin lesions in pairs over all of his body. Eventually it was determined that these were burns produced by a heated cooking fork. "The mother, who had no medical background, denied that the child had any other chronic illness."

Despite the fact that there are other such examples, an argument can be made that cases such as these are merely inappropriate uses of the term *MSBP* that managed to find their way into the literature. The series of cases published by Godding and Kruth[84] offers a more serious challenge to the definitional boundaries of MSBP. These authors surveyed a pediatric asthma practice and determined that 17 children merited the diagnosis of MSBP. To characterize these children they extended the definition of MSBP to include families where noncompliance with treatment and illness exaggeration resulted in children receiving inadequate or inappropriate care. Meadow,[25] in a commentary following their article, maintains that he had faith his colleagues were correctly identifying situations in which the extent of noncompliance and exaggeration reached the level of child abuse. However, he observed, "In a clinic in which more than 2,000 children with asthma are seen I would expect most to be noncompliant to some extent. Similarly a large proportion will exaggerate symptoms or overuse treatment for other reasons. Such behavior is normal."

In fact, by 1995 Meadow felt compelled to write an article titled "What Is, and What Is Not, Munchausen Syndrome by Proxy?"[6] He wrote, "However in the last ten years the label of Munchausen syndrome by proxy (pseudonyms: factitious illness by proxy, Meadow's syndrome) has been applied to a wide variety of abusive behaviour by parents simply because of the way that a parent has lied and deceived professional staff, or because of the weird, calculated, or manipulative way in which a parent has harmed a child." He went on to list a number of behaviors that he labeled "not quite Munchausen syndrome by proxy."

In conclusion, despite many efforts by experts such as Meadow, more and more conditions have come to be called MSBP. We are continually reminded of the lack of a clear definition about what is meant by the term.

How Important Is the Motivation of the Perpetrator?

In his initial paper Meadow called attention to a particular quality in the parents of the 2 children he described. He discussed how curious it seemed that that the 2 mothers were involved intensely in the medical care their children received. This observation has led to one of the fundamental debates in the field. Simply stated, on one side the motivation of the perpetrator, defined as a desire to meet her need for nurturance, is the sine qua non of the syndrome. On the other side of this debate, the perpetrator's motivation is considered almost irrelevant.

By definition a person who engages in factitious behavior knows what he or she is doing but is unaware of the motivation behind that behavior.[53] A person with conscious awareness of motivation would be said to be malingering. For example, a person who fakes an illness consciously in order to be declared ineligible for military service is malingering. A similar person who has no conscious intent to avoid military service might still have a factitious illness that results in him being disqualified.

If we apply this understanding of the terms to MSBP we can see the dilemma faced by medical care providers. A mother who lies about a child's illness specifically to have him qualify for disability benefits is malingering. However, a mother who falsifies information about her child's health without conscious intent is engaging in factitious illness behavior. If you asked her why she was subjecting her child to unnecessary medical care she would be incapable of stating that her motivation was to, say, gain nurturance from her child's pediatrician. In fact, the usual answer given by parents in such situations is that they are requesting medical care for the good of their child. It is up to the pediatrician to "guess" what the motivation might be. The professional is asked to determine the motivation of a person who does not have conscious awareness of that information. This appears to place an undue burden on the medical practitioner.

In Meadow's[85] second paper about MSBP he went into more detail regarding the motivation of the mothers. "It would be naïve to seek a single cause for the harmful behaviour of these mothers. For some the child's illness brought about a closer relationship with a husband; for others it seemed to provide welcome distraction from personal and home difficulties. Several of the mothers thrived on the children's wards. They seemed to love it, bustling around helping other mothers, helping the nurses, and forming close relationships with the junior medical staff."

Not only is there a disagreement about whether motivation is relevant, those who cite the importance of motivation describe many different motivations that underlie the behavior. For example, Alexander[86] states that some parents engage in MSBP behavior to escape an alcoholic or abusive spouse while others do so to induce a parent to return from military service overseas. Gray and Bentovim[55] suggested, "The seeking of medical assistance may well be a way of maintaining an idealized perception of themselves as parents, avoiding action of a physically abusive nature." In other words, taking her child to the doctor, albeit unnecessarily, might be the parent's way to keep from physically abusing the child. Sheridan and Levin[87] in the summary to their book write, "Motivations of the perpetrator are probably not uniform, and may include components of help-seeking; a delusion that the illness is real; rage at the victim, health-care providers, or significant others; and tangible secondary gain."

Others who affirm the importance of motivation simply acknowledge the difficulty of determining what it might be. "Although many of these caretakers seem to enjoy the attention and sympathy they receive from their child's apparent illness, the motivations of those who induce or fabricate illness are complex and poorly understood."[88]

Rosenberg[62] and Wilson,[89] weighing in on the question separately, both felt that the job of the pediatrician had little to do with determining the motivation of the perpetrator. Rosenberg did not include motivation in her original criteria[5] and subsequently wrote that the perpetrator's intent is "diagnostically immaterial."[62] She said this in the context of the pediatrician making the diagnosis that the child is being abused. She went on to say that intent is something that was better served as a legal issue.[44] Wilson stated, "A child's doctor is not required to clarify whether inappropriate parental care is due to mental illness, deprivation, distorted views of science, or persisting over anxiety before acting to promote the welfare of the child."[89]

Fisher,[90] a psychiatrist, stated categorically that he had no way of determining the motivation of perpetrators of MSBP. He went on to comment that being able to apply a *DSM-IV* diagnosis really doesn't take us very far in understanding why parents would abuse their children. He pointed out the similarities between parents who commit MSBP abuse and other types of child abuse. "It is very common for parents who have perpetrated abuse to disclose that they felt uncared for, not close to their parents, never good enough, left out, or unwanted. The same appears to be true for MBP parents."

Schreier, also a psychiatrist, made the motivation of the perpetrator a central feature of his book and subsequent writings. He wrote, "We have come to see the mother as involved in a perverse sadomasochistic relationship with the pediatrician, the infant serving as an 'object in the service of controlling the physician.' "[91] In his more recent writings he continues to maintain that motivation of the parent is distinctly different in MSBP from that of other forms of child abuse. "The primary motivation seems to be an intense need for attention from, and manipulation of, powerful professionals, most frequently, but not exclusively a physician."[57]

Regarding MSBP, motivation of the perpetrator is something about which people remain curious but there is no consensus about what it might be or even if we can possibly discern it.

What Is the Prevalence of This Syndrome, and How Serious Is It?

When describing an illness, the epidemiology of that condition is usually reported. How frequently does it occurs in the population? What is the incidence and prevalence of the illness? Authors disagree widely about how commonly MSBP occurs. Some state it is "…a rare but serious form of child abuse."[92] Others say that it is "fairly common."[51] "We can safely say that the disorder is far from rare, and that it is frequently missed."[46] One author declared, "Munchausen by proxy may be the single most complex—and lethal—form of maltreatment known today."[93]

A first step in determining the frequency of occurrence is to have a clear definition of what constitutes the illness. As we have seen, a definition of MSBP has yet to be agreed on. It has not been established whether the diagnosis should be given to the child or to the adult. To establish prevalence we need to determine the number of children (or adults) with the condition within a particular population. This becomes the numerator of the equation. The denominator is the total number of children (or adults) available as potential victims or perpetrators of MSBP.

The first attempt to determine how prevalent or how serious MSBP might be is represented by Rosenberg's *Web of Deceit* paper.[5] She gathered 117 cases reported in the literature from 1966 to 1987. She then described shared characteristics of these cases. For example, she stated that 9% of the children died. Obviously, having 10 of 117 children die seems a staggering number. Many readers of her paper have concluded that the mortality rate for MSBP is 9%.[12,94–103] This has given rise to such conclusions as, "Given the 9% mortality rate cited in this disorder, it is imperative that steps be taken to protect the child immediately, even before proceeding with further evaluation."[104]

It is widely accepted that children given the diagnosis of MSBP present with any number of different medical problems or symptoms. Obviously, different symptom presentations differ in degrees of lethality. Hence, a series of patients who have been smothered or poisoned, for example, would be much more likely to have high rates of death than a group of patients with exaggerated asthma symptoms, such as those reported by Godding and Kruth.[85]

Another mortality rate occasionally cited[105] is derived from a paper by Alexander et al[11] who documented 5 children that they felt met criteria for MSBP. The authors looked at the siblings of their index cases, determined which of them also had been victims of MSBP, counted the number of children who died (4/13), and came up with a mortality rate of 31%. Two of the 4 deaths involved suffocation and the other 2 were the result of arsenic poisoning.

Among the 117 cases described by Rosenberg were a number of cases involving smothering and poisoning previously published by Meadow. In fact, he wrote a letter to the editor in response to the "Web of Deceit" paper stating, "The article provides excellent qualitative information about the syndrome but extreme caution should be applied to its quantitative aspects and, in particular, to some of the figures which are summarized in the abstract, such as the mortality rate of 9% and the long-term morbidity rate of 8%."[106]

There have been several additional attempts to determine prevalence rates of MSBP. Schreier and Libow[91] sent a questionnaire to neurologists and gastroenterologists in the United States asking for examples of MSBP cases. The 2 specialties were chosen because it was felt that factitious illness was more likely to be found in the patient populations treated by these doctors. As the authors freely admit, the study has significant methodological limitations, and conclusions are difficult to draw. There was a relatively low return rate for the questionnaire, and the total number of potential victims (the denominator) is not reported. Among the conclusions they drew from this survey was that specialists were able to identify cases of MSBP that had not been reported elsewhere.

Godding and Kruth[84] used as the denominator in the prevalence equation the total number of patients in their practice. "In three years of joint consultations about 1,648 (17/1,648) patients with asthma we found management of asthma that constituted child abuse in some 1% of asthmatic patients and their families."

The study conducted by McClure and colleagues[107] in England represented a significant improvement in methodology over any previous effort. The group collected reports of founded cases of MSBP, primarily suffocation, and poisoning, using child protection records. To be included the child had to be referred to child protection services, be investigated, and be declared a founded case. This study obviously selected for the more severe cases that result in reports of abuse requiring protection of the child. They identified 127 cases over a 2-year period and by using the total number of children in the geographic area served by the child protection agencies they determined an approximate prevalence rate of 0.5 in 100,000 children.

A similar attempt to establish prevalence in New Zealand used a somewhat different method.[108] All the pediatricians in the country were surveyed for possible cases of MSBP. There was a 95% return rate on the initial questionnaire. Identified cases were investigated further to avoid duplication. The authors concluded that 2 in 100,000 children met their criteria for MSBP.

Mortality rates of 9% or higher continue to be cited to justify the seriousness of MSBP. Ayoub et al[109] reported a group of mothers who demanded their children be treated for attention-deficit/hyperactivity disorder and be given special educational services despite no deficits being documented by psychological testing and classroom observation. The authors introduced the seriousness of their concern by citing high mortality rates for MSBP.

We are approaching some confidence in determining the prevalence of fatal or near fatal suffocation and poisoning of children through the work of McClure and his group[107] and Denny and colleagues.[108] However, we are not even close to being able to say anything about the frequency of occurrence of other types of MSBP presentations.

Is There a Profile That Can Be Used to Identify Potential Perpetrators of MSBP?

There have been numerous attempts to list characteristics of potential perpetrators that would be of use to physicians, investigators, and child protection officials.[85,110–117] The ability to identify a potential perpetrator before she could hurt a child would be of great value to society. Factors such as being employed in the medical profession, seeming to know more about the child's illness than the treating physicians, hovering over the child while in the hospital, and having an absent husband have all found their way onto such "profiles."

Ostfeld and Feldman[118] present a particularly detailed list of warning signs of FDP. They include 20 items, such as the mother grows anxious if the child improves and medical observations yield information that is inconsistent with parental reports. After saying that MSBP is a borderline diagnosis between pediatrics and child psychiatry, Skau and Mouridsen[119] presented a list of warning signals adapted from Meadow that listed perpetrator characteristics.

Artingstall,[48] a police detective, used profiling the way a criminal investigator would. She explained the limits of the technique, emphasized the need to recognize exceptions, and then proceeded to repeat many of the characteristics mentioned above.

Morley[8] commented as early as 1995 that profile criteria being used to diagnose Munchausen syndrome by proxy were nonspecific. Sanders and Bursch[120] acknowledged the value that profiles and checklists bring by increasing awareness of professionals about the potential for MSBP child abuse. Nevertheless, they concluded, "There is no consistent psychological profile of someone who has engaged in MBP behaviors." They systematically review evidence of all the commonly cited characteristics and note that none of them are specific to perpetrators of MSBP abuse.

Rogers[24] points out that the current state of the field uses a policy of diagnosis by exclusion. Each case is considered independently and requires that all other potential diagnoses be ruled out. He notes that if we had a profile procedure to use as a screening tool that had a 95% predictive value, and assumed a prevalence rate of 1 per 100 we would still not be able to identify perpetrators correctly 5 out of 6 times. Obviously, if we assume prevalence rates approximating 0.5 to 2 in 100,000, as cited previously, identifying potential perpetrators from such a profile would be essentially impossible.

As helpful as it would be to have a profile procedure we could use for screening, efforts made to date do not even begin to address the complexity of the problem.

Is Treatment of MSBP Possible?

This, of course, is an extremely important question. If MSBP is a serious, life-threatening illness, then finding an effective treatment is of the highest priority. There has been a general opinion that MSBP is extremely difficult to treat. Alexander[86] writes, "The willingness to exploit the child is especially dehumanizing, and in forms of child abuse resembles only the seduction of children by pedophiles in terms of intent. Not surprisingly, some observers consider pedophilia and MSBP to be among the least treatable types of child abuse." McGuire and Feldman[97] stated they had not experienced successful treatment of a mother. Babcock and colleagues said, "There is no reported effective psychiatric therapy for the caregivers manifesting this behavior."[121] Ludwig wrote, "As yet, there have been no proven therapies for MBP."[110]

In fact, there is a recurrent theme in the literature that the only reasonable treatment is total separation from the parent. Here is an example: "The only current cure is to completely remove the child from the perpetrator. The court should therefore be requested to allow absolutely no unsupervised contact. This means even for a few seconds. Sometimes the court will not allow the perpetrator to even touch the child. These orders need to be carried out completely."[65] And another: "No evidence exists that their behavior is amenable to psychiatric treatment, or that protective intervention is reliably effective short of severing physical contact and parental rights."[122]

Most authors weighing in on the question of the difficulty of treatment do not define what constitutes treatment. Is the treatment for the child, the caretaker, or the family? What constitutes success? Are we treating child abuse, or are we treating a psychological illness in a caretaking parent? Does treatment consist of undoing any harm caused by medical treatment? Or does it consist of preventing any further unnecessary medical treatment? Can treatment be considered successful if the child and abusive parent are not living in the same home? These are some of the questions that need to be addressed in any discussion of possible treatment.

In fact, some authors have been asking and answering these questions for many years. Perhaps the earliest successful treatment documented was by Nicol and Eccles[123] in 1985. They quite specifically identified they were treating child abuse, used individual psychotherapy, and helped a mother who admitted that she had poisoned her child to come to terms with what she had done. In another early case, a mother who lied about her medical history was referred to a psychiatrist for treatment.[124] The psychiatrist determined that this woman's 3 children were also being medically abused and began psychotherapy. "Up to one year none of the four has been readmitted to hospital, and the children appeared to have escaped further physical harm."

Griffith[125] wrote a thoughtful description from a family systems perspective of 2 families with issues involving MSBP. He discussed intergenerational patterns that gave value to somatic symptoms and their function within the family dynamic and outlined a family therapy–based treatment process.

The only report of a number of cases being treated with a specific treatment protocol is given by Berg and Jones.[125] They chose their cases carefully and demonstrated that children, in specific cases, can be returned to their family of origin, and that parents can learn how to more appropriately read medical cues from their children.

Regarding treatment of MSBP, it would appear that the news is either good or very bad.

Conclusion

More than 3 decades have passed since the introduction of the MSBP concept. As we can see, there are few clear answers about what this thing might be. Given the confusion of the professional community, it is no wonder that legal authorities, journalists, and even parents accused of MSBP feel justified in reflecting back to the medical community their negative feelings. If a large group of pediatricians and child psychiatrists cannot come to agreement, why should we expect the community at large to understand what we are trying to identify, treat, and prevent?

Let's just call it child abuse.

References

1. Boros SJ, Ophoven JP, Andersen R, Brubaker LC. Munchausen syndrome by proxy: a profile for medical child abuse. *Aust Fam Physician.* 1995;24(5): 768-769, 772-763
2. Kempe CH. Sexual abuse, another hidden pediatric problem: the 1977 C. Anderson Aldrich lecture. *Pediatrics.* 1978;62(3):382-389
3. Jenny C, Hymel KP, Ritzen A, Reinert SE, Hay TC. Analysis of missed cases of abusive head trauma. *JAMA.* 1999;281(7):621-626
4. Asher R. Munchausen's syndrome. *Lancet.* 1951;1:339-341
5. Rosenberg DA. Web of deceit: a literature review of Munchausen syndrome by proxy. *Child Abuse Negl.* 1987;11(4):547-563
6. Meadow R. What is, and what is not, 'Munchausen syndrome by proxy'? *Arch Dis Child.* 1995;72(6):534-538
7. Krener P. Factitious disorders and the psychosomatic continuum in children. *Curr Opin Pediatr.* 1994;6(4):418-422

8. Morley CJ. Practical concerns about the diagnosis of Munchausen syndrome by proxy. *Arch Dis Child.* 1995;72(6):528-529; discussion 529-530
9. Anderson J, McKane JP. Munchausen syndrome by proxy. *Br J Hosp Med.* 1996;56(1):43-45
10. Bools CN, Neale BA, Meadow SR. Co-morbidity associated with fabricated illness (Munchausen syndrome by proxy). *Arch Dis Child.* 1992;67(1):77-79
11. Alexander R, Smith W, Stevenson R. Serial Munchausen syndrome by proxy. *Pediatrics.* 1990;86(4):581-585
12. Barker LH, Howell RJ. Munchausen syndrome by proxy in false allegations of child sexual abuse: legal implications. *Bull Am Acad Psychiatry Law.* 1994;22(4):499-510
13. Meadow R. The history of Munchausen syndrome by proxy. In: Levin AV, Sheridan MS, eds. *Munchausen Syndrome by Proxy: Issues in Diagnosis and Treatment.* New York, NY: Lexington Books; 1995:3-11
14. Gomez De Terreros I, Gomez De Terreros M, Serrano Santamaria M, Jimenez Giron AV, Sanchez Salas M, Salazar Espadero N. [Recurrent ingestion of foreign bodies. Unusual presentation of Munchausen by Proxy syndrome]. *Child Abuse Negl.* 1996;20(7):613-620
15. Sheridan MS. The deceit continues: an updated literature review of Munchausen syndrome by proxy. *Child Abuse Negl.* 2003;27(4):431-451
16. Szajnberg NM, Moilanen I, Kanerva A, Tolf B. Munchausen-by-proxy syndrome: countertransference as a diagnostic tool. *Bull Menninger Clin.* 1996;60(2):229-237
17. Libow JA. Munchausen by proxy victims in adulthood: a first look. *Child Abuse Negl.* 1995;19(9):1131-1142
18. Rosenberg DA. Munchausen syndrome by proxy. In: Reece RM, Ludwig S, eds. *Child Abuse: Medical Diagnosis and Management.* 2nd ed. Philadelphia, PA: Lippincott Williams and Wilkins; 2001:363-383
19. Meadow R. Different interpretations of Munchausen syndrome by proxy. *Child Abuse Negl.* 2002;26(5):501-508
20. American Psychiatric Association. *Diagnostic and Statistical Manual of Mental Disorders, Fourth Edition.* Washington, DC: American Psychiatric Association; 1994
21. Fisher GC, Mitchell I. Is Munchausen syndrome by proxy really a syndrome? *Arch Dis Child.* 1995;72(6):530-534
22. Allison DB, Roberts MS. *Disordered Mother or Disordered Diagnosis? Munchausen by Proxy Syndrome.* Hillsdale, NJ: The Analytic Press; 1998
23. Mart E. *Munchausen's Syndrome by Proxy Reconsidered.* Manchester, NH: Bally Vaughn Publishing; 2002
24. Rogers R. Diagnostic, explanatory, and detection models of Munchausen by proxy: extrapolations from malingering, and deception. *Child Abuse Negl.* 2004;28:225-238

25. Meadow R. Commentary. *Arch Dis Child*. 1991;66:960
26. Raspe RE. *The Surprising Adventures of Baron Munchausen*. New York, NY: Peter Pauper; 1944
27. Burman D, Stevens D. Munchausen family. *Lancet*. 1977;2:456
28. Ackerman N, Strobel C. Polle syndrome: chronic diarrhea in Munchausen's child. *Gastroenterology*. 1981;81:1140-1142
29. Casavant MJ. Polle's syndrome (Munchausen by proxy). *Pediatr Emerg Care*. 1995;11(4):264
30. Clark GD, Key JD, Rutherford P, Bithoney WG. Munchausen's syndrome by proxy (child abuse) presenting as apparent autoerythrocyte sensitization syndrome: an unusual presentation of Polle syndrome. *Pediatrics*. 1984;74(6): 1100-1102
31. Liston TE, Levine PL, Anderson C. Polymicrobial bacteremia due to Polle syndrome: the child abuse variant of Munchausen by proxy. *Pediatrics*. 1983;72(2):211-213
32. Rosen CL, Frost JD Jr, Bricker T, Tarnow JD, Gillette PC, Dunlavy S. Two siblings with recurrent cardiorespiratory arrest: Munchausen syndrome by proxy or child abuse? *Pediatrics*. 1983;71(5):715-720
33. Verity CM, Winckworth C, Burman D. Polle syndrome: children of Munchausen. *Br Med J*. 1979;2:422-423
34. Mehl AL, Coble L, Johnson S. Munchausen syndrome by proxy: a family affair. *Child Abuse Negl*. 1990;14(4):577-585
35. Meadow R, Lennert T. Munchausen by proxy or Polle syndrome: which term is correct? *Pediatrics*. 1984;74(4):554-556
36. Money J, Werlwas J. Folie a Dieu in the parents of psychosocial dwarfs: two cases. *Bull Am Acad Psychiatry Law*. 1976;4:351-361
37. Money J. *The Kaspar Hauser Syndrome of "Psychosocial Dwarfism."* Buffalo, NY: Prometheus Books; 1992
38. Sneed RC, Bell RF. The dauphin of Munchausen: factitious passage of renal Stones in a child. *Pediatrics*. 1976;58:127-129
39. Lazoritz S. Munchausen by proxy or Meadow's syndrome? *Lancet*. 1987;2(8559):631
40. Warner JO, Hathaway MJ. Allergic form of Meadow's syndrome (Munchausen by proxy). *Arch Dis Child*. 1984;59(2):151-156
41. Rubin L, Angelides A, Davidson M, Lanzkowsky P. Recurrent sepsis and gastrointestinal ulceration due to child abuse. *Arch Dis Child*. 1986;61:903-905
42. Libow JA, Schreier HA. Three forms of factitious illness in children: when is it Munchausen syndrome by proxy? *Am J Orthopsychiatry*. 1986;56(4):602-611
43. Waring WW. The persistent parent. *Am J Dis Child*. 1992;146(6):753-756
44. Rosenberg DA. Munchausen syndrome by proxy: medical diagnostic criteria. *Child Abuse Negl*. 2003;27(4):421-430

45. Levin AV, Sheridan MS, eds. *Munchausen Syndrome by Proxy: Issues in Diagnosis and Treatment*. New York, NY: Lexington Books; 1995
46. Schreier HA, Libow JA. *Hurting for Love: Munchausen by Proxy Syndrome*. New York, NY: The Guilford Press; 1993
47. Parnell TF, Day DO, eds. *Munchausen by Proxy Syndrome*. Thousand Oaks, CA: Sage; 1998
48. Artingstall K. *Practical Aspects of Munchausen by Proxy and Munchausen Syndrome Investigation*. Boca Raton, FL: CRC Press; 1999
49. Morris R. Munchausen's syndrome and factitious illness. *Cur Opin Psychiatry*. 1991;4:225-230
50. Feldman MD, Eisendrath SJ, eds. *The Spectrum of Factitious Disorders*. Washington, DC: American Psychiatric Press, Inc.; 1996
51. Ayoub CC, Alexander R, Beck D, et al. Position paper: definitional issues in Munchausen by proxy. *Child Maltreat*. 2002;7(2):105-111
52. von Hahn L, Harper G, McDaniel SH, Siegel DM, Feldman KW, Libow JA. A case of factitious disorder by proxy: the role of the health-care system, diagnostic dilemmas, and family dynamics. *Harv Rev Psychiatry*. 2001;9(3):124-135
53. Taylor S, Hyler SE. Update on factitious disorders. *Int J Psychiatry Med*. 1993;23(1):81-94
54. Bools C. Factitious illness by proxy. Munchausen syndrome by proxy. *Br J Psychiatry*. 1996;169(3):268-275
55. Gray J, Bentovim A. Illness induction syndrome: paper I—a series of 41 children from 37 families identified at The Great Ormond Street Hospital for Children NHS Trust. *Child Abuse Negl*. 1996;20(8):655-673
56. Schreier HA, Ayoub CC. Casebook companion to the definitional issues in Munchausen by proxy position paper. *Child Maltreat*. 2002;7(2):160-165
57. Schreier H. Munchausen by proxy defined. *Pediatrics*. 2002;110(5):985-988
58. Meadow R. Unnatural sudden infant death. *Arch Dis Child*. 1999;80(1):7-14
59. Eminson M, Jureidini J. Concerns about research and prevention strategies in Munchausen syndrome by proxy (MSBP) abuse. *Child Abuse Negl*. 2003;27(4):413-420
60. Wrennal L. Munchausen syndrome by proxy/fabricated and induced illness: does the diagnosis serve economic vested interests, rather than the interests of children? *Med Hypotheses*. 2007;68(5):960-966
61. Bools C. *Fabricated or Induced Illness in a Child by a Carer: A Reader*. Oxford, UK: Radcliffe Publishing; 2007
62. Rosenberg DA. From lying to homicide: the spectrum of Munchausen syndrome by proxy. In: Levin AV, Sheridan MS, eds. *Munchausen Syndrome by Proxy: Issues in Diagnosis and Treatment*. New York, NY: Lexington Books; 1995:13-37

63. Rosenberg DA. Munchausen syndrome by proxy: currency in counterfeit illness. In: Helfer MD, Kempe RS, Krugman R, eds. *The Battered Child*. 5th ed. Chicago, IL: University Of Chicago Press; 1997:413-430
64. Ford CV. Ethical and legal issues in factitious disorders: an overview. In: Feldman MD, Eisendrath SJ, eds. *The Spectrum of Factitious Disorders*. Washington DC: American Psychiatric Press, Inc.; 1996:51-63
65. Bosch JJ. Munchausen syndrome by proxy. *J Pediatr Health Care*. 1997;11(5): 242, 252-244
66. Rand DC, Feldman MD. Misdiagnosis of Munchausen syndrome by proxy: a literature review and four new cases. *Harv Rev Psychiatry*. 1999;7(2):94-101
67. Davis PM, Sibert JR. Munchausen syndrome by proxy or factitious illness spectrum disorder of childhood. *Arch Dis Child*. 1996;74(3):274-275
68. Schreier HA. The perversion of mothering: Munchausen syndrome by proxy. *Bull Menninger Clin*. 1992;56(4):421-437
69. Schreier HA. Repeated false allegations of sexual abuse presenting to sheriffs: when is it Munchausen by proxy? *Child Abuse Negl*. 1996;20(11):1135-1137
70. Sigal MD, Altmark D, Carmel I. Munchausen syndrome by adult proxy: a perpetrator abusing two adults. *J Nerv Ment Dis*. 1986;174(11):696-698
71. Ben-Chetrit E, Melmed RN. Recurrent hypoglycaemia in multiple myeloma: a case of Munchausen syndrome by proxy in an elderly patient. *J Intern Med*. 1998;244(2):175-178
72. Yorker BC. Hospital epidemics of factitious disorder by proxy. In: Feldman MD, Eisendrath SJ, eds. *The Spectrum of Factitious Disorders*. Washington, DC: American Psychiatric Press, Inc.; 1996:157-174
73. Sheridan MS. Munchausen syndrome by proxy in context II: professional proxy and other analogs. In: Levin AV, Sheridan MS, eds. *Munchausen Syndrome by Proxy: Issues in Diagnosis and Treatment*. New York, NY; Lexington Books; 1995:85-101
74. Tucker HS, Finlay F, Guiton S. Munchausen syndrome involving pets by proxies. *Arch Dis Child*. 2002;87(3):263
75. Feldman MD. Canine variant of factitious disorder by proxy. *Am J Psychiatry*. 1997;154(9):1316-1317
76. Tofler IR, Knapp PK, Drell MJ. The achievement by proxy spectrum in youth sports. Historical perspective and clinical approach to pressured and high-achieving children and adolescents. *Child Adolesc Psychiatr Clin N Am*. 1998;7(4):803-820
77. Meadow R. False allegations of abuse and Munchausen syndrome by proxy. *Arch Dis Child*. 1993;68(4):444-447
78. Rand DC. Munchausen syndrome by proxy: integration of classic and contemporary type. *Issues in Child Abuse Accusations*. 1990;2:83-89

79. Feldman MD, Bibby M, Crites SD. 'Virtual' factitious disorders and Munchausen by proxy. *West J Med*. 1998;168(6):537-539
80. Ernst TN, Philp M. Severe iron deficiency anemia. An example of covert child abuse (Munchausen by proxy). *West J Med*. 1986;144(3):358-359
81. Senocak ME, Turken A, Buyukpamukcu N. Urinary obstruction caused by factitious urethral stones: an amazing manifestation of Munchausen syndrome by proxy. *J Pediatr Surg*. 1995;30(12):1732-1734
82. Somani VK. Witchcraft's syndrome: Munchausen's syndrome by proxy. *Int J Dermatol*. 1998;37(3):229-230
83. Johnson CF. Dermatologic manifestations. In: Levin AV, Sheridan MS, eds. *Munchausen Syndrom by Proxy: Issues in Diagnosis and Treatment*. New York, NY: Lexington Books; 1995:189-200
84. Godding V, Kruth M. Compliance with treatment in asthma and Munchausen syndrome by proxy. *Arch Dis Child*. 1991;66(8):956-960
85. Meadow R. Munchausen syndrome by proxy. *Arch Dis Child*. 1982;57(2):92-98
86. Alexander R. The Munchausen by proxy family. In: Levin AV, Sheridan MS, eds. *Munchasen Syndrome by Proxy: Issues in Diagnosis and Treatment*. New York, NY: Lexington Books; 1995:479
87. Sheridan MS, Levin AV. Summary. In: Levin AV, Sheridan MS, eds. *Munchausen syndrome by Proxy: Issues in Diagnosis and Treatment*. New York, NY: Lexington Books; 1995:433-443
88. Hall DE, Eubanks L, Meyyazhagan LS, Kenney RD, Johnson SC. Evaluation of covert video surveillance in the diagnosis of Munchausen syndrome by proxy: lessons from 41 cases. *Pediatrics*. 2000;105(6):1305-1312
89. Wilson RG. Fabricated or induced illness in children. Munchausen by proxy comes of age. *BMJ*. 2001;323(7308):296-297
90. Fisher GC. Etiological speculations. In: Levin AV, Sheridan MS, eds. *Munchausen Syndrome by Proxy: Issues in Diagnosis and Treatment*. New York, NY: Lexington Books; 1995:39-57
91. Schreier HA, Libow JA. Munchausen syndrome by proxy: diagnosis and prevalence. *Am J Orthopsychiatry*. 1993;63(2):318-321
92. Main DJ, Douglas JE, Tamanika HM. Munchausen's syndrome by proxy. *Med J Aust*. 1986;145(6):300-301
93. Feldman MD. Foreword. In: *Sickened: The Memoir of a Munchausen by Proxy Childhood*. New York, NY: Bantam Books; 2003:V-IX
94. Gunter M. Induction, identification or folie a deux? Psychodynamics and genesis of Munchausen syndromes by proxy and false allegations of sexual abuse in adolescents. *Med Law*. 1998;17(3):359-379
95. Hyman PE, Bursch B, Beck D, DiLorenzo C, Zeltzer LK. Discriminating pediatric condition falsification from chronic intestinal pseudo-obstruction in toddlers. *Child Maltreat*. 2002;7(2):132-137

96. Magnay AR, Debelle G, Proops DW, Booth IW. Munchausen syndrome by proxy unmasked by nasal signs. *J Laryngol Otol.* 1994;108(4):336-338
97. McGuire TL, Feldman KW. Psychologic morbidity of children subjected to Munchausen syndrome by proxy. *Pediatrics.* 1989;83(2):289-292
98. Ostfeld BM, Feldman MD. Factitious disorder by proxy: awareness among mental health practitioners. *Gen Hosp Psychiatry.* 1996;18(2):113-116
99. Berkowitz CD. Pediatric abuse. New patterns of injury. *Emerg Med Clin North Am.* 1995;13(2):321-341
100. Griffiths H, Cuddihy PJ, Marnane C. Bleeding ears: a case of Munchausen syndrome by proxy. *Int J Pediatr Otorhinolaryngol.* 2001;57(3):245-247
101. Klebes C, Fay S. Munchausen syndrome by proxy: a review, case study, and nursing implications. *J Pediatr Nurs.* 1995;10(2):93-98
102. Mills RW, Burke S. Gastrointestinal bleeding in a 15 month old male. A presentation of Munchausen's syndrome by proxy. *Clin Pediatr (Phila).* 1990;29(8):474-477
103. Sheridan MS. Munchausen syndrome by proxy. *Health Soc Work.* 1989;14(1):53-58
104. Mian M. A multidisciplinary approach. In: Levin AV, Sheridan MS, eds. *Munchausen Syndrome by Proxy: Issues in Diagnosis and Treatment.* New York, NY: Lexington Books; 1995:271-286
105. Volz AG. Nursing interventions in Munchausen syndrome by proxy. *J Psychosoc Nurs Ment Health Serv.* 1995;33(9):51-58
106. Meadow R. Letter to the editor. *Child Abuse Negl.* 1990;14:289
107. McClure RJ, Davis PM, Meadow SR, Sibert JR. Epidemiology of Munchausen syndrome by proxy, non-accidental poisoning, and non-accidental suffocation. *Arch Dis Child.* 1996;75(1):57-61
108. Denny SJ, Grant CC, Pinnock R. Epidemiology of Munchausen syndrome by proxy in New Zealand. *J Paediatr Child Health.* 2001;37(3):240-243
109. Ayoub CC, Schreier HA, Keller C. Munchausen by proxy: presentations in special education. *Child Maltreat.* 2002;7(2):149-159
110. Ludwig S. The role of the physician. In: Levin AV, Sheridan MS, eds. *Munchausen Syndrome by Proxy: Issues in Diagnosis and Treatment.* New York, NY: Lexington books; 1995:287-294
111. Souid AK, Keith DV, Cunningham AS. Munchausen syndrome by proxy. *Clin Pediatr (Phila).* 1998;37(8):497-503
112. Leonard KF, Farrell PA. Munchausen's syndrome by proxy. A little-known type of abuse. *Postgrad Med.* 1992;91(5):197-204
113. Mercer SO, Perdue JD. Munchausen syndrome by proxy: social work's role. *Soc Work.* 1993;38(1):74-81
114. Pasqualone GA, Fitzgerald SM. Munchausen by proxy syndrome: the forensic challenge of recognition, diagnosis, and reporting. *Crit Care Nurs Q.* 1999;22(1):52-64; quiz 90-51

115. Baldwin MA. Munchausen syndrome by proxy: neurological manifestations. *J Neurosci Nurs.* 1994;26(1):18-23
116. Schreier HA, Libow JA. Munchausen by proxy syndrome: a modern pediatric challenge. *J Pediatr.* 1994;125(6 Pt 2):S110-S115
117. Reece RM. Unusual manifestations of child abuse. *Pediatr Clin North Am.* 1990;37(4):905-921
118. Ostfeld BM, Feldman MD. Factitious disorder by proxy: clinical features, detection, and management. In: Feldman MD, Eisendrath SJ, eds. *The Spectrum of Factitious Disorders.* Washington, DC: American Psychiatric Press, Inc.; 1996:83-108
119. Skau K, Mouridsen SE. Munchausen syndrome by proxy: a review. *Acta Paediatr.* 1995;84(9):977-982
120. Sanders MJ, Bursch B. Forensic assessment of illness falsification, Munchausen by proxy and factitious disorder, NOS. *Child Maltreat.* 2002;7:112-124
121. Babcock J, Hartman K, Pedersen A, Murphy M, Alving B. Rodenticide-induced coagulopathy in a young child. A case of Munchausen syndrome by proxy. *Am J Pediatr Hematol Oncol.* 1993;15(1):126-130
122. Kinscherff R, Famularo R. Extreme Munchausen syndrome by proxy: the case for termination of parental rights. *Juv Fam Court J.* 1991:41-53
123. Nicol AR, Eccles M. Psychotherapy for Munchausen syndrome by proxy. *Arch Dis Child.* 1985;60(4):344-348
124. Black D. The extended Munchausen syndrome: a family case. *Br J Psychiatry.* 1981;138:466-469
125. Griffith JL. The family systems of Munchausen syndrome by proxy. *Fam Process.* 1988;27(4):423-437
126. Berg B, Jones DP. Outcome of psychiatric intervention in factitious illness by proxy (Munchausen's syndrome by proxy). *Arch Dis Child.* 1999;81(6):465-472

Chapter 2

Medical Child Abuse

None can doubt that these two children were abused, but the acts of abuse were so different in quality, periodicity, and planning from the more usual non-accidental injury of childhood that I am uneasy about classifying these sad cases as variants of non-accidental injury. —Meadow, 1977[1]

Introduction

We start from a simple premise: We are talking about child abuse, a different presentation of child abuse, but abuse just the same. We go back to that point in 1977 when Roy Meadow[1] described his 2 cases and say that many of the difficulties of the past 30 years concerning Munchausen syndrome by proxy (MSBP) ensue from starting down the wrong road. He suggested we were looking at something that was *not* a "variant of non-accidental injury."

At the time he made that observation the medical evaluation of child abuse was in its infancy. From what professionals have learned over the years about abuse in general and about this type of abuse, we have no problem seeing that what has been called MSBP is, indeed, a type of non-accidental injury. In fact, if we focus on the child being harmed, and call what happens to the child *abuse*, we can allow the rest to follow logically. For us to proceed, we need a name for it. We call it simply *medical child abuse*.

Definition of Medical Child Abuse

Medical child abuse occurs when a child receives unnecessary and harmful or potentially harmful medical care at the instigation of a caretaker. As we shall see, this is not a particularly new idea. It has been in the making for many years. Support for this way of understanding child abuse within the medical care environment comes from many sources. The only mystery is why it has taken so long to arrive at the point of replacing the term *MSBP* with a straightforward description of child abuse.

At first consideration it may seem inconsequential to define a type of child maltreatment as medical child abuse. Yet it really does represent a conceptual shift. As is usually the case, the paradigm shift we advocate greatly simplifies things. For example, with this definition it is not necessary to determine the parent's motivation to know that a child is being harmed and that the abuse should stop. This step alone makes the evaluation and treatment of this type of abuse much less complicated.

This is not to say that the motivation of the perpetrator is irrelevant. It is just as relevant as it is in any other type of child abuse. This is the theme that we will develop in this chapter. Medical child abuse is similar in most ways to other types of child maltreatment. Determining that a child has been abused and stopping it comes first. Examining the motivation of the perpetrator of the abuse comes later. Our responsibility is to determine if the child is being harmed. Once the presence or absence of abuse has been established, we can factor in motivational considerations while considering the ongoing safety of the child.

Child maltreatment is the term that includes all the ways children can be hurt. Caretakers can harm children through acts of omission or commission. To survive and thrive children need food, shelter, love, appropriate developmental stimulation, and protection from dangers in their environment. If people who have been entrusted to provide these basic needs, their caretakers, fail to do so, we say the child is the victim of neglect. Neglect is an act of omission.

Physical neglect has its counterpart in physical abuse. Physical neglect is characterized by not protecting a child from physical harm; physical abuse is characterized by actually causing physical harm. Psychological neglect is paired with psychological abuse. In psychological or emotional neglect, a parent or caretaker fails to provide for the basic emotional needs of the child. In psychological abuse the caretaker systematically attacks the child using psychological means. A child who grows up in a toxic psychological atmosphere of constant criticism, threats, and belittling comments can find it extremely difficult to cope with everyday stresses in life. Usually we do not consider sexual abuse to be matched with "sexual neglect" but a case could certainly be made. For example, a caretaker might be deemed sexually neglectful if he or she were to deny the emerging sexual physical changes and emotional experiences of an adolescent.

On the other hand medical neglect is a well-established concept. It refers to a parent or other caretaker not getting needed medical care for a child entrusted to his or her supervision.[2] There can be many perfectly understandable reasons why a parent might not take a child for needed medical services. The parent might not know the services are available. He or she might be a recent immigrant, unable to speak English, or might be developmentally disabled. There might be financial reasons for not seeking care. While all of these potential motivations will be explored at some point, the first consideration of society and the medical care establishment is to determine if the child is being neglected medically.

Medical neglect is defined as a child being deprived of necessary medical care. Medical child abuse happens when a caretaker is responsible for a child getting too much medical care, care that the child does not need and that is harmful or potentially harmful.

Child maltreatment is not an illness in the traditional sense. It is something that happens in the life of a child. To be sure, child abuse can result in a child *having* an illness. The child can experience emotional or physical harm that results in a medical condition that meets criteria for a specific illness. For example, emotional abuse can result in long-term psychological damage in the form of depression. Sexual abuse can cause physical or psychological harm. Long-term effects of sexual abuse can include sterility from sexually transmitted infections, pregnancy, or human immunodeficiency virus infection. In the emotional realm survivors of child sexual abuse have higher risks of drug and alcohol abuse, depression, and anxiety disorders.[3] By the same token, physical abuse and medical child abuse, in addition to possible emotional consequences, can both cause life-threatening sequelae, crippling disability, or death.

It is appropriate here to note that medical child abuse refers only to unnecessary, harmful, or potentially harmful medical care. A child smothered with a pillow until she stops breathing and dies is the victim of a deadly assault. Likewise, a child given salt in his formula who expires in the midst of a convulsion caused by high sodium levels in the bloodstream has been poisoned to death. These are both examples of fatal, physical child abuse. It is medical child abuse if the child survives the attack, is hospitalized, and undergoes diagnostic tests that would not be necessary if it were known she was purposefully smothered or poisoned. It is medical child abuse when a parent claims falsely that her child had a seizure and the child is put on anti-seizure medication. When a child receives multiple diagnostic tests, including needle sticks, x-rays, and procedures based on persistently exaggerated claims by the parent, the child experiences medical abuse. A child can be harmed just as effectively with an inappropriately applied hypodermic needle as he or she can by being hit with a baseball bat.

We have presented this definition of medical child abuse at numerous professional meetings. Pediatricians, family practice physicians, and other primary care providers seem to have no difficulty understanding what constitutes medical child abuse. However, occasionally a child abuse professional has expressed apprehension that the term *medical child abuse* might imply children being abused by medical professionals. Even the inclusion in the definition that the abuse occurs "at the instigation of a caretaker" does not seem to assuage this concern.

We know that some children receive unnecessary care, and sometimes harmful care initiated by physicians. We call this *malpractice*. Medical child abuse, as we define it, is quite distinct from malpractice. It is the product of medical care that is delivered in good faith, by concerned medical professionals, for the express benefit of the child. It is care that meets the standards of practice generally agreed on by the medical community given the signs and symptoms demonstrated by the child or asserted by the caretaker. It is also medical care that would not be given if it were not for the improper actions of the child's caretaker.

If someone hits a child with a stick we do not blame the stick. We place responsibility with the person who wields the stick. In medical child abuse, medical care is the stick, the implement of the abuse. The physician may prescribe the medical care, but the primary responsibility lies with the adult caretaker who violates the treatment contract by giving false or misleading information regarding the need for medical treatment. Clearly, the physician is not an unthinking stick and maintains responsibility for the treatments prescribed. However, this does not absolve the caretaker from his or her basic responsibility to the child.

Evidence for Building a Consensus

We first presented the concept of *medical child abuse* at the annual meeting of the American Professional Society on the Abuse of Children (APSAC) in

Tucson, AZ, in 1995. In the last dozen years we have lectured many times at local and national meetings explaining the concept. But we have not been alone in using the term. Long before we began using *medical child abuse*, Fleischer and Ament[4] referred to *medicinal abuse*. In the same year we presented in Tucson, Libow[5] also made reference to *medical abuse*. So did Boros and colleagues.[6] They not only used the term but suggested MSBP be retired. In her chapter written in 1996, Rand[7] advocated protecting the child "from physical, emotional, and medical abuse." Feldman and Allen[8] wrote about a judge commenting from the bench that factitious disorder by proxy "is a form of medical child abuse." Bryk,[9] in her courageous paper in *Pediatrics* published in 1997, described her experience as a child victim. She told of her mother repeatedly striking her with a hammer to cause injuries that would require medical care. In the abstract to the paper we find, "This article chronicles the actual experiences of an MBPS victim through 8 years of medical abuse at the hands of her mother…." Other uses of the terms *medical abuse* and *medical child abuse* show up in the literature more recently.[10,11]

These authors used *medical abuse* as a synonym for MSBP. Rather than using the term as a convenient synonym for MSBP, factitious disorder by proxy, pediatric condition falsification, or some other variation, we have advocated simply calling this class of child maltreatment what it really is, child abuse.

In doing so we have echoed many professionals who have expressed discomfort with the MSBP label, including Meadow, who gave us the name in the first place. We have already referred to Meadow[12] commenting as early as 1991, "at times I have regretted coining it." There has been a steady stream of commentators who advocated diagnosing a specific illness, or describing the effects of the abuse in place of making a diagnosis of MSBP. Fisher and Mitchell[13] in 1995 wrote, "It is recommended that paediatricians abandon making a diagnosis of Munchausen syndrome by proxy or factitious illness by proxy and instead diagnose the specific fabricated or induced medical illness(es) or condition(s) they encounter."

Also in 1995 Morley[14] said, "The diagnosis of Munchausen syndrome by proxy gives no indication about what happened to the child. As a substitute I suggest that the exact nature of the problem should be stated: suffocation, poisoning, putting blood in the urine, falsely reporting fits, or whatever is the problem."

Davis and Sibert[15] wrote, "Just as with other medical terms in the past, which have entered into public usage and changed their meaning (such as mongolism, idiocy, cretinism, etc), Munchausen syndrome by proxy has come to mean something else and has lost its value. We believe factitious illness spectrum disorder of childhood would be an appropriate substitute. We should always try and qualify this however by defining exactly what abuse was perpetrated and what the harm was to the child."

As yet another example that sentiment against the use of MSBP has been evident for many years we quote from Donald and Jureidini[16]: "We suggest a more rigorous approach to Munchausen syndrome by proxy, with explicit acknowledgment that it is abuse and that the medical system is critical to its genesis. This leads us to question the broadness with which the label is applied (eg, in cases of imposed upper airway obstruction) and to argue for management strategies closer to those accepted for other forms of child maltreatment."

In the last chapter we documented the general confusion in the field regarding MSBP. Against this backdrop there is an emerging consensus that use of *MSBP* is not helpful. As an example, Meadow[17] has recently commented that the term *MSBP* is seldom used in court anymore in Great Britain. He explained that courts have found it much more useful to understand exactly what harm the child has experienced and whether or not the child needs protection from future harm. In the last few years he and others have referred to MSBP as Munchausen syndrome by proxy *abuse*.[18-20] Recognized experts have found it necessary to systematically attach "abuse" to MSBP presumably to maintain a primary focus on the "act" rather than the "actor."

In the same vein, Eminson and Jureidini[20] recently wrote, "The use of a label like MSBP establishes that child abuse is an issue and that the medical system is involved.... But categorization of the parent as the perpetrator of MSBP or the child as a victim of MSBP abuse provides clinicians with little further guidance as to what psychological and physical management is appropriate for this particular child."

Wilson,[21] commenting in an editorial in the *British Medical Journal* on the recently released government report regarding "fabricated or induced illness in children by carers," concurred that it was time to abandon the term. He concluded, "Munchausen by proxy has had an honourable life and valuable effects beyond its own confines."

Similarities With Other Forms of Child Maltreatment

In the conclusion to his original paper Meadow[1] wrote that despite the fact that the 2 children he described were the victims of abuse, he felt it necessary to draw a distinction, and not categorize them as "variants of non-accidental injury." He felt it necessary to set them apart from other victims of child abuse based on "quality, periodicity, and planning" on the part of the perpetrator. But in the last 3 decades, as we have gained more experience with child maltreatment in general, the differences from other types of child abuse have lessened and the similarities have become more apparent. As an obvious example, who engages more in the planning of child abuse than a predatory pedophile who might spend years grooming a particular victim?

A central feature that supposedly distinguished MSBP from other types of child abuse was the perpetrator giving false information regarding how the child became ill.[22,23] Yet in other types of child abuse, getting a truthful account of how a child was abused is rare and deceit is commonplace. Jones[24] commented, "It appears that as each variety of child abuse is explored the density of denial becomes described by successive groups of clinicians. Yet denial was clearly described in the earliest accounts of physical abuse and has constituted a central part of many of the cases." In fact, lying about how one's child came to harm almost seems natural because telling the truth in such circumstances has potentially dire consequences for the perpetrator of that harm.

Another feature medical child abuse shares with other types of child maltreatment is the wide variety of possible abusive events. These acts of abuse can vary in both kind and severity. Abusive events can happen one time or many times. One child can be exposed to many different kinds of abusive events.

In each of the categories of abuse and neglect experienced by children there is a continuum of behavior from mild to severe. The events can be trivial or life-threatening. As an example, let us look at corporal punishment. The range of possible corporal punishment behavior stretches from threatening a spanking, to a light tap on the bottom, to a vigorous spanking with the hand, to beating with an object causing disfigurement or death.

Sexual abuse can range from inappropriate sexual comments to repeated rape. Likewise, medical child abuse presents as a continuum from over-anxious parenting to induction of illness requiring life-threatening surgery.[25]

This understanding, that child abuse and neglect fall along a continuum of behaviors, leads to another similarity between medical child abuse and other forms of child maltreatment. In all forms of child abuse and neglect there is a process of determining when a certain threshold has been met that results in a child requiring protection. At some point on the continuum, behavior experienced by a child impresses the larger community as being potentially harmful. This line, which when crossed constitutes abuse, is determined by a number of factors. The threshold is defined by culture and locale. Any form of corporal punishment is against the law in Sweden. Spanking in Sweden, even with an open hand, is a form of physical child abuse. In the United States, in most jurisdictions, corporal punishment is legal and not considered abusive as long as it does not result in marks on the skin of the child. And in many developing countries punishment with a stick, with the accompanying welts, is considered normal child-rearing behavior.

What constitutes abuse changes over time and exists in a cultural context. What is physical abuse today in the United States was normal parenting a century ago. Whether a specific behavior "crosses the line" is not a medical question per se. Medical care providers are part of their culture and, reflecting the mores of that culture, are qualified to render an opinion about the possibility that the threshold has been reached whereupon a child needs protection. But the real determiner of fact is the courts and, by extension, the child protection system. These together represent the systematic expression of society's beliefs and desires about what constitutes good enough parenting and what represents potentially harmful child-rearing.

There are several references to the concept of "crossing the line" in the MSBP literature. As early as 1989 Meadow[26] addressed the threshold issue directly. "Anxious parents may worry needlessly that their healthy child is ill. A mother who is inexperienced, under stress, lonely, or herself ill is all the more likely to perceive symptoms in her child that others do not observe. The child is taken to doctors, perhaps on many occasions, if she cannot be reassured. Often the child will have unpleasant investigations and treatments because of the mother's insistence. Most doctors, however, would not classify this process as child abuse unless the mother's persistence and refusal to accept normal results was excessive and the quality of the child's life was being seriously impaired." Here, the author is using a 2-part commonsense rule, the mother not listening to medical advice and "the child's life was being seriously impaired," as the threshold defining abuse.

Godding and Kruth[27] concluded that 17 patients in their practice of asthma and allergy were victims of MSBP. "The abuse consisted mainly of neglect, in that necessary treatment was not given. In some cases a more direct form of abuse was observed, when useless and sometimes harmful investigations and treatment were given." They recognized that behavior of the parents of the 17 children was seen in many other parents in their practice but felt that treatment by the parents of these particular children exceeded a perceived standard that, for them, constituted abuse. They proceeded to call this abuse MSBP.

One of the justifications used for separating victims of medical child abuse from their caretakers is the presumed high fatality rate in this type of abuse. The implication is that a parent who exaggerates symptoms will proceed to fabrication of symptoms and eventually to induction of illness. The presumption is that, given a continuum of behavior from mild to severe, a perpetrator will proceed along that path eventually resulting in the child experiencing fatal child abuse. What we actually see, not surprisingly, is a pattern common with other types of child abuse. The fact that a continuum exists in all forms of child maltreatment does not necessarily imply that a perpetrator will escalate along that continuum. A parent who spanks a child with her hand does not necessarily go on to beat her child with a stick. Discovering that a child has been exposed to inappropriate nudity by his parents does not necessarily mean the child will be sexually fondled or forced to have intercourse. Yet, it sometimes happens. The mother of the boy who eventually ended up having multiple acute life-threatening events in the hospital that we described in the introduction started by exaggerating symptoms. This was a clear example of medical abuse where the parent actually did proceed along the continuum from illness exaggeration, to fabrication, and to life-threatening illness induction. In this regard, medical child abuse once again shares a general characteristic with other forms of child maltreatment. Some cases show patterns of escalating harmful behavior, and others do not.

It is commonly accepted that children exposed to one kind of abuse or neglect are often exposed to other forms. Roughly one-quarter of children evaluated for sexual abuse also meet criteria for having experienced physical abuse.[28] Children with histories of physical abuse often have experienced neglect. We see this as well with victims of medical child abuse who have experienced other forms of maltreatment. From the earliest examples this has been the case. In 1968 Pickering and Ellis[29] reported on a child they felt was the victim of accidental salicylate poisoning due to lack of knowledge on the part of the mother. The same child was admitted to the hospital 8 years later "…after being assaulted by her mother; her head had been beaten against the wall, producing extensive bruising, and her legs were widely bruised from trauma produced by a leather belt."[30] On the basis of this subsequent example of physical abuse, and from information about the intervening years, the authors revised their earlier assumption and concluded that the mother had purposefully poisoned her child in infancy with aspirin. They concluded that the infant was a victim of "the battered child syndrome" with the "battering" being chemical rather than physical.

While others have reported similar findings,[31,32] Bools and colleagues[33] were especially effective in documenting other forms of abuse in victims of medical child abuse and their siblings. They found that 73% of the 56 children who had been victims of what they referred to as *fabricated illnesses* had an additional history of non-accidental injury, failure to thrive (FTT), inappropriate medication administration, or neglect. Also, 17% of their siblings had been diagnosed with FTT, neglect, non-accidental injury, or were receiving inappropriate medication.

Children abused medically have often been maltreated in other ways. Likewise, parents who commit different types of maltreatment may have common characteristics. As Fisher[34] says, "No two abusive parents are the same, yet a careful study of physically, sexually, and emotionally abusive parents reveals common patterns of past histories and life experiences—and many of these histories are shared with parents who fabricate or induce illnesses in their children. Unfortunately, and probably because of the dramatic and sensational reports of MBP in the literature and recently in the media, I believe there has been a tendency for MBP to be considered radically different from the better-known and understood types of child abuse."

The APSAC Taskforce on Munchausen by Proxy, Definitions Working Group[35] divided MSBP into 2 parts that they called *factitious disorder by proxy*, a diagnosis given to the perpetrator, and *pediatric condition falsification*, a diagnosis assigned to the child. The group specifically addressed the problem of how to use *Diagnostic and Statistical Manual of Mental Disorders, Fourth Edition* and *International Classification of Diseases, Ninth Revision (ICD-9)* diagnostic classifications. This is not a trivial matter as receiving compensation for evaluation and treatment services is dependent on having an appropriate diagnostic code to attach to a request for payment. The group concluded that pediatric condition falsification be coded as "…Child Abuse-V61.21 when focus is on perpetrator, Child Abuse-995.5, when focus is on victim…."[35] Code 995.5 refers to "child maltreatment syndrome." Specific types of child abuse can be designated with a fifth number. For example, code 995.50 represents child abuse, unspecified, while code 995.51 is child abuse, emotional/psychological abuse. Code 61.21 indicates that the perpetrator was a parent. It is entirely appropriate to code medical child abuse as *ICD-9* code 995.5 and it seems equally appropriate that if we are going to code it as child abuse that we call it *child abuse* instead of *pediatric condition falsification*.

In the last chapter we highlighted the controversy regarding treatment of MSBP. On the one hand, professionals stated that it was not treatable. On the other, there were claims that it responded to treatment. This seeming contradiction dissolves if one considers that what has been called MSBP is really child abuse and therefore would be expected to respond to treatment just as successfully as other types of child abuse. Once again, we are only asserting what others have suggested previously. Meadow[36] in one of his earliest papers wrote about children with seizures either fabricated or induced by their caretakers: "When it was proved, or extremely probable, that the epilepsy was false it was usual for the child to be protected in the same way as for other forms of child abuse, the social services department was notified, a case conference convened, and very often a court order imposed for the safety of the child."

Basically the same treatment strategy has been advocated on a number of occasions.[37–41] The general treatment plan involves identifying the abuse, stopping it, making sure that it does not reoccur, ameliorating the consequences of the abuse, and doing this in the least restrictive environment, which includes dealing with the perpetrator.

What Makes Medical Child Abuse Unique

Different types of child abuse share many features. Deception on the part of the perpetrator, or unwillingness to take responsibility for the abuse, is common to all. Each type has many different ways in which it can present. There is usually a continuum of behavior from mild to severe. A determination of abuse is triggered by a community perception that a certain threshold has been reached that distinguishes harmful from adequate parenting. Having a range of behaviors from mild to severe allows for the possibility that a caretaker might escalate to committing more severe abuse, but this is not always the case. Children abused in one manner often find themselves experiencing other forms of child maltreatment. And the same general treatment process applies to all forms of child abuse.

What distinguishes one type of abuse from another is the form the abuse takes. In sexual abuse the abusive act includes sexual activities. Physical abuse implies physical harm done to the body. Psychological abuse affects the psyche. Medical abuse requires a medical environment. According to Donald and Juridini,[16] it is differentiated from the other forms of child abuse "…only by the active engagement with the medical profession in the production of morbidity."

There is some evidence that medical abuse occurs more frequently in families that put a high value on somatic symptoms and medical treatment.[42] This hypothesis will need to be tested in further research but it stands to reason that people who grow up going to doctors for reasons that might not have much to do with need for medical care might be more likely to involve their children in unnecessary medical care. Fisher[34] wrote, "It is very common for parents who have perpetrated abuse to disclose that they felt uncared for, not close to their parents, never good enough, left out, or unwanted." For parents who commit medical abuse we might want to add "a tendency to pay special attention to somatic complaints."

One issue that may distinguish medical child abuse from other types of abuse and neglect is a concern that it is primarily a phenomenon of developed countries. The prevalence of sexual abuse has been found to be remarkably consistent across cultures. If one uses a definition such as, "unwanted physical contact with the genitals between a child 14 years or younger and someone at least 4 years older," there are similar percentages of adults describing such contact in countries from many continents.

Concern regarding medical abuse, however, has been expressed in countries with the best-developed medical systems. Most reports come from the United States, Great Britain, Australia, New Zealand, and Western Europe. Does there need to be a well-established medical care delivery system for medical child abuse to exist? And more specifically, does Western-style medicine, with its reliance on multiple diagnostic tests and subspecialty referrals provide an environment where children are more likely to be abused in this way? There have been reported cases in the literature from other countries but such reports are few and far between.[43–45] Feldman and Brown[46] reviewed the literature from developing countries and concluded that factitious disorder by proxy could be said to be a product of Western medicine.

Putting the New Concept Into Practice

At the beginning of this chapter we stated that using the term *medical child abuse* represents a major change in our thinking that simplifies evaluation and treatment. We have discussed how the term *medical child abuse* fits into the framework of our existing child maltreatment structure. Now we would like to review how the use of the term *medical child abuse* clarifies the problems identified in Chapter 1.

For a new theoretical concept to have usefulness it must take existing information and pieces of data that did not fit in an old theoretical construct, and allow them to fall into place easily. The questions discussed in Chapter 1 offer multiple pieces of data that do not fit well within the theoretical framework of MSBP or one of its synonyms. Let's take the issues one at a time and see how the medical child abuse framework explains them.

1. **Is this really a syndrome?**
    No. The behavior commonly called MSBP is a form of child abuse that takes place in a medical setting. Child abuse is not an illness or a syndrome in the traditional sense but an event that happens in the life of the child. The consequences of medical abuse can lead to both emotional and physical disease in children. The definition for *medical child abuse* is: A child receiving unnecessary and harmful or potentially harmful medical care at the instigation of a caretaker.

2. **What should we call it?**
   Medical child abuse. Using this term ensures that we focus on the fact that a child is being abused, and that the abuse takes place within a medical setting. The term *medical child abuse* implies that medical care is being used to harm children. To determine who is responsible for the maltreatment one must identify who initiates the harmful medical care. If the doctor initiates the treatment, we call it *malpractice*. If a parent or caretaker instigates the treatment, we call it *medical child abuse*.

3. **If MSBP is an illness, to whom is the diagnosis assigned?**
   Medical child abuse is not an illness. However, it is clear that the recipient of the abuse is a child. For reimbursement purposes it is appropriate to use *ICD-9* codes identifying child abuse (995.5).

4. **How far does the MSBP concept extend?**
   Medical child abuse is defined as a child receiving unnecessary and harmful or potentially harmful medical care. It would not be appropriate to use the term for someone other than a child or for behavior that does not take place as part of medical care. Adults mistreated by other adults do not experience child abuse. Animals subjected to abuse by their owners are more properly identified by language including cruelty to animals. Children receiving unnecessary sexual abuse evaluations at the instigation of a parent are clearly victims of medical child abuse because repeated, unwarranted medical examinations and sexual abuse interviews are abusive. Children prescribed psychotropic medications solely because their caretaker repeatedly reports symptoms of attention-deficit/hyperactivity disorder (ADHD) that turn out not to be observed by an objective third party are victims of medical child abuse. However, if parents insist their children suffer from ADHD but the children receive no psychotropic medications, or other unnecessary medical care, it would not be appropriate to use the medical child abuse designation.

5. **How important is the motivation of the perpetrator?**
   Just as important as it is for any other type of child abuse or neglect. The motivation of the perpetrator is not necessary to make the determination of medical child abuse but is quite useful in answering management questions such as, "Can the child remain safely in the custody of the caretaker?"

6. **What is the prevalence of this syndrome, and how serious is it?**
   Until we have used the definition consistently in a number of jurisdictions we cannot know what the prevalence might be. Once having said that medical child abuse is a child receiving unnecessary and harmful or potentially harmful medical care, it remains to be seen what various communities consider surpassing the threshold or crossing the line. We all have a general idea of what represents unnecessary medical care but this is a decision to be made by representatives of the community at large in courtrooms and child protection offices.

   It is easier to say how serious it is. Medical child abuse is just as serious as other forms of child abuse. We can say there are mild, moderate, and severe presentations just as there are for psychological abuse, sexual abuse, and physical abuse. At the mild end of the spectrum, children experience only mild harm. An example might be missing several weeks of school each year attending unnecessary doctor visits. At the other end of the spectrum, medical child abuse can result in death.

7. **Is there a profile that can be used to identify potential perpetrators of MSBP?**
   No. There is no more specificity in identifying perpetrators of medical child abuse than there is for other types of child abuse. Perpetrators of child abuse have been shown to come from all ethnic backgrounds, walks of life, and economic strata. To date, there are no studies that show perpetrators of medical child abuse to be significantly different from any other type of child abuse perpetrator with the exception that perpetrators of medical child abuse tend toward somatization in their own lives.[42] Keep in mind, however, that most adults who tend to over-interpret their own physical symptoms do not exaggerate, fabricate, or induce illness in their children.

8. **Is treatment of MSBP possible?**
   Medical child abuse is clearly treatable if one defines treatment the same way one defines other types of child abuse treatment. It is possible to identify the abuse, to stop it, to prevent it from reoccurring, to treat the consequences of the abuse, and to do this in the least restrictive environment.

In summary, medical child abuse, as an organizing model, allows for clear straightforward answers to the basic questions that have confounded the field. The concept *medical child abuse* allows us to see what needs to be done and how to do it. We can use the existing legal and social service structures to protect children. There is an educational process that needs to take place similar to what police, prosecutors, and judges experienced when learning about physical and sexual abuse of children several decades ago. But the most difficult work will be within the medical profession itself as it sorts out its role in children being abused within the medical environment. Before we can address this question we need to look at how we got where we are today.

References

1. Meadow R. Munchausen syndrome by proxy. The hinterland of child abuse. *Lancet.* 13 1977;2(8033):343-345
2. Jenny C. Recognizing and responding to medical neglect. *Pediatrics.* 2007;120(6):1385-1389
3. Beitchman JH, Zucker KJ, Hood JE, daCosta GA, Akman D, Cassavia E. A review of the long-term effects of child sexual abuse. *Child Abuse Negl.* 1992;16(1):101-118
4. Fleisher D, Ament ME. Diarrhea, red diapers, and child abuse: clinical alertness needed for recognition; clinical skill needed for success in management. *Clin Pediatr.* 1977;16:820-824
5. Libow JA. Munchausen by proxy victims in adulthood: a first look. *Child Abuse Negl.* 1995;19(9):1131-1142
6. Boros SJ, Ophoven JP, Andersen R, Brubaker LC. Munchausen syndrome by proxy: a profile for medical child abuse. *Aust Fam Physician.* 1995;24(5):768-769, 772-763
7. Rand DC. Comprehensive psychosocial assessment in factitious disorder by proxy. In: Feldman MD, Eisendrath SJ, eds. *The Spectrum of Factitious Disorders.* Washington, DC: American Psychiatric Press; 1996:109-133
8. Feldman MD, Allen DB. "False-positive" factitious disorder by proxy. *South Med J.* 1996;89(4):452-453
9. Bryk M, Siegel PT. My mother caused my illness: the story of a survivor of Munchausen by proxy syndrome. *Pediatrics.* 1997;100(1):1-7
10. Rand DC, Feldman MD. An explanatory model for Munchausen by proxy abuse. *Int J Psychiatry Med.* 2001;31(2):113-126
11. von Hahn L, Harper G, McDaniel SH, Siegel DM, Feldman MD, Libow JA. A case of factitious disorder by proxy: the role of the health-care system, diagnostic dilemmas, and family dynamics. *Harv Rev Psychiatry.* 2001;9(3):124-135

12. Meadow R. Commentary. *Arch Dis Child.* 1991;66:960
13. Fisher GC, Mitchell I. Is Munchausen syndrome by proxy really a syndrome? *Arch Dis Child.* 1995;72(6):530-534
14. Morley CJ. Practical concerns about the diagnosis of Munchausen syndrome by proxy. *Arch Dis Child.* 1995;72(6):528-529; discussion 529-530
15. Davis PM, Sibert JR. Munchausen syndrome by proxy or factitious illness spectrum disorder of childhood. *Arch Dis Child.* 1996;74(3):274-275
16. Donald T, Jureidini J. Munchausen syndrome by proxy. Child abuse in the medical system. *Arch Pediatr Adolesc Med.* 1996;150(7):753-758
17. Meadow R. Different interpretations of Munchausen syndrome by proxy. *Child Abuse Negl.* 2002;26(5):501-508
18. Meadow R. Munchausen syndrome by proxy abuse perpetrated by men. *Arch Dis Child.* 1998;78(3):210-216
19. Southall DP, Plunkett MC, Banks MW, Falkov AF, Samuels MP. Covert video recordings of life-threatening child abuse: lessons for child protection. *Pediatrics.* 1997;100(5):735-760
20. Eminson M, Jureidini J. Concerns about research and prevention strategies in Munchausen syndrome by proxy (MSBP) abuse. *Child Abuse Negl.* 2003;27(4):413-420
21. Wilson RG. Fabricated or induced illness in children. Munchausen by proxy comes of age. *BMJ.* 2001;323(7308):296-297
22. Rosenberg DA. Web of deceit: a literature review of Munchausen syndrome by proxy. *Child Abuse Negl.* 1987;11(4):547-563
23. Sheridan MS. The deceit continues: an updated literature review of Munchausen syndrome by proxy. *Child Abuse Negl.* 2003;27(4):431-451
24. Jones DP. The syndrome of Munchausen by proxy. *Child Abuse Negl.* 1994;18(9):769-771
25. Ludwig S. The role of the physician. In: Levin AV, Sheridan MS, eds. *Munchausen Syndrome by Proxy: Issues in Diagnosis and Treatment.* New York, NY: Lexington Books; 1995:287-294
26. Meadow R. ABC of child abuse. Munchausen syndrome by proxy. *BMJ.* 1989;299(6693):248-250
27. Godding V, Kruth M. Compliance with treatment in asthma and Munchausen syndrome by proxy. *Arch Dis Child.* 1991;66(8):956-960
28. Roesler TA, McKenzie N. Effects of childhood trauma on psychological functioning in adults sexually abused as children. *J Nerv Ment Dis.* 1994;182(3):145-150
29. Pickering D, Ellis H. Neonatal hypoglycaemia due to salicylate poisoning. *Proc R Soc Med.* 1968;61(12):1256
30. Pickering D. Letter: salicylate poisoning as a manifestation of the battered child syndrome. *Am J Dis Child.* 1976;130(6):675-676

31. Mitchell I, Brummitt J, DeForest J, Fisher G. Apnea and factitious illness (Munchausen syndrome) by proxy. *Pediatrics.* 1993;92(6):810-814
32. Gray J, Bentovim A. Illness induction syndrome: paper I—a series of 41 children from 37 families identified at The Great Ormond Street Hospital for Children NHS Trust. *Child Abuse Negl.* 1996;20(8):655-673
33. Bools CN, Neale BA, Meadow SR. Co-morbidity associated with fabricated illness (Munchausen syndrome by proxy). *Arch Dis Child.* 1992;67(1):77-79
34. Fisher GC. Etiological speculations. In: Levin AV, Sheridan MS, eds. *Munchausen Syndrome by Proxy: Issues in Diagnosis and Treatment.* New York, NY: Lexington Books; 1995:39-57
35. Ayoub CC, Alexander R, Beck D, et al. Position paper: definitional issues in Munchausen by proxy. *Child Maltreat.* 2002;7(2):105-111
36. Meadow R. Fictitious epilepsy. *Lancet.* 1984;2(8393):25-28
37. Senner A, Ott MJ. Munchausen syndrome by proxy. *Issues Compr Pediatr Nurs.* 1989;12(5):345-357
38. Kravitz RM, Wilmott RW. Munchausen syndrome by proxy presenting as factitious apnea. *Clin Pediatr (Phila).* 1990;29(10):587-592
39. Baldwin MA. Munchausen syndrome by proxy: neurological manifestations. *J Neurosci Nurs.* 1994;26(1):18-23
40. Masterson J, Wilson J. Factitious illness in children: the social worker's role in identification and management. *Soc Work Health Care.* 1987;12(4):21-30
41. Eminson DM, Postlethwaite RJ. *Munchausen Syndrome by Proxy Abuse: A Practical Approach.* London, UK: Arnold; 2001
42. Bools C, Neale B, Meadow R. Munchausen syndrome by proxy: a study of psychopathology. *Child Abuse Negl.* 1994;18(9):773-788
43. Bappal B, George M, Nair R, Khusaiby SA, De Silva V. Factitious hypoglycemia: a tale from the Arab world. *Pediatrics.* 2001;107(1):180-181
44. Al-Ateeqi W, Shabani I, Abdulmalik A. Child abuse in Kuwait: problems in management. *Med Princ Pract.* 2002;11(3):131-135
45. Ifere OA, Yakubu AM, Aikhionbare HA, Quaitey GE, Taqi AM. Munchausen syndrome by proxy: an experience from Nigeria. *Ann Trop Paediatr.* 1993;13(3):281-284
46. Feldman MD, Brown RM. Munchausen by proxy in an international context. *Child Abuse Negl.* 2002;26(5):509-524

Chapter 3

How Did We Get Here?

Munchausen syndrome by proxy often is managed differently from other forms of child maltreatment, although it is differentiated from them only by the active engagement with the medical profession in the production of morbidity. —Donald and Jureidini, 1996[1]

Introduction

To explain how we got where we are today, we must return to 1977 when Meadow[2] published, "Munchausen Syndrome by Proxy: The Hinterland of Child Abuse." Actually, we need to begin earlier. In 1951 Asher[3] wrote, in 3 pages, a paper giving an account of several patients who severely overused medical services. He made light of the fact that he was "dedicating the new illness" to the Baron von Munchausen whose name had become synonymous with exaggerated stories through a series of books filled with tall tales. He gave 3 case histories, made some comments, and said, "That is a general outline; and few doctors can boast that they have never been hoodwinked by the condition." He struck a responsive chord among his medical colleagues. Physicians had dealt with patients who malingered or fabricated symptoms for as long as the profession has existed. Still, the notion that certain patients could get hospitalized on numerous occasions for factitious reasons, thereby wasting important medical resources, caused considerable attention among Asher's colleagues. Doctors responded with letters to the editor acknowledging that they too had been "hoodwinked" and calls were made to establish a registry of patients who fabricated symptoms to get themselves admitted to the hospital.

Asher accentuated the part about the physician being manipulated by his patient. Meadow[2] referred to the deceitful acts of the parent but at the same time correctly identified this behavior as child abuse. He cited C. Henry

Kempe's[4] work on the battered child in a way that firmly placed his observations within the realm of protection of abused children. However, in his closing comments he said he did not feel comfortable calling the children victims of non-accidental injury. With these words he essentially said that what he called Munchausen syndrome by proxy (MSBP) was different from child abuse. If not non-accidental injury, then what was it?

We begin by looking at the time before Meadow's first paper to see how contemporaries were conceptualizing new presentations of child abuse. We see that a number of investigators were documenting alternate forms of child maltreatment, particularly examples of non-accidental poisoning. In the subsequent 5 years (1977–1982) the MSBP concept gradually came to be more widely applied. The next 4 years (1983–1987), ending in the publication of "Web of Deceit" by Rosenberg,[5] were marked by the appearance of fascinating case reports about how children could be harmed in the medical setting. In taking this historical journey we hope to discover how we got off the track.

The Years before 1977: Uncommon Manifestations and Non-accidental Poisoning

Prior to the publication of "The Battered Child Syndrome"[4] in 1962 there was little direct role for pediatricians in protecting children from abuse.[6] Social agencies in large cities responded to situations of severe neglect but physicians did not consider it part of their role to develop medical evidence demonstrating maltreatment. In fact, when Kempe presented his paper in 1961 as a workshop at the American Academy of Pediatrics, and later published his findings, he experienced a mixed response from the medical community.[6] Doctors found it difficult to believe that parents would beat their children on multiple occasions to cause the kinds of injuries Kempe and his colleagues were reporting. Ten years later he followed his work on physical abuse with a description of children who had been sexually abused in their families.[7] In both cases his scholarly approach and his status as chair of the Department of Pediatrics at the University of Colorado gave permission for a new generation of pediatricians to consider child abuse as a major factor affecting the lives of their patients.

In his original paper, Kempe and colleagues[4] described the battered child in very general terms. In fact, the original representation was so all-inclusive that just about any form of physical abuse would qualify as battered child syndrome. "In an occasional case the parent or parent substitute may also have assaulted the child by administering an overdose of a drug or by exposing the child to natural gas or other toxic substances."[4] The authors said the syndrome could vary from very mild to extremely severe. It was only later that battered child syndrome came to be identified with the classic features resulting from multiple beatings. In 1975 he published "Uncommon Manifestations of the Battered Child Syndrome"[8] as an editorial comment to several child abuse papers published in the same issue of the journal. He listed 11 symptom presentations that should alert physicians to possible child abuse, including hypernatremic dehydration resulting from a parent withholding water and non-accidental poisoning with barbiturates or other tranquilizing substances. He concluded the brief paper saying, "Readers are invited to submit additional examples in order to improve our clinical acumen in this difficult field."

The next year Pickering[9] answered with, "Salicylate Poisoning As a Manifestation of the Battered Child Syndrome." He began his paper by saying, "Kempe has asked for case reports of drug poisoning as a manifestation of the battered child syndrome." He discussed a child seen at age 19 days with aspirin poisoning. At that time it was unclear whether this was an accidental or non-accidental poisoning. However, when the child returned years later covered with bruises from being beaten Pickering felt comfortable reassessing his original diagnosis.

Dine[10] has the distinction of being one of the first physicians to publish a detailed case description of non-accidental poisoning as child abuse. He described a 19-month-old child admitted 5 times in 4 months with episodes of prolonged sleep. His mother offered vague reports of head injury to explain the sleepiness but there were never any confirmatory findings. The mother was questioned specifically on several occasions regarding the child ingesting something accidentally but consistently denied that he had received any substances that might make him sleep. However, his physicians continued to believe he might have been poisoned and, because of this, kept him in the hospital for 7 days during which time he had no difficulties. On the seventh hospital day his mother visited him in his room and gave him ice cream. A half an hour later he became unconscious. The psychotropic medication, perphenazine, a phenothiazine sold as Trilafon, was found in his urine.

When confronted with this evidence and the information that the hospital staff knew she possessed a prescription for this medication the mother continued to deny she had done anything to her child. However, she did get herself admitted to a psychiatric facility and her child was sent home in the custody of his father under supervision of child protective services. In additional comments the author adds that this youngster had previously been treated for iron deficiency anemia, frequent pneumonias, and failure to thrive. He states that the child's mother had been prescribed the psychotropic medication she used to poison her child after receiving a diagnosis of postpartum psychosis. She had made several suicide attempts.

We discuss this case in such detail because it is prototypical of literally hundreds of case reports made over the next 40 years. This account was published in *Pediatrics* in 1965, 3 years after Kempe's battered child article and 12 years before Meadow's MSBP paper. Dine comments directly on similar features of this type of child abuse with those published by Kempe that dealt with physical abuse. He also points out differences, such as the abuse continued while in the hospital. He called attention to the child experiencing neglect from iron deficiency anemia and failure to thrive. He also commented on the perpetrator of the abuse refusing to acknowledge or cooperate with the investigation as being similar to the parents who batter their children. The child received unnecessary medical care including numerous diagnostic tests and a trial of phenobarbital for seizures that were caused by the serial drug overdoses. His mother gave false medical history. In the discussion of the mother's behavior on the hospital ward Dine wrote that she acted in a manner consistent with that reported by Fontana and associates,[11] "Many of these patients do give the outward impression of devotion to their children. They may present the disarming attitude of over protectiveness, cooperativeness, and neatness."

When Dine and McGovern[12] next published a review of cases of intentional poisoning of children they were able to acknowledge Meadow's contribution. Yet they continued to document cases of poisoning as a response to Kempe's call for reporting of uncommon examples of child abuse. The 48 cases they assembled had been published in 28 different scientific publications by different authors. As an example, they cited Lansky,[13] "An Unusual Case of Childhood Chloral Hydrate Poisoning." The child had come to the hospital in a coma on 4 different occasions after the mother gave gastric tube feedings.

They also included the work of Rodgers and colleagues[14] from the Hospital for Sick Children in London. This group published a paper titled, "Nonaccidental Poisoning: An Extended Syndrome of Child Abuse." The authors describe 7 cases of poisoning. The substances used included salt, diuretics, Tuinal, methaqualone, dihydrocodeine, and phenformin. The case histories read very much like Dine's original article. The children were described as having experienced other forms of child abuse such as being treated at the age of 2 months for a scald burn and black eyes. Two of these children had siblings who died under unusual circumstances. Several of the mothers were hospitalized in psychiatric facilities after being confronted by medical staff. The authors offered these comments regarding their involvement in the cases: "We and other clinicians diagnosing this form of child abuse almost invariably found it difficult to be objective in assessing the significance of the known facts related to these children. This emotional barrier has been recognized as a problem in the diagnosis of conventional forms of child abuse and must be overcome if such children are to be adequately protected. Once the validity of the diagnosis has been accepted in some cases subsequent cases were easier to assess objectively." This paper was published in the *British Medical Journal* in 1976.

Others heeded Kempe's call. Berger[15] described 2 children with multiple episodes of suffocation. Jones[16] wrote about a mother who produced factitious skin lesions on both her and her baby. Mortimer[17] titled his paper, "Acute Water Intoxication As Another Unusual Manifestation of Child Abuse." Kempe's influence was clearly obvious in the following quote from the paper, "Kempe listed some of the rarer manifestations of this disorder and asked that others should be reported so as to improve clinical acumen in this difficult field." The case Mortimer reported involved a 4-year-old boy admitted to the hospital in a coma after having been forced to drink water from a garden hose as punishment for soiling.

In 1981 Shnaps and colleagues[18] published, "The Chemically Abused Child." In it they described an 18-month-old girl poisoned by her mother with chlorpromazine. The authors summarized 15 other cases of non-accidental poisoning, many of which were included in the larger series later published by Dine. They discussed how non-accidental poisoning was different from physical battering and observed that the abuse may go on longer and the parents may be more mentally disturbed. They acknowledged Meadow's article and the MSBP concept but, like Dine publishing a year later, followed

Kempe in describing non-accidental poisoning as an unusual type of child abuse. Two years later, Baugh and colleagues[19] reported a case of severe salt poisoning in a 5-year-old boy they referred to as "chemical abuse." The boy had burn scars on his feet and ankles from previous abuse. He was given salt as a punishment for enuresis.

By 1983 Fischler[20] was able to document 222 cases in his paper titled, "Poisoning: A Syndrome of Child Abuse." He discussed several kinds of parent behavior that resulted in children being poisoned including MSBP, which he said accounted for 20 of the cases he was reporting. Among his examples of poisoning were parental use of alcohol and other medicines to sedate a child inappropriately and use of toxic doses of vitamins or other substances that were originally intended for healthy purposes.

During the same general time, without making reference to Kempe (or Meadow), pediatricians reported cases of parents injecting insulin to produce hypoglycemia,[21–23] water intoxication,[24] polymicrobial sepsis,[25] recurrent suffocation,[26] malnutrition from cult diets,[27] and various other types of non-accidental poisoning.[28] None of these authors, including those publishing after 1977, described the children as victims of MSBP.

The cases just cited of uncommon manifestations of child abuse involved parents inducing or fabricating illness, children presenting for medical treatment on multiple occasions resulting in multiple medical procedures, denial of knowledge by the perpetrator as to the etiology of the child's illness, and symptoms abating in the absence of the perpetrator. In other words, these cases meet criteria according to Rosenberg[5] for MSBP. There were many motivations ascribed to parents.

Growing Acceptance of MSBP: 1977–1982

The year 1977 saw the publication of "Munchausen Syndrome by Proxy: The Hinterland of Child Abuse."[2] In his paper Meadow introduced a new element, namely, the motive of the parent, the purpose for which the abuse was committed. With Meadow and MSBP, caretakers are said to possess a motivation to deceive the medical care establishment to meet a specific personal need of the parent. This became a prism through which future cases of uncommon manifestations of child abuse in a medical care setting were viewed. Between 1977 and 1982, as we have seen, new cases of child abuse were portrayed primarily as unusual manifestations of the battered child syndrome. But this was about to change.

For example, in 1978 Hvizdala and Gellady[29] published, "Intentional Poisoning of Two Siblings by Prescription Drugs: An Unusual Form of Child Abuse." A mother poisoned one child with barbiturates, resulting in ataxia, and a second with warfarin, causing a bleeding disorder. The authors stated that Meadow had recently reported a similar case but also cited Schmitt and Kempe.[30] In 1979 Lee[31] gave an account of twins whose mother simulated bleeding with her own blood, but also was caught pricking the lip of her 4-month-old. She was found guilty of assault and her children were placed in the care of social services. The author referred to this as a case similar to that having been recently described by Meadow but stated that it seemed that the mother felt incapable of raising the children and was using the hospital as a refuge for them. The author evidently felt it important to comment on the motivation of the parent but inferred a motivation different from that suggested by Meadow. In 1981 Outwater and colleagues[32] published a case involving a child with hematuria (blood in the urine). They used minor blood group typing to determine that the blood came from the patient's mother. They cited Meadow's original paper and commented that it included a case of factitious hematuria.

In 1982 Hodge and colleagues[33] published, "The Bacteriologically Battered Baby: Another Case of Munchausen by Proxy." They cited both Kempe and Meadow, described a child with polymicrobial sepsis induced by her mother, identified it as child abuse, and characterized it as a case of MSBP. They observed in the discussion that only 9 other cases had been referred to in the literature as MSBP prior to their writing. Note the title and the debt it owes to "the battered child syndrome." When Halsey et al[34] and Liston and colleagues[35] published their single case reports of polymicrobial sepsis in 1982 and 1983 they characterized them as MSBP (although Liston and colleagues used the term *Polle syndrome*).

Meadow has described the interest generated during those years by his initial paper among his colleagues in Great Britain. He wrote a letter to the editor in 1982,[36] saying he had received information regarding more than 60 children whose parents fabricated symptoms of epilepsy or induced seizures in their child. Also that year he published a series of 19 cases summarizing his experience over the preceding few years.[37]

These cases give a much more detailed description than offered previously of what Meadow meant by MSBP. Meadow said he only included children in this case series where there was "...clear evidence of massive and persistent fabrication by a parent of both the history and the signs." He wrote that he did not include children where there was suspected or mild fabrication "...nor did he include the slightly more common instances of children who were poisoned by a parent. However if poisoning occurred as well as other fabricated acts by the parent the child is included." From these comments and from the references cited we must assume that Meadow was not only aware of the growing literature regarding non-accidental poisoning, but felt that he could distinguish MSBP from these other acts of child abuse by considering the quality of parental behavior.

The children he described suffered through multiple medical evaluations, hospitalizations, trials of medication, and diagnostic procedures that were, for the most part, completely unnecessary but carried out because of the false information provided by parents. The author included fascinating details of the lengths to which parents went to medicalize their child. Meadow said of one boy, "He was prescribed and given the following drugs for the alleged illness: prednisolone, hydrocortisone, ACTH, intravenous methylprednisolone, cyclophosphamide, azathioprine, ampicillin, penicillin, cephaloridine, erythromycin, co-trimoxizole, fusidic acid, cimetidine, metoclopramide, propantheline, prochlorperazine, trimeprazine, chlorpromazine, trifluoperazine, hydralaxine, methyldopa, frusemide, naproxen, aspirin, paracetamol, pethidine, and phenylbutazone. At the time the deception was revealed he was being considered for plasmaphoresis [kidney dialysis]."

What did the new prism mean for practicing physicians? Not only were pediatricians to determine that abuse was occurring in the medical environment, that their own medical treatments might in fact be unnecessary and harmful, but it was also incumbent on them to determine the parent's motive for perpetuating the abuse. The next few years (1983–1987) represented the height of pediatric reporting of fascinating and bizarre cases of MSBP. This was a watershed time for MSBP. Meadow set the example but he soon had many peers.

The Golden Age of Case Reports: 1983–1987

The fascinating case reports from this era introduced issues that we still struggle with today. For example, in 1983 Rosen et al[38] published, "Two Siblings with Recurrent Cardiorespiratory Arrest: Munchausen Syndrome by Proxy or Child Abuse?" Here is how the perpetrator is described: "The mother never took the children anywhere without resuscitation equipment. She reported that some days she didn't even have time to get dressed in the morning; she just went from child to child performing resuscitations. She confided that her husband, who was a minister, could not cope with the children's problems; he had left the medical responsibilities up to her and had become immersed in his work." The mother was subsequently observed on videotape smothering the younger of the 2 children. On being shown the videotape she initially denied that she had done anything, then admitted that she had smothered the child on one occasion. Soon after being confronted she attempted suicide and was hospitalized. Psychological testing done at the time indicated she suffered from a narcissistic personality disorder. The title of the paper suggests that the confusion existing today, whether to call this child abuse or MSBP, was present at that time as well.

Palmer and Yoshimura[39] published a case study in 1984 of polymicrobial sepsis in the *Journal of the American Academy of Child Psychiatry*. The authors cited references that included 24 patients described in the literature prior to their publication as having MSBP. Of note, a significant portion of those patients were described by their authors as non-accidental poisoning or other forms of child abuse and not MSBP. In other words, Palmer and Yoshimura retroactively redefined children who were poisoned by caretakers and treated by other physicians as having experienced MSBP. It is unclear if they felt they were able to determine the motivation of the perpetrator or just included all cases of non-accidental poisoning in the new MSBP category.

The patient they described was a 9-year-old girl who began going to the hospital in her first weeks of life and continued to have numerous medical difficulties until she was removed from the home at age 2½. The mother was suspected of having poisoned her child the year previously, and firm evidence was discovered of non-accidental poisoning when the child was 21 months of age. Between the ages of 2½ and 5 the child lived in foster care and thrived. Her developmental delays completely resolved but she did continue to show psychiatric difficulties. "While Lynn was in foster care, her parents divorced, her father was incarcerated for sexually abusing her older sister, and her mother attempted suicide and was hospitalized." The child was returned to her mother at the age of 5 against the advice of her physician and the department of social services.

Once back with her mother she began experiencing recurrent urinary tract infections. At age 9 she was admitted to the hospital in septic shock. After a thorough workup of all possible causes for sepsis, the treatment team decided the illness was caused by the child's mother and moved to have the child put in protective custody. In their discussion of the case the authors also detailed illnesses the mother fabricated in herself.

They discussed the management issues including factors that predispose for successful treatment. This statement represents the central tenet of their advice: "Medical treatment of the child is the first priority and often is only possible on separation from the parent. The second task is to create an umbrella of protection, including the mobilization and coordination of pediatric, psychiatric, social and legal services."

Here we have a child who began going to doctors inappropriately in the first weeks of life. She experienced numerous types of child abuse including potentially fatal poisoning that began while she was a toddler. She thrived while in foster care and once again began showing recurrent patterns of illness when returned to her mother. The case points out the long-term nature of the problem. The conclusion the authors come to is that, given the long-standing, complex, potentially life-threatening nature of the situation, the intervention needs to be broad-based, multidimensional, and permanent.

Warner and Hathaway[40] reported a series of cases in which mothers falsely believed their children were allergic to foods, and because of the allergies the children experienced significant behavioral and other symptoms. "Cases 10 and 11 were also submitted to extreme aero-allergen avoidance. This included their mother insisting on them sleeping on the back of an upturned wardrobe, wrapped in toilet paper and silver foil rather than blankets." They described another mother writing lengthy letters regarding her obsessions with allergic substances. Meadow[41] wrote a commentary following this paper in which he questioned whether exaggerated, obsessive belief systems in parents met criteria for MSBP but acknowledged that he did feel the behavior described had stretched beyond the line where it should be considered abusive. This idea, that there is a line that, when crossed, represents child abuse is consistent with the evaluation of all other types of child abuse and neglect.

Guandolo[42] recounted the story of treating a 5-year-old child for many years in an outpatient setting for illnesses in numerous organ systems. The child made more than 250 outpatient pediatric visits for illnesses that never amounted to significant disease. He discussed the frustration of the primary care pediatrician and introduced the term *the medical game*. He states that for many years the treating physician was playing by one set of rules while his patient's mother was playing by an entirely different set.

When the child was 1½ years old, because of frequent complaints of ear infections and colds reported by his mother, he received a consultation from an otolaryngologist. "His report read (in its entirety): 'Diagnosis: normal ear, nose and throat examination; Treatment: with the history of recurrent otitis media and normal ear examination today, I suggested adenoidectomy as an adjunct to hyposensitization.'" In other words, in the presence of a completely normal examination surgery was recommended based on history received from the patient's mother.

The boy was placed on phenobarbital therapy for seizures despite normal electroencephalogram findings. He was treated for migraine headaches and numerous other illnesses totally based on symptoms reported by his mother. The years passed. Eventually the mother told the office staff that she was a law student, that she had passed the bar examination, and that she was interested in "negligence law." She also stated that she had been offered a position as a faculty member in the Russian history department at a local university. At this point the treating physician called the woman's husband who was, in fact, a lawyer who had studied Russian history, although neither of these accomplishments could be attributed to his wife. The husband confirmed that the child was basically healthy and that much of what the mother had been relating over a period of 4 years was completely false.

This case provides a good reminder that to practice good medicine one must confirm early impressions by collecting information from multiple sources including alternate history sources, the physical examination, and results of laboratory tests. Physicians have been taught this for generations but still need to be reminded.

That same year (1985) Malatack et al[43] discussed a patient who had recurrent episodes of unexplained gastrointestinal bleeding. To determine the source of the bleeding the child received the following diagnostic tests: a Meckel's scan, air contrast barium enema, colonoscopy, gastroduodenoscopy (which visualized the site of a previously healed small bowel biopsy), complete coagulation evaluation, technetium scan, and mesenteric angiography. The patient received daily transfusions. An exploratory laparotomy was normal, but due to continuing symptoms he went back to the operating room 3 more times before eventually a transverse colostomy was performed. Between procedures he never appeared very ill. The staff commented on how happy he looked. He received many transfusions of packed red blood cells during his 93 consecutive days in the hospital. Toward the end of his hospital stay a hospital staff member discovered the mother with her child in the bathroom and blood in the wastebasket. She had been withdrawing blood from the infant's central venous line and discarding it, or placing it in his diapers, colonoscopy bag, or nasogastric tube.

In one of the most imaginative presentations of child abuse ever published a mother managed to have her child be diagnosed and treated for cystic fibrosis (CF) for a number of years. Orenstein and Wasserman,[44] a pediatrician and child psychiatrist team, related the story in 1986. The mother fabricated chloride sweat tests, and added fat to stool samples. She signed releases for other hospitals to provide information, and then called the hospitals to withdraw the permission. She called the hospital bacteriology laboratory and claimed to be a medical student who, while visiting the laboratory, had noticed that the child had grown out specific bacteria prior to someone throwing away the plates.

And that's not all. To get a sputum sample of a child who actually suffered from CF, the perpetrator called the local Cystic Fibrosis Foundation and asked for the name of a young person who could be a support for her child who, she maintained, had been recently diagnosed with CF. She then called this teenager and said that she needed a sputum sample for a research project, met him in the hospital parking lot, retrieved a sputum sample, and delivered it to her child's doctors saying that it came from her son. The foundation had attempted to call her back only to find the number did not exist. The hospital had no record of a recently diagnosed child. With this information the treatment team was able to demonstrate effectively the extent of the parent's fabrication and protect the child.

With access to medical records, the authors determined that, a year previously, the false nature of the CF diagnosis had been uncovered at another hospital. This was the reason for the parent's refusal to allow the hospitals to share information. The child was placed in the custody of grandparents and immediately got significantly better. After 6 months he was returned to his parents against medical advice. The family moved and had not been located by the local agency that provides child protection services. Among other things this case highlights the importance of obtaining prior medical records.

Web of Deceit: 1987

Cases like these produced the material from which Rosenberg[5] extracted the 117 examples of MSBP she reported in "Web of Deceit: A Literature Review of Munchausen Syndrome by Proxy" published in *Child Abuse & Neglect* in 1987. Pediatricians continued to publish descriptive case accounts of fascinating examples of child abuse in the medical environment. Indeed, they continue to appear today.[45] However, with the publication of "Web of Deceit" we entered a new phase in the history of MSBP.

We would venture to say, without having actually counted, that "Web of Deceit" is the second most frequently cited paper in the field after Meadow's original work. (Science Citation Index notes that Meadow's original paper[2] has been quoted 360 times in the medical literature, and Rosenberg's "Web of Deceit"[5] paper 177 times.) Rosenberg was the first to specify criteria describing the syndrome. Hers was the first attempt to collect in one place all of the various case reports being produced. From these reports she extracted general conclusions such as a 9% mortality rate for children suffering from MSBP. She also cited a long-term morbidity rate of 8% and stated that confronting the perpetrator was associated with death of the child in 20% of cases. As we have seen, numerous subsequent authors have relied on these numbers.

As influential as this paper has been, it has not been without its detractors.[1] We noted that Meadow wrote a letter to the editor of *Child Abuse & Neglect*[46] stating that these numbers were too high. He pointed out, for example, that in his experience, in only 1 case in 100 when a parent was confronted with the abuse did harm come to the child. Looking back at "Web of Deceit" from this vantage point, it is easy to see its value in galvanizing interest in this form of child abuse. It is just as easy to see its methodological flaws. By analyzing data from 117 published cases of extreme presentations, Rosenberg gained an understanding of those particular cases. Just how much this information could be generalized remained to be seen.

In the long run it is more important that Rosenberg, in writing "Web of Deceit," helped set the tone for the debate that has ensued regarding the motive of the perpetrator as a central feature of the syndrome. We have emphasized that Rosenberg did not include motivation of the perpetrator in her 4 defining characteristics of MSBP. However, in the title of her paper she makes reference to the perpetrator's motive to deceive. She represents that perpetrators of this form of child abuse set out to weave a "web of deceit" that captures unwary physicians and makes them complicit in the abuse of innocent children. Two of the 4 diagnostic criteria she specified refer to deceit on the part of the caretaker. The first characteristic of her syndrome is the faking of symptoms and the third is the denial on the part of the caretaker of the cause of the illness. A result of this tone is the introduction of moral judgment, physicians judging the possible immoral motivation of caretakers, into the discussion that will lead to significant difficulties in the future.

Meanwhile, at about the same time, researchers and clinicians continued to work evaluating and defining unusual manifestations of child abuse. Cases reported as MSBP began clustering according to the symptom presentations. As an example, after a few cases of falsified seizures were published, soon a series of many cases was available for study.[36] In the next chapter we look at the major groups of illnesses that have been characterized as having features of MSBP.

References

1. Donald T, Jureidini J. Munchausen syndrome by proxy. Child abuse in the medical system. *Arch Pediatr Adolesc Med.* 1996;150(7):753-758
2. Meadow R. Munchausen syndrome by proxy. The hinterland of child abuse. *Lancet.* 1977;2(8033):343-345
3. Asher R. Munchausen's syndrome. *Lancet.* 1951;1:339-341
4. Kempe CH, Silverman FW, Steele BF, Droegemueller W, Silver H. The battered child syndrome. *JAMA.* 1962;181:17-24
5. Rosenberg DA. Web of deceit: a literature review of Munchausen syndrome by proxy. *Child Abuse Negl.* 1987;11(4):547-563
6. Radbill SX. A history of child abuse and infanticide. In: Helfer RE, Kempe CH, eds. *The Battered Child.* Chicago, IL: University of Chicago Press; 1974:3-21
7. Kempe CH. Sexual abuse, another hidden pediatric problem: the 1977 C. Anderson Aldrich lecture. *Pediatrics.* 1978;62(3):382-389

8. Kempe CH. Uncommon manifestations of the battered child syndrome. *Am J Dis Child.* 1975;129:126-128
9. Pickering D. Letter: salicylate poisoning as a manifestation of the battered child syndrome. *Am J Dis Child.* 1976;130(6):675-676
10. Dine MS. Tranquilizer poisoning: an example of child abuse. *Pediatrics.* 1965;36(5):782-785
11. Fontana VJ, Donovan D, Wong R. The "maltreatment syndrome" in children. *N Engl J Med.* 1963;269:138-139
12. Dine MS, McGovern ME. Intentional poisoning of children—an overlooked category of child abuse: report of seven cases and review of the literature. *Pediatrics.* 1982;70(1):32-35
13. Lansky LL. An unusual case of childhood chloral hydrate poisoning. *Am J Dis Child.* 1974;127(2):275-276
14. Rogers D, Tripp J, Bentovim A, Robinson A, Berry D, Goulding R. Non-accidental poisoning: an extended syndrome of child abuse. *Br Med J.* 1976;1(6013):793-796
15. Berger D. Child abuse simulating "near-miss" sudden infant death syndrome. *J Pediatr.* 1979;95(4):554-556
16. Jones DP. Dermatitis artefacta in mother and baby as child abuse. *Br J Psychiatry.* 1983;143:199-200
17. Mortimer JG. Acute water intoxication as another unusual manifestation of child abuse. *Arch Dis Child.* 1980;55(5):401-403
18. Shnaps Y, Frand M, Rotem Y, Tirosh M. The chemically abused child. *Pediatrics.* 1981;68(1):119-121
19. Baugh JR, Krug EF, Weir MR. Punishment by salt poisoning. *South Med J.* 1983;76(4):540-541
20. Fischler RS. Poisoning: a syndrome of child abuse. *Am Fam Physician.* 1983;28(6):103-108
21. Bauman WA, Yalow RS. Child abuse: parenteral insulin administration. *J Pediatr.* 1981;99(4):588-591
22. Scarlett JA, Mako ME, Rubenstein AH, et al. Factitious hypoglycemia. Diagnosis by measurement of serum C-peptide immunoreactivity and insulin-binding antibodies. *N Engl J Med.* 1977;297(19):1029-1032
23. Mayefsky JH, Sarnaik AP, Postellon DC. Factitious hypoglycemia. *Pediatrics.* 1982;69(6):804-805
24. Crumpacker RW, Kriel RL. Voluntary water intoxication in normal infants. *Neurology.* 1973;23(11):1251-1255
25. Kohl S, Pickering LK, Dupree E. Child abuse presenting as immunodeficiency disease. *J Pediatr.* 1978;93(3):466-468
26. Minford AM. Child abuse presenting as apparent "near-miss" sudden infant death syndrome. *Br Med J (Clin Res Ed).* 1981;282(6263):521

27. Roberts IF, West RJ, Ogilvie D, Dillon MJ. Malnutrition in infants receiving cult diets: a form of child abuse. *Br Med J.* 1979;1(6159):296-298
28. Volk D. Factitious diarrhea in two children. *Am J Dis Child.* 1982;136:1027
29. Hvizdala EV, Gellady AM. Intentional poisoning of two siblings by prescription drugs: an unusual form of child abuse. *Clin Pediatr.* 1978;17(6):480-482
30. Schmitt BD, Kempe CH. The pediatrician's role in child abuse and neglect. *Curr Probl Pediatr.* 1975;5(5):3-47
31. Lee DA. Munchausen syndrome by proxy in twins. *Arch Dis Child.* 1979;54(8):646-647
32. Outwater KM, Lipnick RN, Luban NL, Ravenscrotf K, Ruley EJ. Factitious hematuria: diagnosis by minor blood group typing. *J Pediatr.* 1981;98(1):95-97
33. Hodge D III, Schwartz W, Sargent J, Bodurtha J, Starr S. The bacteriologically battered baby: another case of Munchausen by proxy. *Ann Emerg Med.* 1982;11(4):205-207
34. Halsey NA, Frentz JM, Tucker TW, Sproles T, Redding J, Daum RS. Recurrent nosocomial polymicrobial sepsis secondary to child abuse. *Lancet.* 1983;2(8349):558-560
35. Liston TE, Levine PL, Anderson C. Polymicrobial bacteremia due to Polle syndrome: the child abuse variant of Munchausen by proxy. *Pediatrics.* 1983;72(2):211-213
36. Meadow R. Munchausen syndrome by proxy and pseudo-epilepsy. *Arch Dis Child.* 1982;57(10):811-812
37. Meadow R. Munchausen syndrome by proxy. *Arch Dis Child.* 1982;57(2):92-98
38. Rosen CL, Frost JD Jr, Bricker T, Tarnow JD, Gillette PC, Dunlavy S. Two siblings with recurrent cardiorespiratory arrest: Munchausen syndrome by proxy or child abuse? *Pediatrics.* 1983;71(5):715-720
39. Palmer AJ, Yoshimura GJ. Munchausen syndrome by proxy. *J Am Acad Child Psychiatry.* 1984;23(4):503-508
40. Warner JO, Hathaway MJ. Allergic form of Meadow's syndrome (Munchausen by proxy). *Arch Dis Child.* 1984;59(2):151-156
41. Meadow SR. Commentary. *Arch Dis Child.* 1984;59:156
42. Guandolo VL. Munchausen syndrome by proxy: an outpatient challenge. *Pediatrics.* 1985;75(3):526-530
43. Malatack JJ, Wiener ES, Gartner JC Jr, Zitelli BJ, Brunetti E. Munchausen syndrome by proxy: a new complication of central venous catheterization. *Pediatrics.* 1985;75(3):523-525
44. Orenstein DM, Wasserman AL. Munchausen syndrome by proxy simulating cystic fibrosis. *Pediatrics.* 1986;78(4):621-624
45. Tamay Z, Akcay A, Kilic G, et al. Corrosive poisoning mimicking cicatricial pemphigoid: Munchausen by proxy. *Child Care Health Dev.* 2007;33(4):496-499
46. Meadow R. Letter to the editor. *Child Abuse Negl.* 1990;14:289

Chapter 4

Uncommon Manifestations of Battered Child Syndrome

A child's doctor is not required to clarify whether inappropriate parental care is due to mental illness, deprivation, distorted views of science, or persisting over anxiety before acting to promote the welfare of the child. —Wilson, 2001[1]

Introduction

It is possible to speculate where we would be today had the Munchausen syndrome by proxy (MSBP) concept not been introduced when it was. In the period from 1975 to 1985, when MSBP was taking hold, the interest in new forms of child abuse was well established. People were calling attention to specific illnesses that offered the possibility for abuse when caretakers reported symptoms inaccurately. It is likely that, absent the fascination with caretaker motivation, the field would have developed a body of information about these illnesses just as it was expanding knowledge of conditions like sexual abuse and shaken baby syndrome.

We documented in the last chapter how Dine and McGovern[2] gathered numbers of cases of non-accidental poisoning into an impressive series. Others collected examples of other diseases involving a parent initiating harmful medical care. In addition to non-accidental poisoning, researchers and clinicians identified factitious seizures, extreme illness exaggeration, recurrent suffocation, polymicrobial sepsis, and chronic recurrent pseudo-obstruction of the bowels of young children as specific disease entities that could be used to abuse children in a medical environment. All of these conditions have been described as separate illness entities and in the context of MSBP. We next review these disease conditions that have been identified as associated with MSBP; what Kempe[3] would call "uncommon manifestations of the battered child syndrome."

False Epilepsy

Much of the work describing epilepsy as a disease that can be used to abuse children has been done by Meadow.[4,5] Among the spate of responses he received after publication of his first paper were inquiries from physicians about parents who misrepresented their children as having seizures or actually induced seizures in their children. He published an article[5] that gave data on 32 children treated for epilepsy who did not have the disease.

Epilepsy provides fertile ground for abuse. The illness is frightening by itself and, when it occurs in a child, generates intense emotional reactions from parents. Epilepsy can vary from a one-time phenomenon associated with elevated temperature in an infant to a severe debilitating condition. Actual seizures can be remarkably variable consisting of anything from a few seconds staring off into space to full-blown grand mal events. A seizure can occur spontaneously in a completely random manner or in response to an insult to the brain from trauma, suffocation, or chemical means. The result is that parents can be afraid their child is having a seizure, pretend their child is having a seizure, actually cause the seizure, or truly observe a real electrical seizure event. Add to this the possibility that older children can learn to simulate a convulsion and develop a pattern of having pseudoseizures either with conscious or unconscious motivation.

These factors make seizure diagnosis and management in children a difficult proposition. The result is that doctors need to rely heavily on the report of parents and caretakers. Treatment is often initiated based on the history given by the parent. It is extremely rare that a child whose mother reports having seizures will oblige with a fit in the office that a physician can actually observe. Although electroencephalogram (EEG) evidence is usually sought, it is sometimes equivocal or not diagnostic. Twenty-four hour videotaped EEGs have proven helpful in making a diagnosis, but even this test is not definitive. Given all these considerations it is notable that more pediatricians have not remarked on the possibility of abuse.

Among the 32 children Meadow[5] described, parents fabricated symptoms in 23 of them. They told physicians the child had had seizures when that was not true. In 11 cases parents had induced a seizure through suffocation or drug intoxication. The children had endured from months to years of evaluations and treatments of nonexistent illness or seizures directly induced by a parent. In addition to the treatment of factitious seizures, these children often experienced other forms of child abuse including other fabricated symptoms. We commented earlier that Meadow discussed treatment of these children by saying that each child was protected using the same means as other abused children. He described making a notification to child protective services and getting court involvement when necessary.

Extreme Illness Exaggeration

Warner and Hathaway[6] were early proponents of the idea that severe illness exaggeration by parents and belief in nonexistent allergy could cause harm to children. They reported on 17 children from 13 families where they felt the parental belief system reached such an extreme degree that it constituted child abuse. We cited previously the case they described where a mother had her children sleep on a wardrobe wrapped in toilet paper and silver foil to avoid allergens.

Masterson et al[7] did not report on a series of children but did add to the discussion of extreme belief in allergy. They described the evaluation and treatment experience of a large number of patients with asthma at National Jewish Hospital in Denver, CO. Treatment of a chronic, remitting disease with a spectrum of presentation from mild to severe, such as asthma, offers an opportunity for parents to exaggerate or distort the reporting of symptoms to such a degree that harmful medical treatment can result. "Our experience has been that inpatient hospitalization with a multidisciplinary team approach affords the most efficient and comprehensive opportunity to identify 'illness exaggerating' cases and that the primary dissimilarity between these cases and the typical Munchausen by proxy cases is the presence of clinically verified, but mild, disease."

Godding and Kruth[8] contributed 17 cases. In the introduction to their paper they maintained that they considered severe illness exaggeration and severe non-adherence to treatment as MSBP. They stated that anywhere from 10% to 50% of patients do not adhere to treatment. They singled out a tiny percentage of these patients who met their criteria for parents who were committing child abuse. "In one case a 10-year-old boy had had three acute episodes of type III alveolitis (pigeon fancier's lung). He had developed severe symptoms of weight loss (6 kg), high fever, and dyspnea, and had spent a long time in hospital before he recovered. The parents, who owned some 40 pigeons that lived in their home, had been informed on several occasions about the etiology of their son's disease. They had stated that all their birds had been given away, when all the time they were hiding the 40 pigeons in the room next to the patient's room, and this was only discovered when the hospital social worker was sent to visit the house after the third acute attack." Non-adherence to treatment is a common problem and in its more severe forms can certainly be considered medical neglect or medical child abuse.

Roesler et al,[9] also writing from National Jewish Hospital, described 11 cases of children, aged 3 years or younger, with failure to thrive (FTT) based on a parent's belief in overwhelming food allergy. The children in this series had been subjected to many months of severely restricted diets, in some cases eating only 2 or 3 foods, in an effort to avoid foods to which the children were later found not to be allergic.

The uniting feature of these cases, with the exception of extreme non-adherence to treatment, is the fervor with which the parent believes in his or her approach to the medical illness. It is so strong and illogical in many cases that an independent observer would have a hard time construing this as an attempt to deceive the doctor. As in the example of the children wrapped in toilet paper and aluminum foil, the story often strains credulity. For this reason this particular form of parental behavior, while an unusual manifestation of child abuse, has generally not been considered under the designation of MSBP. When Gray and Bentovim[10] reported 41 cases, including 5 children whose parents withheld food due to belief in food allergies, they made a specific attempt to distinguish "illness induction syndrome" from MSBP or factitious disorder by proxy. They wanted to be clear that they felt no need to invoke MSBP. They were offering examples of child abuse.

Recurrent Suffocation

Recurrent suffocation is a symptom presentation that has received much attention. Berger[11] reported 2 cases in 1979. In both the child had recurrent episodes of apnea that occurred only in the presence of the mother. In one case, "Further study of the patient's history showed that the episodes occurred both day and night and that all episodes (home or hospital) occurred only when the mother was present. The father asked if the patient might be 'allergic' to the mother." This child had had 2 older siblings die of sudden infant death syndrome (SIDS).

It is for good reason that recurrent suffocation has received notice. It is an extremely lethal form of child abuse. Many of the deaths blamed on MSBP are the result of suffocation. In Rosenberg's[12] literature review she reported 10 deaths, 4 of which were from children being smothered by their mother. Two of the 4 children who died in the report from Alexander et al[13] of serial MSBP were smothered.

Smothering is simple to do. It only takes a few minutes with a pillow or a cupped hand held over the face of the child to cause anoxia, unconsciousness, seizures, or death. It is impossible to detect with any known diagnostic test. In many instances there are no postmortem findings that distinguish it from SIDS. It can be repeated many times before a child actually dies. Smothering a child is like playing Russian roulette. Only occasionally is there a bullet in the chamber that makes the act irrevocable.

We related an early report by Rosen et al[14] involving siblings smothered by their mother with the act caught on videotape. Rosen and colleagues[15] followed up with a review of 17 children with apnea and multiple resuscitations. They evaluated records of 81 families receiving home monitoring for apnea and identified, retrospectively, 17 children with multiple episodes of resuscitation at home or in the hospital. They divided these 17 children into 3 groups defined by who had witnessed the apneic episode. The group that generated most interest involved children who were solely in the presence of their mother when the episode began. Six of the 17 children met this criterion. These were children who clearly were experiencing anoxia as witnessed by a third party. They were not children whose mother merely claimed to have seen them turn blue. In fact, they had real respiratory difficulty as witnessed by someone other than the mother. However, the anoxia began only in the presence of the mother. Two of these 6 children were observed on videotape being smothered. For a third there was other convincing evidence of smothering. These 3 children were removed from their mothers and experienced no further spells. The remaining 3 children were sent home with their parents and all died within a month of leaving the hospital. The authors describe these 6 children as being representative of MSBP.

In 1987 Southall[16] published his first 2 cases of covert video surveillance involving recurrent suffocation. This began a long debate in the British medical literature regarding the ethical appropriateness of videotaping children in the care of their mothers without the mothers' knowledge.

Mothers had been seen before on videotape deliberately harming their children. However, the behavior was caught during videotaping for another purpose, such as continuous EEG monitoring.[14] Southall and colleagues[16] suspected that children with recurrent apnea were being smothered by mothers but had no proof. They purposefully established a condition whereby the child could be monitored without the mother's knowledge.

Meanwhile, the next significant series describing suffocated children was published by Meadow in 1990.[17] If not obvious before, this article single-handedly established the deadly seriousness of recurrent suffocation. He reviewed the cases of 27 children from 27 different families, all of whom had experienced confirmed suffocation. Nine children died and one had severe brain damage. In the 27 families there had been 33 siblings born before the index child was suffocated. Of those 33 older children, 18 had died suddenly and unexpectedly in early life. In the 27 families there were a total of 60 children (not counting younger siblings of index patients) of whom 27 had died suddenly.

Suffocation in confirmed cases occurred not only in the home but also in the hospital. The perpetrator in almost every case was a mother. "After discovery and in the period surrounding court proceedings, at least eight mothers threatened to kill themselves; none did, but five mothers took small overdoses of drugs or injured themselves. In the months that followed two husbands killed themselves."

A considerable time after the event, 5 mothers remembered the hatred that they had felt for their child. Meadow noted, "The hatred was occasioned by the child's seeming so happy and healthy, when they themselves were miserable or when they had themselves had had such an unhappy childhood. Seven acknowledged that they were using suffocation as a means of getting into contact with friendly and helpful medical and social services, but when challenged why it was necessary to go to the length of suffocating their child to achieve that goal (when all they needed to do was make up a story of illness for the child), they said that there must have been a stronger feeling of hostility toward the child than they had realized."

The conclusion one must draw from this study is that children who get repeatedly suffocated have a significant chance of dying. And if mothers are motivated to assume the sick role by proxy, a significant portion of them also admit to having strong negative feelings for the baby they are smothering.

Samuels et al,[18] a group that included Southall, reported on a series of 157 infants who had received mouth-to-mouth resuscitation. The research team attempted to determine the cause of the respiratory difficulty that would necessitate resuscitation. They admitted the children to the hospital, monitored them physiologically and, in many cases, also sent them home with monitoring equipment. They were able to reach a final diagnosis in about half of the children (77/157). They described a pattern they could observe on the monitor tracings that they felt was suggestive of suffocation. This pattern included vigorous physical activity and increased heart rate before the onset of hypoxia. They said they felt this might represent the child struggling to get air while being smothered. A total of 18 children met the criteria for having evidence of suffocation.

Children suspected of being suffocated were considered for covert video surveillance. In fact, of the 18 children, 14 were later observed being suffocated.[19] From the original sample of 157 children, an additional 7 children were categorized as victims of child abuse due to fabricated information from the parents that could not be confirmed by physiological measurements. These children were referred to as representing MSBP. Hence, as early as 1992 Samuels and colleagues[19] were restricting the use of the term *MSBP* to cases of fabrication of symptoms not associated with actual suffocation, and not using it to describe recurrent suffocation.

This report followed the publication "Munchausen Syndrome by Proxy" by Samuels and Southall.[20] However, when Southall and colleagues[21] next published a significant series of patients, they titled the paper "Covert Video Recordings of Life-threatening Child Abuse: Lessons for Child Protection." They reported on 39 children, including the 14 previously described, undergoing covert video surveillance after suspicion of smothering by a parent. Thirty of the 39 children were observed on videotape being smothered. Three other children experienced physical abuse while being observed, and poisonings were also documented. The authors acknowledged that intentionally suffocating children to induce illness is a behavior called *MSBP*. They said, however, that as they observed multiple forms of child abuse, they were avoiding the term *MSBP* "…because it does not describe adequately the range of abuse that occurred; we prefer to describe the actual abuse identified." It is clear that Southall and colleagues, by this publication, wanted to distinguish recurrent suffocation from MSBP by calling it *life-threatening child abuse.*

Meadow's[22] next contribution to the understanding of recurrent suffocation was a report of 81 children who were initially thought to have died from SIDS. The cases were collected over 18 years. In 19 of the 50 families the parents confessed to suffocating their children. Seventy-five of the 81 children had previous unusual or unexplained events reported by the perpetrator including the baby stopping breathing, looking blue, appearing dazed, or having seizures. Fifty-five of the babies were found dead between 11 am and 10 pm (ie, in the middle of the day and early evening as opposed to during the night when one would expect a child to die from SIDS). Nearly half of the children had been discharged from the hospital within the previous week. Usually the child was found to be well in the hospital. Four children died on the anniversary of a previous sibling's death. Seven children had their deaths predicted by the parents. Twenty-seven children had blood in the mouth, nose, or on the face. Forty children had no signs of trauma.

Meadow summarized his feelings regarding the quality of these data by saying, "If a young child was admitted to the hospital as a result of a young, harassed mother from a poor home recounting a startling or unusual event, and the baby is found to be completely normal, it does not mean all is well. When next morning the pathology reports and the x-ray reports come back normal, it would be safer to discharge the hospital notes and normal investigation reports out of the door than the baby. That mother has brought the child to hospital for a reason that we have not understood. There is ample evidence that children suffering recurrent physical abuse, as well as Munchausen syndrome by proxy abuse, have many warning signals and previous hospital encounters before the final event that maims or kills." By 1999 Meadow was using the term *Munchausen syndrome by proxy abuse* almost exclusively. Parenthetically, he said that the term *SIDS* should be abandoned and that we should just say that the death was "unexplained" or "undetermined" rather than pretending it was a natural death from some yet to be identified agent.

A more recent attempt to understand the relationship between SIDS and recurrent suffocation was conducted by Truman and Ayoub.[23] They did a retrospective analysis of 138 children with apparent life-threatening events, unexplained deaths, and SIDS or SIDS-related illnesses. In their analysis they used risk factors for recurrent suffocation such as age, number of events, presence of frank blood around the mouth at autopsy, and siblings with unexplained deaths in infancy. They found that children with presumably true SIDS died at a young age, typically had 1 or 2 events, had few findings on autopsy, and were unlikely to have siblings who had died unexpectedly. Conversely, they identified a "high-risk group" with a high probability of suffocation that had multiple events, at an older age, witnessed only by the parent.

As we look back on the development of our understanding regarding suffocation abuse, 2 things stand out. Recurrent suffocation of infants is a catastrophic form of life-threatening child abuse, and trying to understand whether the perpetrator was motivated to seek the illness role by proxy has become less and less important.

Polymicrobial Sepsis

Polymicrobial sepsis is a serious infectious disease process characterized by finding more than one bacterial organism growing in the bloodstream. Sepsis is almost always caused by only one organism. The frequency of children with positive blood cultures having more than one organism is less than 1%.[24] When 2 or more bacteria are growing in the bloodstream, there is usually a ready explanation. For example, this can occur when there is severe immune compromise. Another explanation is contamination of a central intravenous access line. Over the past several decades there has been a growing awareness that child abuse could be a significant cause of polymicrobial sepsis.

In 1978 Kohl and colleagues[25] described a 4-year-old who was hospitalized with recurrent bacterial infections of skin and soft tissues. She had been getting infections since infancy and by the time of their evaluation had many healed scars from past abscesses and a healed burn scar on her foot. They suspected immunodeficiency disease and, in fact, eventually concluded she had immune system compromise secondary to recurrent infection. The child was in the hospital for 4 months, during which time she had abscesses, pyogenic arthritis of the major joints, and septicemia often with multiple organisms, and many times with organisms that should be responding to antibiotics she was receiving. An investigation revealed that she had therapeutic concentrations of the antibiotics only when they were administered when her mother was not present in the hospital room.

A resident physician walked into the room and found the mother disconnecting the intravenous tubing and pouring antibiotic solution on the floor. The mother denied that she was purposely trying to interfere with treatment. The child was removed from her mother's care, stopped developing infections, and her immune system returned to normal. The child was left with a permanent limp from the recurrent septic arthritis she had experienced. The infections she had suffered over the years had been a result of her mother injecting spit or fecal material into her tissues. This woman was convicted of child abuse defined as preventing her daughter from getting appropriate antibiotics. She was sentenced to 10 years in prison.

The authors commented that, "Even when the child developed symptoms of septic shock and disseminated intravascular coagulation, the mother remained calm, offering solace to the nurses, house staff, and attending physicians." The authors stated they felt it took them so long to make the diagnosis because of "…resistance by attending physicians accepting that an apparently pleasant mother could be performing bizarre acts of abuse on a critically ill child in the hospital. Once this possibility was accepted, appropriate tests and surveillance quickly clarified the situation and allowed therapeutic interventions."

Unlike the report by Kohl and colleagues, the next 3 single cases of polymicrobial sepsis reported in 1982 and 1983[26-28] included discussions of MSBP. Although there are a number of other single case reports of polymicrobial sepsis due to tampering with central lines,[12,29-35] it was not until 15 years later that Feldman and Hickman[36] did a systematic study regarding the relationship between central venous lines and MSBP. They examined all of the children over a many year period who had received central venous lines for any reason at a children's hospital. They excluded all the children who had clear indications for line placement, such as the need to administer chemotherapy for cancer treatment. In the group with no clear indication were 292 children. They found that 10 had been evaluated for MSBP, with 8 children "confirmed" to meet their criteria. They then examined records for all children receiving a diagnosis of MSBP to see if they had received a central venous line. They determined that approximately 1 in 6 children (17%) diagnosed with MSBP also had a central line. Two of the children with both MSBP and a central line died. One of these experienced septic shock from infection acquired through his central line, and the other had air injected through his line causing an air embolus. Over half of the children with MSBP and a central line had infections usually on a recurrent basis.

The placement and maintenance for considerable lengths of time of central venous catheters in children is a relatively recent phenomenon. It represents an advance in medical technology. Several decades ago intravenous sites were predominantly on peripheral locations such as the hands or feet and had to be changed every few days. With the placement of long-term catheters came the possibility that they would be used for abuse. Malatack and colleagues[37] commented on this in 1985, and their prediction has proven to be correct. Hickman, one of the authors of the study regarding central lines and MSBP, was instrumental in the development of central line technology. His contribution was so great that one type of central access catheter is named for him.

Chronic Intestinal Pseudo-obstruction

When Schreier and Libow[38] decided to survey subspecialists regarding MSBP they chose neurologists and gastroenterologists. We assume they felt gastroenterologists would see fabricated or induced cases of vomiting and diarrhea. Instead, a much less common gastrointestinal presentation has been associated with MSBP in recent years: chronic recurrent pseudo-obstruction of the bowel in young children. This is a condition that mimics the classical picture of bowel obstruction. It differs in being episodic and is difficult to diagnose with usual diagnostic procedures such as radiologic films of the bowels. This means that the parent's account of the child's symptoms is often the primary source of information to make the diagnosis.

Several years before Schreier and Libow's survey, Sullivan and colleagues[39] identified pseudo-obstruction as part of a pattern of fabricated illness. Kosmach and colleagues[40] told of a child who received a small bowel transplant after many years of pseudo-obstruction symptoms reported by her mother that turned out to be fabricated. The child had had numerous medical illnesses leading up to the transplant. Once the determination had been made that implicated the mother, the medical team got a court order excluding her from contact with the child. The medical team proceeded to systematically clear up all her medical problems. At the time of their report, they were in the process of discharging her from a psychiatric facility to a medical foster home.

Another group of researchers,[41] evaluating children with chronic intestinal pseudo-obstruction for possible transplant, ruled out surgery for 2 children they felt had MSBP. They felt a child who received surgery, in retrospect, also met criteria for MSBP.

As early as 1995, Hyman[42] recognized that many children with pseudo-obstruction had symptoms fabricated by their parents. Later, he and colleagues[43] reviewed 39 cases of pseudo-obstruction in toddlers and found 8 children who did not meet criteria for the illness. These 8 children they felt were fabricated examples of pseudo-obstruction. They then compared characteristics of those 8 children with the other youngsters who met full criteria. The factors that distinguished the 2 groups were identified. "Clinical features suggesting pediatric condition falsification in toddlers presenting with chronic and severe digestive complaints included (a) daily abdominal pain, (b) illness involving three or more organ systems, (c) an accelerating disease trajectory, (d) a reported history of preterm birth, (e) absence of dilated bowel on x-ray, (f) normal antroduodenal manometry, and (g) no urinary neuromuscular disease."

A group of Italian gastroenterologists[44] reviewed children evaluated for small bowel disease who turned out to have normal manometric studies with an eye to determining if they could decide on an alternate diagnosis. They identified 12 children with normal studies and decided that 4 of them met criteria for MSBP. They confirmed the diagnosis by removing the children from their families and having their symptoms disappear. Another group[45] looked more closely at 32 children found not to have colonic disease and determined that 7 of these met criteria for MSBP. Following separation from parents, these children had no further gastrointestinal symptoms.

We feel Henry Kempe would be proud of the efforts to identify "uncommon manifestations of the battered child." Work continues to characterize specific types of illness that lend themselves to the concomitant diagnosis of medical child abuse.

References

1. Wilson RG. Fabricated or induced illness in children. Munchausen by proxy comes of age. *BMJ*. 2001;323(7308):296-297
2. Dine MS, McGovern ME. Intentional poisoning of children—an overlooked category of child abuse: report of seven cases and review of the literature. *Pediatrics*. 1982;70(1):32-35

3. Kempe CH. Uncommon manifestations of the battered child syndrome. *Am J Dis Child.* 1975;129:126-128
4. Meadow R. Munchausen syndrome by proxy and pseudo-epilepsy. *Arch Dis Child.* 1982;57(10):811-812
5. Meadow R. Fictitious epilepsy. *Lancet.* 1984;2(8393):25-28
6. Warner JO, Hathaway MJ. Allergic form of Meadow's syndrome (Munchausen by proxy). *Arch Dis Child.* 1984;59(2):151-156
7. Masterson J, Dunworth R, Williams N. Extreme illness exaggeration in pediatric patients: a variant of Munchausen's by Proxy? *Am J Orthopsychiatry.* 1988;58(2):188-195
8. Godding V, Kruth M. Compliance with treatment in asthma and Munchausen syndrome by proxy. *Arch Dis Child.* 1991;66(8):956-960
9. Roesler TA, Barry PC, Bock SA. Factitious food allergy and failure to thrive. *Arch Pediatr Adolesc Med.* 1994;148(11):1150-1155
10. Gray J, Bentovim A. Illness induction syndrome: paper I—a series of 41 children from 37 families identified at The Great Ormond Street Hospital for Children NHS Trust. *Child Abuse Negl.* 1996;20(8):655-673
11. Berger D. Child abuse simulating "near-miss" sudden infant death syndrome. *J Pediatr.* 1979;95(4):554-556
12. Rosenberg DA. Web of deceit: a literature review of Munchausen syndrome by proxy. *Child Abuse Negl.* 1987;11(4):547-563
13. Alexander R, Smith W, Stevenson R. Serial Munchausen syndrome by proxy. *Pediatrics.* 1990;86(4):581-585
14. Rosen CL, Frost JD Jr, Bricker T, Tarnow JD, Gillette PC, Dunlavy S. Two siblings with recurrent cardiorespiratory arrest: Munchausen syndrome by proxy or child abuse? *Pediatrics.* 1983;71(5):715-720
15. Rosen CL, Frost JD Jr, Glaze DG. Child abuse and recurrent infant apnea. *J Pediatr.* 1986;109(6):1065-1067
16. Southall DP, Stebbens VA, Rees SV, Lang MH, Warner JO, Shinebourne EA. Apnoeic episodes induced by smothering: two cases identified by covert video surveillance. *Br Med J (Clin Res Ed).* 1987;294(6588):1637-1641
17. Meadow R. Suffocation, recurrent apnea, and sudden infant death. *J Pediatr.* 1990;117(3):351-357
18. Samuels MP, Poets CF, Noyes JP, Hartmann H, Hewertson J, Southall DP. Diagnosis and management after life threatening events in infants and young children who received cardiopulmonary resuscitation. *BMJ.* 1993;306(6876):489-492
19. Samuels MP, McClaughlin W, Jacobson RR, Poets CF, Southall DP. Fourteen cases of imposed upper airway obstruction. *Arch Dis Child.* 1992;67(2):162-170
20. Samuels MP, Southall DP. Munchausen syndrome by proxy. *Br J Hosp Med.* 1992;47(10):759-762

21. Southall DP, Plunkett MC, Banks MW, Falkov AF, Samuels MP. Covert video recordings of life-threatening child abuse: lessons for child protection. *Pediatrics*. 1997;100(5):735-760
22. Meadow R. Unnatural sudden infant death. *Arch Dis Child*. 1999;80(1):7-14
23. Truman TL, Ayoub CC. Considering suffocatory abuse and Munchausen by proxy in the evaluation of children experiencing apparent life-threatening events and sudden infant death syndrome. *Child Maltreat*. 2002;7(2):138-148
24. Mian M, Huyer D. Infection and fever. In: Levin AV, Sheridan MS, eds. *Munchausen Syndrom by Proxy: Issues in Diagnosis and Treatment*. New York, NY: Lexington Books; 1995:161-180
25. Kohl S, Pickering L, Dupree E. Child abuse presenting as immunodeficiency disease. *J Pediatr*. 1978;93:466-468
26. Hodge D III, Schwartz W, Sargent J, Bodurtha J, Starr S. The bacteriologically battered baby: another case of Munchausen by proxy. *Ann Emerg Med*. 1982;11(4):205-207
27. Halsey NA, Frentz JM, Tucker TW, Sproles T, Redding J, Daum RS. Recurrent nosocomial polymicrobial sepsis secondary to child abuse. *Lancet*. 1983;2(8349):558-560
28. Liston TE, Levine PL, Anderson C. Polymicrobial bacteremia due to Polle syndrome: the child abuse variant of Munchausen by proxy. *Pediatrics*. 1983;72(2):211-213
29. Frederick V, Luedtke GS, Barrett FF, Hixson SD, Burch K. Munchausen syndrome by proxy: recurrent central catheter sepsis. *Pediatr Infect Dis J*. 1990;9(6):440-442
30. Clark GD, Key JD, Rutherford P, Bithoney WG. Munchausen's syndrome by proxy (child abuse) presenting as apparent autoerythrocyte sensitization syndrome: an unusual presentation of Polle syndrome. *Pediatrics*. 1984;74(6):1100-1102
31. Seferian EG. Polymicrobial bacteremia: a presentation of Munchausen syndrome by proxy. *Clin Pediatr (Phila)*. 1997;36(7):419-422
32. Boros SJ, Ophoven JP, Andersen R, Brubaker LC. Munchausen syndrome by proxy: a profile for medical child abuse. *Aust Fam Physician*. 1995;24(5):768-769, 772-763
33. DiBiase P, Timmis H, Bonilla JA, Szeremeta W, Post JC. Munchausen syndrome by proxy complicating ear surgery. *Arch Otolaryngol Head Neck Surg*. 1996;122(12):1377-1380
34. Goldfarb J, Lawry KW, Steffen R, Sabella C. Infectious diseases presentations of Munchausen syndrome by proxy: case report and review of the literature. *Clin Pediatr (Phila)*. 1998;37(3):179-185

35. Baron HI, Beck DC, Vargas JH, Ament ME. Overinterpretation of gastroduodenal motility studies: two cases involving Munchausen syndrome by proxy. *J Pediatr.* 1995;126(3):397-400
36. Feldman KW, Hickman RO. The central venous catheter as a source of medical chaos in Munchausen syndrome by proxy. *J Pediatr Surg.* 1998;33(4):623-627
37. Malatack JJ, Wiener ES, Gartner JC Jr, Zitelli BJ, Brunetti E. Munchausen syndrome by proxy: a new complication of central venous catheterization. *Pediatrics.* 1985;75(3):523-525
38. Schreier HA, Libow JA. *Hurting for Love: Munchausen by Proxy Syndrome.* New York, NY: The Guilford Press; 1993
39. Sullivan CA, Francis GL, Bain MW, Hartz J. Munchausen syndrome by proxy: 1990. A portent for problems? *Clin Pediatr (Phila).* 1991;30(2):112-116
40. Kosmach B, Tarbell S, Reyes J, Todo S. "Munchausen by proxy" syndrome in a small bowel transplant recipient. *Transplant Proc.* 1996;28(5):2790-2791
41. Sigurdsson L, Reyes J, Kocoshis SA, et al. Intestinal transplantation in children with chronic intestinal pseudo-obstruction. *Gut.* 1999;45(4):570-574
42. Hyman PE. Chronic intestinal pseudo-obstruction in childhood: progress in diagnosis and treatment. *Scand J Gastroenterol Suppl.* 1995;213:39-46
43. Hyman PE, Bursch B, Beck D, DiLorenzo C, Zeltzer LK. Discriminating pediatric condition falsification from chronic intestinal pseudo-obstruction in toddlers. *Child Maltreat.* 2002;7(2):132-137
44. Cucchiara S, Borrelli O, Salvia G, et al. A normal gastrointestinal motility excludes chronic intestinal pseudoobstruction in children. *Dig Dis Sci.* 2000;45(2):258-264
45. Di Lorenzo C, Flores AF, Hyman PE. Age-related changes in colon motility. *J Pediatr.* 1995;127(4):593-596

Chapter 5

Why Has It Taken So Long?

By focusing on the perpetrator, however, the medical profession fails to recognize its own contribution to the development of MSBP and ignores the victim's perspective. If we as medical professionals do not recognize the cause of symptoms is abuse, we contribute to the damage. —Donald and Jureidini, 1996[1]

Introduction

Thus far, we have delineated the problem and offered a potential solution. We have described the manner in which the pediatric community embraced the Munchausen syndrome by proxy (MSBP) concept, and advanced a notion about how the field might have developed had MSBP never been invented. But, before we proceed to discuss evaluation and treatment of medical child abuse, 2 more questions need to be addressed. The questions go hand-in-hand. The first is, "Why has it taken so long for the professional community to realize that MSBP doesn't work?" The second is, "What about motivation?" We take up these 2 questions in this chapter and the next.

All of the alternative explanations for this particular kind of abusive behavior in the medical setting share a common feature. *Munchausen syndrome by proxy, pediatric condition falsification, factitious disorder by proxy, Meadow's syndrome,* and even the newest and best attempt, *fabricated or induced illness in a child by a carer,* all focus attention on the acts of a caretaker rather than the effects of the actions on a child. As an example, *pediatric condition falsification* acknowledges that there is a pediatric condition, presumably abnormal, but the focus is on the "falsification." All of these terms describe what the adult does rather than what the child experiences.

We have said previously that motivation in this type of child abuse is just as important as it is in any other type of maltreatment. Once it has been established that a child has been harmed, it is important to discover why that harm took place in order to make sure that it does not happen again. But knowledge of the motivation of the perpetrator is not necessary to make the initial determination that a child might need protection. We can decide that a sexually abused child needs protection without knowing whether or not the perpetrator was intoxicated, senile, or had an abnormal sexual attraction to young children. Likewise, we can determine that a child has received nonessential medical treatment that is harmful and decide that it should not happen again without knowing precisely why a parent would want this to happen to her child.

As we have seen, individual authors have put forth this point of view periodically over the last three decades. But the field as a whole has continued to maintain its focus on the perpetrator rather than on the victim. Why is this? Why has it taken so long to get beyond Munchausen syndrome by proxy?

People before us have offered answers to this question. Some maintain that *Munchausen syndrome by proxy* was just too good a name. The sobriquet caught the attention of doctors. It was easy to remember and had a certain mystery about it. Meadow said that it had journalistic value.[2] Some people say that it has become so ingrained that it will not be possible to extirpate it from common usage.[1] Something about the term made us believe that it really represented more than child abuse. While *we* argue that use of the term has set us back many years, others contend that without such a dramatic designation we never would have arrived at our current level of awareness of the multiple ways parents can abuse children in the medical environment.

Still, the explanation that the name is too attractive does not seem adequate. The question is an important one and deserves a much better answer. We have seen evidence that even the most central figures in the field understood many years ago that MSBP was abuse, and that it was best to respond to it using standard techniques for child abuse investigation and treatment. The possibility was there even in the earliest days to recognize it and treat it as we would other emerging forms of child abuse. Instead, each new group of doctors, on finding themselves giving medical care based on false information, returned to the MSBP concept and wrote a case study about this fascinating distortion of maternal behavior.

One thing is certain. The distinguishing feature between medical abuse and other forms of child abuse is the role of the medical community. We have to consider that this unique aspect has something to do with the answer to our question. The community's response to child maltreatment is the charge of a loosely associated group of child abuse professionals. Pediatricians and other medical personnel intersect with the child abuse community when a child is maltreated in a way that might have medical consequences. This represents a small but important portion of a typical pediatrician's practice. Children who have experienced medical child abuse represent a subset of all maltreated children seen in pediatric practices. Because of medicine's involvement in the abuse, the relationship between the medical community and child abuse community is different in this type of maltreatment than it is for any other. Child protection workers, judges, and police by necessity defer to medical people when medical child abuse is considered.

We argue that it has taken so long for doctors and child protection workers to come to a new understanding regarding medical child abuse precisely because the child abuse community has been waiting for doctors to come to terms with their own involvement, however unintentional, in committing harm to children. We think that doctors could not, because of their sense of guilt and shame, bring themselves to admit their complicity, and acknowledge that their benevolently applied treatments were making children ill. Doctors and nurses are blind to the abuse because they are involved and want, more than anything, not to have to look at it.

The Significance of the "Oh, No!" Event

We think the answer to the question, "Why has it taken so long?" stems from the involvement of medical care providers in inadvertently carrying out abuse at the instigation of caretakers. Instead of merely being an observer the physician is a participant. As participants doctors and nurses lose some of their objectivity. Objectivity presumes a degree of neutrality. But medical personnel are not exactly neutral when a child is harmed in the medical setting. As much as they would like to think otherwise, the fact remains that the abuse could not take place without them. And as long as the deception persists, medical caregivers continue to prescribe and treat all the while thinking they are doing their jobs appropriately. However, when the subterfuge ends, medical participants find themselves in a terrible position.

We refer to the time when medical personnel discover that something terribly wrong has taken place as the "Oh, No!" moment. This event includes a flood of new information for the physician, and along with the new knowledge is a profound emotional experience. We think the response to this emotional experience is the basis for why the MSBP concept has lingered.

One of the authors (CJ) remembers vividly an experience 15 years ago with a mother whose child was in the hospital for 300 of 360 days with a number of seemingly unrelated serious illnesses. The child was restricted to a wheelchair. She had a gastric tube and received all feedings through it. She was said to have impaired vision and hearing, and wore eyeglasses and hearing aids. She had a continuous series of episodes of severe dehydration, requiring hospitalization and intravenous therapy. Her primary care pediatrician was widely recognized as one of the kindest practitioners in the community. He specialized in children with special needs. The child's specialty care providers were among the best doctors in a respected academic medical center. Midway through this yearlong process, this author was one of a series of attending physicians who tried to treat the child on the inpatient service and remembers being bullied by the mother who demanded special care for the girl in an angry, hyper-protective fashion. Six months later a careful physician discovered the mother putting spit in the central line of her child. The mother lost custody of the little girl who made a remarkable recovery from her numerous debilitating conditions in the span of a few months. Many of the attending physicians, including this author, shared a sudden feeling of horror that they had contributed to the abuse of the child.

This moment, when the deception is discovered, has considerable import for all concerned. There may be instances when medical personnel respond to the discovery objectively. Just as often, however, the revelation is accompanied by an understandable and intense emotional response. Look again at the description of several groups of authors writing from 25 years ago discussing the response to discovery. Kohl and colleagues[3] talked about overcoming the "…resistance by attending physicians accepting that an apparently pleasant mother could be performing bizarre acts of abuse on a critically ill child in the hospital. Once this possibility was accepted, appropriate tests and surveillance quickly clarified the situation and allowed therapeutic interventions." Dine and McGovern,[4] writing about children who had been poisoned, said, "We and other clinicians diagnosing this form of child abuse almost invariably found it difficult to be objective in assessing the significance of the known facts related to these children. This emotional barrier has been recognized as a problem in the diagnosis of conventional forms of child abuse and must be overcome if such children are to be adequately protected. Once the validity of the diagnosis has been accepted in some cases subsequent cases were easier to assess objectively." Dine says the emotional wall is similar to that which must be overcome in considering other forms of child abuse. We think the barrier is significantly higher and more emotionally difficult to overcome because of the participation of the physician in the abuse.

One of our colleagues had an "Oh No!" moment just recently. We explained to him using his notes from the treatment of one of his patients, a teenager with kidney disease, that he had been prescribing higher and higher doses of more powerful medications resulting in more and more side effects. Regrettably, the patient's mother only gave the child the medicine occasionally, but told the doctor emphatically that she was following prescribed treatment. When we tried to give the teenager the medicine in the hospital as prescribed, the child became very ill from the medicine. Our friend looked at the laboratory results and said, "Oh my God! What have I been doing to this boy?"

Medical personnel reaching the "Oh, No!" moment experience a sudden, wrenching reversal from seeing their actions in a positive light to a negative one. Doctors and nurses make a conscious decision to dedicate their careers to helping people. They feel good when their patients get better. Professionals who take care of children take pride in seeing children grow up to be healthy individuals. Their self-esteem is bolstered by the sense that they are administering health-giving treatments. It is no wonder that they feel bad when they discover they have taken part in care that results in real or potential harm. What they do with that discomfort has allowed the MSBP phenomenon to continue.

In the "Oh, No!" moment doctors and nurses who thought they had an agreement with the mother, an agreement to work together for the well-being of the child, find out this is not the case. They feel betrayed. To feel betrayed is to feel threatened and vulnerable. Anger is the emotional response best suited to generating a sense of protection. Anger helps people to deal with threats, either physical or emotional. But getting angry is not the only thing people do in the middle of the "Oh, No!" instant. Medical personnel are trained not to get angry with their patients. Partly because of this, in addition to getting angry at this critical time doctors try to make sense out of what just happened to them. They try to come up with an explanation. They look for a rationalization.

For the doctor evaluating a child for potential sexual abuse or physical abuse the primary questions focus around the child. What happened? Are there physical or emotional sequelae? Does the child need to be protected? In contrast, doctors and nurses involved in medical child abuse often first need to examine their own participation. Many times the opening question they ask when they discover the deception is not, "What happened to the child and how can I make sure it doesn't happen again?" Quite reasonably, the first question is likely to be, "How did I get in this position of hurting a child that I set out to help?"

We think the perpetuation of the MSBP concept is a direct outcome of doctors trying to understand how they got involved in being the instrument of medical child abuse. The doctor asks, "Why me?" This is the motivation question the physician really wants answered. As much as one might want to think otherwise, it *is* personal.

Declaring the Mother Ill as a Rationalization for Participation in Medical Abuse

A useful rationalization for someone in this predicament is to describe the person who betrayed you as ill. After all, medical personnel treat people with medical illness. In response to feeling betrayed a person can get angry and act against all his or her medical training, or define the situation in a way that allows treatment to be offered. This is what we have done. Despite studies that indicate no clear pattern of mental illness in perpetrators of medical child abuse, the notion persists that people who abuse their children in a medical environment suffer from a specific mental illness called *factitious disorder by proxy* or *MSBP*. The mental illness is defined in whole or in part based on the motivation of the person being diagnosed. Remember, the motivation question most doctors want answered is, "Why me?" So the question being asked of the perpetrator with respect to motivation is, "Why did you choose me as an instrument in your plan?" Asked in this way the question selects for answers involving the perpetrator's relationship with the medical establishment.

The name of the possible illness has varied over time. In the beginning mothers who harmed their children in this way were felt to be psychotic. Over the years the focus has shifted to describing them as suffering from a personality disorder. More descriptively, as Schreier and Libow[5] put it, the perpetrator of medical child abuse is said to be, "hurting for love." Because of deprivation experienced in her childhood, a woman seeks out a physician with whom she can have a special relationship that provides nurturing for her and involves her physician in giving care to her child whether or not the child actually needs it.

Here is Meadow[6] commenting on Schreier and Libow: "I do think there is some truth in it. As I said to them, I don't think they are right in saying it is all to do with an unsatisfactory relationship these mothers had with their fathers. I think much more relevant is the unsatisfactory relationship they have had with their mothers. They lacked love and respect from their mothers. That is a much more positive finding from most of our research. But they have had tough childhoods. I do accept that a minority are literally in love with their paediatricians and doctors. It is a minority, but I have several letters the paediatricians have shown me which are in fact love letters and the mothers were doing anything to get contact. I think it is with a caring person, rather than sexual lust."

In other words, Meadow does not agree with the specific hypothesis of Schreier and Libow but does feel comfortable giving an explanation that includes having the physician function to replace a psychological loss experienced by the perpetrator. It is as if there is some compensation for having been involved in harming a child if in doing so the physician has made up for a lack of love and respect of the perpetrator's mother.

This feels very different from the situation faced by the physician evaluating sexual abuse. Physicians commonly do not spend much time contemplating the psychological makeup of adults who are sexually attracted to children when deciding if a child should be protected from being molested. Most would agree that having a primary sexual preference for young children is far from "normal" and might stem from a distorted parent-child relationship. However, little time is spent establishing whether or not the perpetrator is mentally ill before instituting child protection measures.

Yet the mental illness explanation does provide an answer to the question, "How did I get involved in committing abuse?" Diagnosing the person behind the abuse deflects blame from the physician. If the mother of the child was mentally ill it is clearly not fair to blame the doctor. The doctor didn't know he was treating the wrong patient. The physician can be excused for not reading the situation correctly. The person he or she was dealing with, the mother, did not follow the rules in the treatment process because of her mental illness. We make allowances for people suffering from illness, including mental illness. This answer to the motivation question meets, in some ways, the needs of the physician, and also the needs of the perpetrator, but does not address what the child requires. In some cases it may also be true.

A second response to the answer to the question, "How did I get involved in this?" is to look for and sometimes find that one has been the victim of fraud. Weston and Morelli[7] explained that their colleagues did numerous unnecessary surgeries on a child with a benign skin condition by saying the mother "…could only receive free public housing, food stamps, and medications if she had a disabled child." The fact that the mother was perpetrating fraud is used to soften the realization that surgery was performed repeatedly on a skin condition that rarely if ever requires treatment. Other examples include parents lying about a child having cancer to get funds donated to buy a television and other material goods,[8] a mother faking symptoms in her child to get medications that she then sold,[9] and a mother who wanted a second child to receive a feeding tube to qualify for additional state funding.[10] Of note, Kathy Bush, who subjected her child to numerous unnecessary surgeries and hospitalizations, was eventually found guilty of insurance fraud.[11]

Here, then, are 2 possible motivations of the perpetrator that at least partially explain why the medical care provider should be held blameless from causing harm to the child while trying to be therapeutic. In the first explanation a secret, previously undiagnosed illness in the perpetrator misleads the physician. In the second the medical care provider is the victim of illegal activity. With both of these explanations it is possible to rationalize how the doctor was deceived into being the instrument of abuse.

Once again, we cannot claim to have discovered a new truth. Others have described the confusing, frustrating, and painful position of the physician or nurse waking up to his or her role in medical child abuse. Mian[12] wrote, "For the health care givers to entertain the possibility of MBP may also require an admission and recognition that they unwittingly caused some or all of the morbidity in a child. Further, it involves admitting to having been duped. It is difficult to face the possibility of having been a harmful fool." As early as 1987 Zitelli and colleagues[13] introduced the term *professional participant* to refer to doctors, legal professionals, nurses, and social workers who find themselves becoming unwitting collaborators.

Too often the response to the discovery of complicity in hurting a child has been to look around in confusion and stumble on the MSBP concept as an explanation. Logically, it doesn't make much sense. It seems improbable that every time a doctor gives improper medical care based on false information from a caretaker that the reason he did so was because the parent suffers from the same ill-defined syndrome. There could be many other explanations but in the emotional moment, in the rush to find an explanation, this has happened all too frequently. This does not have to happen but it is completely understandable when it does. As Dine pointed more than 25 years ago, once you've been in the situation, and overcome the emotional barriers, it is easier the second time to step back and respond less passionately.

If MSBP Does Not Exist, Does That Mean There Was No Abuse?

One attempt to get rid of the diagnosis of MSBP is represented by Allison and Roberts'[14] book, *Disordered Mother or Disordered Diagnosis? Munchausen by Proxy Syndrome*. Previously we quoted the dedication. "This book is dedicated to those mothers who have been wrongly accused of criminal abuse and neglect because they suffered from a nonexistent disorder." If we are to eliminate the diagnosis of MSBP, does this mean that we have to agree that mothers have been wrongly accused of criminal abuse and neglect? How can we do this when we know that some parents have committed unspeakably horrible acts against their children? Do we have to throw the baby out with the diagnosis?

We can cite a dozen published examples of mothers diagnosed as MSBP giving their children ipecac, a strong stomach irritant, in order to make them vomit.[15-26] In many cases the child vomited for months or years before the repeated intentional poisoning was discovered. These children were hospitalized countless times and underwent numerous diagnostic procedures that were potentially harmful and totally unnecessary. In addition to being poisoned they were the victims of medical child abuse. Should we say that their mothers (most of the perpetrators were mothers) were wrongly accused of criminal abuse because they were diagnosed with a nonexistent disorder? Or should we say that they poisoned their children, subjected them to harmful medical care, and also were misdiagnosed as having a poorly defined mental illness?

For a long time ipecac was sold over the counter. Mothers kept it in the medicine cabinet with the understanding that making a child vomit after an accidental poisoning might save the child's life. Ipecac had its over-the-counter status revoked in the United States in 2003 on the recommendation of an advisory panel to the US Food and Drug Administration and can now be obtained only by prescription.[27] Gradually, pediatricians and emergency department physicians came to realize that ipecac was more dangerous than the ingestions it was being used to treat.

Recently, in our hospital a mother locked herself and her daughter in her child's bathroom. As they emerged from the bathroom the child abuse physician, having been called by concerned nursing staff, asked if she could look in the mother's purse. The mother refused. The child threw up. The vomitus was sent to the laboratory and was found to contain ipecac. The child was put under protective custody. Family court, taking into account the relevant facts of the case, found that this mother had poisoned her little girl and the court placed the child in a secure foster home.

In this instance, we agree with Allison and Roberts that the mother should not be diagnosed with a nonexistent disorder. We also agree with the court that the child needs protection from the criminal abuse committed by her mother. We do not need to posit a mental illness specific to perpetrators of medical child abuse but we do still need to protect the child victims. The abuse is real.

In addition to poisoning them with ipecac, parents do other terrible things to their children while involving the medical care system. Here are some examples. (1) A child in Italy, whose parents fabricated symptoms of hypoglycemia, received a subtotal pancreatectomy before her physicians discovered the deception.[28] (2) A father claimed on multiple occasions that his infant daughter had stopped breathing[29] resulting in numerous emergency department evaluations. Finally, emergency response personnel were called once again to transport the child from home to the hospital. They discovered a dead baby with a balloon in her throat. Forensic investigators found semen on the balloon that matched her father's DNA type. (3) Another child was admitted on multiple occasions for apnea.[30] While in the hospital his mother injected naphtha, a petroleum product, into his intravenous line. He survived but was left developmentally delayed, with cerebral palsy, and blindness. (4) A child received a small bowel transplant to treat pseudo-obstruction diagnosed on parent report of symptoms that turned out to be falsified.[31]

In cases such as these children suffer from the actions of their parents but also from the actions of physicians and other health care personnel. Medical care providers are active if unwitting participants in the abuse. In other types of abuse doctors and nurses get involved after the fact. They see the results of the abuse and are active in treating the effects. In medical child abuse, medical care providers find themselves squarely in the middle of the abuse process. They do not cause the abuse. That responsibility rests with the parents who inaccurately present their children for unnecessary treatment. But they do carry out the medical aspect of the abuse.

What Should Doctors Do?

We maintain that an unconscious unwillingness to deal with their complicity in medical child abuse has blinded members of the medical community from understanding that children need protection from this type of child abuse just as much as they would from other forms of child maltreatment. This blindness contributes to delayed identification of children at risk and a muddled response by the child protection community. Instead of invoking a rationalization such as MSBP or the presence of fraud, what should physicians and other medical care providers be doing?

We think they should do the same as they would with other forms of child maltreatment. They should help the community identify children who may be harmed, diagnose the medical consequences of maltreatment, and introduce remediation. They should perform their function as medical experts to help children avoid potentially damaging maltreatment. In many forms of child maltreatment doctors have a role. However, that role is not to be judge or jury. It is not to investigate crimes or otherwise to perform a police function. It is to help identify children who may be at risk and contribute to the efforts of the professional community that offers protection.

When physicians find themselves in the truly uncomfortable situation where they have given harmful and unnecessary medical treatment to a child, they need to resist the impulse to react angrily out of self-protection. As much as one can understand such actions, a self-protective reaction really gets in the way of their primary function, to provide the appropriate medical care, which may involve protecting the child from caretakers. If a parent has committed fraud then the properly delegated authorities can investigate. This does not fall under the job description of medical care providers. It can be argued that identifying and diagnosing mental illness in the parents of a child under his or her care might be part of a pediatrician's responsibility. However, as the physician caring for the child, the primary treatment responsibility is to the child, and treatment of the adult requires a second treatment contract.

The danger, as we see it, is that physicians who wake up during the "Oh, No!" moment may decide that their responsibility to the child ends when they discover a parent has not been giving accurate information. They may declare an end to the treatment relationship because the parent has violated an aspect of the treatment contract. It is true that a parent who gives false information in the treatment context makes accurate treatment much more difficult. Obviously, medical treatment of a child with a cooperative, well-meaning, and honest parent is much more liable to result in a good outcome. Having a parent who gives false information makes treatment considerably more difficult, but does not invalidate the physician's responsibility to care for the child.

Implications for Treatment

In the second half of this book we take up treatment of medical child abuse in considerable detail. Still, some thoughts about treatment strategies are appropriate as we address the question, Why has it taken so long? What does the realization that one has been providing medical care based on false information mean when it comes to deciding on future treatment? Basically, there appears to be 3 options. The first represents the danger mentioned previously. The physician or medical care team may decide to stop treatment altogether. The second option is to do what many have done: diagnose an illness in the parent and attempt to treat this illness while hopefully benefiting the child at the same time. The third option is to move directly to protecting the child as one would with any other form of child maltreatment.

Chapter 5
Why Has It Taken So Long?

Here is an example of a pediatric ward struggling with a child being starved by his mother.[32] The author gives a thoughtful account of the use of MSBP concepts to attempt treatment. The treatment approach labels the mother with a mental illness while attempting to avoid having the mother feel rejected and blamed.

The baby gained weight easily when fed by nurses in the hospital. The nursing staff concluded that the mother had been feeding the child with watered down formula even after demonstrating she knew the correct technique for formula preparation. The staff decided that it was ethical and necessary for the protection of the baby to allow the mother to assume full responsibility for the child's nutrition for several days. They suspected the mother would resume her pattern of starving her baby. The staff encouraged the mother to care for her child as she would at home including preparation of formula. Samples of the formula prepared by the mother were sent to the laboratory and were found to be 5 times more dilute than indicated. Before, during, and after this trial feeding period the nurses agonized over whether they were allowing the child to be harmed while in their care. After proving the child was being starved, the staff confronted the mother with their knowledge. They explained to the mother what they knew about MSBP and suggested the diagnosis of postpartum depression "…in part to 'save face' since Jenny's trust and cooperation were needed if treatment were to succeed." They encouraged the mother to see herself as mentally ill in order to justify not only what the mother did to the child but what they as health care providers had allowed her to do. After an initial period of anger and denial the mother agreed to be hospitalized along with her infant in a mental health unit where she received intensive treatment for 4 months before returning home with her child.

This case had a good outcome and represents successful treatment. The nursing personnel were able to maintain their therapeutic relationship with the mother and use it to encourage her to get needed treatment. The woman in this case report accepted the invitation by the staff to see herself as needing mental health treatment. Note how conflicted the staff feels about sharing their knowledge that the perpetrator is harming the child. They feel it necessary to allow the mother to "save face."

Should we conclude from this account that declaring a perpetrator mentally ill is a necessary step in treatment? It did seem to be helpful in this case.

However, in other situations the accused parent might not experience receiving a mental illness diagnosis as a benevolent act. In fact, she might respond by looking on the Internet under *Munchausen syndrome by proxy* and discovering the Mothers against Munchausen by Proxy Allegations (MAMA) Web site. In this event she could read:

> The motives of the accusers [doctors] can be multi-faceted. Often, allegations are used by a doctor or institution to evade a medical malpractice lawsuit, or to simply rid themselves of a troublesome mom when frustrated and unable to diagnose a child's condition. EVERY PARENT who is seriously advocating for their child is in imminent danger of this cruel and ridiculous allegation! Mothers are emotionally raped, publicly slandered, criminally charged and jailed. Even if their child is returned, they will suffer a lifetime from the trauma and may be tens or hundreds of thousands of dollars in debt from the legal fees!

We said that the moment of discovery of the subterfuge has import for everyone. It is not only a significant event for doctors and medical personnel, but also for the parent who has been distorting the truth. At the point of discovery the parent might not respond to being given a medical diagnosis with thankful acceptance. Instead, the perpetrator might feel attacked, or perhaps even betrayed. One result of medical personnel attempting to medicalize the situation can be the creation of a mutually antagonistic struggle, with each side feeling attacked by the other. When this happens the biggest potential loser is the child.

Fortunately, there are alternatives to the approach given above. We think it is more difficult for medical personnel learning they have been implicated in abusive behavior to react objectively than it is when discovering other forms of child abuse. This is especially true the first time. However, once we come to terms with the notion that parents are not always trustworthy, then we can approach the situation much as we would with other forms of child maltreatment.

Let us illustrate the third option with the use of a common procedure employed by child abuse specialists investigating physical abuse of a child. The approach involves using the available facts and presenting them as dispassionately and professionally as possible. The situation results when a child has been badly injured and admitted to the hospital. It is obvious that the injuries are the result of physical child abuse. No one is admitting responsibility for causing harm to the child. The specialist approaches the parent and attempts to obtain a history of what happened in the home. The parent becomes angry and denies that he or she did anything to hurt the child. The doctor, after being called names, carefully explains that the injuries did not occur in the course of normal childhood activity. The injuries, based on a thorough medical evaluation, were the result of a violent action that could have resulted in death. The doctor is interested in protecting the child from future harm and any help the parent can give in understanding what happened will aid in ensuring the child's safety. "Your child almost died! Someone did something very bad to this child. I need your help keeping your child safe."

This treatment strategy allows the physician to be therapeutic. A parent may respond in any of a number of ways. He or she may continue to deny any involvement, admit guilt, identify another potential perpetrator, or offer an alternative narrative. Regardless, the next steps in the therapeutic process can proceed. That process involves identifying a child at risk, and stopping the potential abuse. The physician need not diagnose the parent or terminate the treatment. It is possible the parent may terminate the treatment with this provider but this becomes part of the investigation regarding the need to protect the child from that parent.

The same strategy works with children suspected of having been abused medically. If the physician suspects a child may be the victim of medical abuse, he or she can consult with colleagues to confirm that medical treatment was offered that was not necessary and may be harmful. Following this, he or she can approach the parent and say that treatment given previously was not necessary and that from this point forward treatment will proceed in a new direction. The doctor can enlist the help of the caretaker in shifting the treatment in the appropriate direction. The caretaker may concur with the new treatment or obstruct it. In either case the physician is living up to his or her responsibility to provide the best medical care for the child. If at this point the child must be protected from the parent insisting on harmful medical care, the child protection community can be involved as it would with any other form of child maltreatment.

Conclusion

It has taken 30 years to get to the point where we can accept harm caused by a caretaker in a medical environment as medical child abuse. Doctors have feelings, and it is understandable that they feel terrible when they discover they have been used to hurt a child. Their well-meaning attempt to respond to their own feelings of shame and guilt have led them to do what they do best, make another diagnosis, this time of the adult caretaker perpetrating abuse. Unfortunately, as often as not, this approach has been unsuccessful. It would be much better if professionals worked harder to recognize when they are being lied to, changed the medical care given, and reversed the harmful effects, rather than trying to understand how they got involved. Hopefully, the next 30 years will be much better for the children affected by this form of maltreatment, and for the medical personnel who want to protect them.

Of course, medical personnel should also try to understand how they were deceived into ordering unnecessary tests or scheduling unnecessary surgery. Studying ways parents deceive physicians can result in fewer children harmed by medical abuse. However, after 30 years of continuing surprise that doctors and other medical care personnel have been used in this way, we can finally say, "It happens!" and, " Let's get on with the task of protecting children from further harm."

References

1. Donald T, Jureidini J. Munchausen syndrome by proxy. Child abuse in the medical system. *Arch Pediatr Adolesc Med.* 1996;150(7):753-758
2. Meadow R. The history of Munchausen syndrome by proxy. In: Levin AV, Sheridan MS, eds. *Munchausen Syndrome by Proxy: Issues in Diagnosis and Treatment.* New York, NY: Lexington Books; 1995:3-11
3. Kohl S, Pickering L, Dupree E. Child abuse presenting as immunodeficiency disease. *J Pediatr.* 1978;93:466-468
4. Dine MS, McGovern ME. Intentional poisoning of children—an overlooked category of child abuse: report of seven cases and review of the literature. *Pediatrics.* 1982;70(1):32-35
5. Schreier HA, Libow JA. *Hurting for Love: Munchausen by Proxy Syndrome.* New York, NY: The Guilford Press; 1993
6. Meadow SR. Munchausen syndrome by proxy. *Med Leg J.* 1995;63(Pt 3):89-104
7. Weston WL, Morelli JG. "Painful and disabling granuloma annulare": a case of Munchausen by proxy. *Pediatr Dermatol.* 1997;14(5):363-364

8. Kahan BB, Yorker BC. Munchausen syndrome by proxy. *J Sch Health.* 1990;60(3):108-110
9. Eberle AJ. Munchausen by proxy. *J Am Acad Child Adolesc Psychiatry.* 1997;36(11):1491-1492
10. Kwasman A. Munchausen syndrome by proxy. *Arch Pediatr Adolesc Med.* 1997;151(2):211-212
11. Tumolo J. Making children sick. Munchausen's syndrome by proxy. *Adv Nurse Pract.* 2001;9(6):103-106
12. Mian M. A multidisciplinary approach. In: Levin AV, Sheridan MS, eds. *Munchausen Syndrome by Proxy: Issues in Diagnosis and Treatment.* New York, NY: Lexington Books; 1995:271-286
13. Zitelli BJ, Seltman MF, Shannon RM. Munchausen's syndrome by proxy and its professional participants. *Am J Dis Child.* 1987;141(10):1099-1102
14. Allison DB, Roberts MS. *Disordered Mother or Disordered Diagnosis? Munchausen by Proxy Syndrome.* Hillsdale, NJ: The Analytic Press; 1998
15. Sutphen JL, Saulsbury FT. Intentional ipecac poisoning: Munchausen syndrome by proxy. *Pediatrics.* 1988;82(3 Pt 2):453-456
16. Berkner P, Kastner T, Skolnick L. Chronic ipecac poisoning infancy: a case report. *Pediatrics.* 1988;82:384-386
17. McClung HJ, Murray R, Braden N, Fyda J, Myers R, Gutches L. Intentional ipecac poisoning in children. *Am J Dis Child.* 1988;142:637-639
18. Colletti RB, Wasserman RC. Recurrent infantile vomiting due to intentional ipecac poisoning. *J Pediatr Gastroenterol Nutr.* 1989;8(3):394-396
19. Johnson JE, Carpenter BL, Benton J, Cross R, Eaton LA Jr, Rhoads JM. Hemorrhagic colitis and pseudomelanosis coli in ipecac ingestion by proxy. *J Pediatr Gastroenterol Nutr.* 1991;12(4):501-506
20. Sugar JA, Belfer M, Israel E, Herzog DB. A 3-year-old boy's chronic diarrhea and unexplained death. *J Am Acad Child Adolesc Psychiatry.* 1991;30(6):1015-1021
21. Schreier HA. The perversion of mothering: Munchausen syndrome by proxy. *Bull Menninger Clin.* 1992;56(4):421-437
22. Goebel J, Gremse DA, Artman M. Cardiomyopathy from ipecac administration in Munchausen syndrome by proxy. *Pediatrics.* 1993;92(4):601-603
23. Schneider DJ, Perez A, Knilamus TE, Daniels SR, Bove KE, Bonnell H. Clinical and pathologic aspects of cardiomyopathy from ipecac administration in Munchausen's syndrome by proxy. *Pediatrics.* 1996;97(6 Pt 1):902-906
24. Goldfarb J. A physician's perspective on dealing with cases of Munchausen by proxy. *Clin Pediatr (Phila).* 1998;37(3):187-189
25. Cooper C, Kilham H, Ryan M. Ipecac—a substance of abuse. *Med J Aust.* 1998;168(2):94-95

26. Bader AA, Kerzner B. Ipecac toxicity in "Munchausen syndrome by proxy." *Ther Drug Monit.* 1999;21(2):259-260
27. Shannon M. The demise of ipecac. *Pediatrics.* 2003;112(5):1180-1181
28. Caruso M, Bregani P, Di Natale B, D'Arcais A. [Induced hypoglycemia. A unusual case of child battering]. *Minerva Pediatr.* 1989;41(10):525-528
29. Milroy CM. Munchausen syndrome by proxy and intra-alveolar haemosiderin. *Int J Legal Med.* 1999;112(5):309-312
30. Saulsbury FT, Chobanian MC, Wilson WG. Child abuse: parenteral hydrocarbon administration. *Pediatrics.* 1984;73(5):719-722
31. Kosmach B, Tarbell S, Reyes J, Todo S. "Munchausen by proxy" syndrome in a small bowel transplant recipient. *Transplant Proc.* 1996;28(5):2790-2791
32. Facey S. Munchausen syndrome by proxy. *Nurs Times.* 1993;89(4):54-56

Chapter 6

So, Why *Do* They Do It?

We take a different stance, that the explanation of MSBP abuse, in common with more usual patterns of physical and sexual abuse, belongs properly in the epistemology of sociology, not of medicine. —Eminson and Jureidini, 2003[1]

Introduction

We recently lectured on medical child abuse at the University of California-Davis Child Abuse and Neglect Conference. At the end of the talk several respected colleagues approached us with comments. They had heard us define medical child abuse and describe its place in the overall context of child maltreatment. They understood the necessity to maintain the focus on the child needing treatment and they agreed that medical child abuse represented a significant improvement over past ways of describing Munchausen syndrome by proxy (MSBP) behavior. But they still felt compelled to ask, "So, why *do* they do it?" These same professionals deal with physical, sexual, and psychological abuse every day and have first-hand experience of parents doing terrible things to children. Yet they still questioned if there was something unique about the motivation of these particular parents. It is a question that continually calls for an answer.

Our colleagues' question has 2 parts. The first involves why would a parent do something to harm her child? The second part is why would a parent choose the medical setting, or involve their physicians, to harm a child? The first part of the question is common to all aspects of child maltreatment. The second is specific to medical child abuse. In the last chapter we suggested that the persistent concern about motivation in medical child abuse has roots in the underlying question, "Why me?" We feel the motivation question is not so much "Why do they do it?" but more specifically, "Why did that mother do it to me?" Nonetheless, we feel it is appropriate to give more general answers to the motivation question. The answers to both are to be found in explanations regarding how people act toward one another, or treat one another. These are behavioral or sociological questions, not medical ones.

The concept of motivation implies that there is a discernible reason why a person would act in a certain way. Generally speaking, the reason does not have to be "rational" but it does have to make sense to an objective observer. Here, we are asking why a parent would behave in an abusive manner toward her child. Over the years, a number of theories have been advanced to explain the abusive behavior of parents. In this chapter we will consider theories put forth specifically to explain abusive behavior in a medical setting. In his recent book, Bools[2] covers much of the same ground as we do here and the reader may want to compare discussions. Psychological explanations are available from various theoretical perspectives. From a sociological standpoint the question is approached through consideration of what is generally referred to as *illness behavior*. Finally, we will examine features of the doctor-patient relationship in an effort to answer conclusively the question, "So, why *do* they do it?"

Some General Thoughts About Motivation

Most of the time people understand in a commonsense way why one person treats another in a particular manner. The behavior of one human being toward another follows generally predictable patterns that are influenced by, among other things, temperament, defined roles, previous experience, belief systems, and various cultural influences. These are some of the factors that make up motivation. There is the thought that if one knows enough about a person one can predict how he or she will act toward other people in any particular situation. People say things like, "She's a good mother," and assume that they have a common understanding—that a good mother is nurturing, attentive, and responsive to her children while all the time keeping them safe from harm. A "good mother" would never abuse her child or allow her child to be abused. Of course, it is not as simple as that and people are often surprised by how other people behave.

One likes to think that most mothers are "good mothers." Generally, abusive parenting is thought to be abnormal. There has been significant resistance to even considering the notion that a parent would harm her child purposefully. In fact, as each new type of child abuse has come to conscious awareness in the community, the possibility that parents could do such harm has been met with skepticism and disbelief. When Kempe and colleagues[3] described the battered child syndrome, they commented, "Many physicians find it hard to believe that such an attack could have occurred and they attempt to obliterate such suspicions from their minds, even in the face of obvious circumstantial evidence." There was a similar response to understanding the true prevalence of child sexual abuse.

With medical child abuse early investigators assumed the parents must be insane. In 1970 Pickel et al[4] described 3 children whose mothers withheld water to the point of severe dehydration. Although he offered no objective psychiatric evidence he assumed these mothers must be psychotic to do such a thing. He portrayed one of the mothers in these terms, "Apparently his mother disliked changing diapers and thirsted the child. The mother stated that the bruises occurred secondary to a fall, but their distribution did not seem consistent with the history. The grandfather claimed the child was beaten with a rubber hose. In view of the active child neglect and abuse, arrangements were made to have him placed in a foster home." There is nothing psychologically specific about this description. It sounds like thousands of other abuse presentations. However, for this physician the only way to explain how a parent could withhold water to such a significant degree was that she was "psychotic or near psychotic."

Another early attempt to determine the motivation of perpetrators of medical abuse was made in 1977 by Fleischer and Ament[5] (1 month after Meadow published his first paper). They depicted 3 children given laxatives by their mothers to cause diarrhea. They described all 3 mothers as depressed. Even after stating that studies of child-abusing parents indicated a wide range of psychiatric disorders, including no psychiatric illness, they said, "In contrast, the pattern of medicinal abuse in the present cases could *only* result from psychotic thought processes that allow inappropriate affects, attitudes, and behavior." The conclusion from this paper was that a parent could physically batter a child for any of a number of reasons but could give laxatives causing serious medical problems only by way of "psychotic thought processes."

As adamant as professionals have been in seeking and finding mental illness in perpetrators of medical abuse, they have had difficulty identifying what it might be. In a review paper, Souid and colleagues[6] wrote, "The perpetrator, by definition, suffers from a serious emotional disorder that impairs judgment. The emotional disorder is not diagnosable; its pathology is culturally invisible and masked by social adaptation (eg, overreacting to the child's illness and emotional hunger)." Needless to say, it seems improbable that mothers who commit medical child abuse have a serious emotional disorder that cannot be diagnosed.

In a similar vein Rosenberg[7] wrote, "Despite the fact that the mothers who perpetrate MSBP are frequently described as 'normal' psychiatrically, this is obviously not the case. Clearly the behavior is biologically abnormal, though its origins are, as yet, abstruse." In the same paper she also declared, "Occasionally, the distinction in clinical practice between MSBP and intentional poisoning, infanticide, pathological doctor shopping, extreme parental anxiety, or parental thought disorder is not entirely clear (probably because the underlying psychopathology overlaps)."

The implication of this statement to us seems to be that what might differentiate these dissimilar types of behavior is the difference in "underlying psychopathology." If we could only understand the underlying psychopathology, and if they did not overlap so much, then we could distinguish one behavior from another and diagnose MSBP separately from intentional poisoning. If we only knew why they did it then perhaps we would be able to tell one type of behavior from another.

Of course, another way of interpreting the situation is to say that one expression of psychopathology could lead to many different behaviors, and many different psychopathologies could lead to the same behavior. For example, a mother who experienced early childhood deprivation could act in a variety of ways toward her children. In response to her own unfortunate upbringing she could poison her child, ignore her child, hire a nanny to make up for her lack of child-rearing abilities, or lavish loving attention to compensate for what she did not receive. Likewise, a mother lacking in intelligence (developmentally disabled), depressed (affectively disordered), deprived in her early childhood (attachment disordered), or wanting to start a career that required her to be childless (selfish) could intentionally poison her child.

Perhaps, as some have indicated, medical child abuse will eventually follow the pattern of other forms of child maltreatment. Mercer and Purdue[8] said,

"Most people probably do not believe that a parent would intentionally induce illness in a child. These behaviors seem as outrageous today as child abuse or incest seemed 20 years ago." In other words, as we develop the capacity to identify medical abuse more easily and become more familiar with it, we may not have to reach as far to characterize the actions of the perpetrator.

Psychological Explanations Why Parents Medically Abuse Children

So, how have we tried to explain MSBP behavior? In the 1980s theorists searching for a psychological explanation generally turned to psychoanalytic theory. Several papers referred to an article by Stern[9] written in 1948 describing "the Medea complex" as an explanation of why a mother would kill her child. In Greek mythology Medea killed her son because he might grow up to be the rival to her husband. This explanation of infanticide, however, only partially explained the numerous ways parents might harm children.

A succinct psychoanalytic formulation for MSBP was given in a letter to the editor by Lesnik-Oberstein[10] in 1986:

> The Munchausen by proxy mother's childhood is characterized by severe emotional deprivation. Her needs for care, warmth, affection, and attention were ignored and neglected. As a result, she experienced these needs as extremely painful/anxiety provoking and split-off/repressed them. At some point in her childhood it is likely that she may have been hospitalized and experienced for the first time, in the hospital setting, care and affection. Later on she may have chosen nursing as a way of returning to a hospital setting and, as a way of solving her emotional problems, giving to others the care and affection that she craves. But the solution fails. She marries a man who fails to meet her emotional needs, and that solution also fails. When she has a child, she projects on her child (via projective identification) her unconscious split-off/repressed "needy self," and the child, from whom she is poorly differentiated, becomes the representative of her needy self. As such a representative, the child is caused to be hospitalized in order to provide for mother the vicarious

satisfaction, by proxy, of her emotional needs which are also more directly met for mother's involvement in the pediatric ward. The painful and dangerous consequences for the child of mother's behavior are dealt with by denial.

As referred to previously, Schreier and Libow, in their book, *Hurting for Love*,[11] and in other writings,[12,13] advance the theory that the mother perpetrating MSBP uses her child as a fetishistic object to meet her psychological needs. While not significantly different from the account offered by Lesnik-Oberstein, Schreirer and Libow go into considerable detail to explain their position. Others have given psychoanalytically oriented theoretical prescriptions for MSBP behavior.[14,15]

Attachment theory, as an outgrowth of classical analytic thought, has been used as a theoretical construct that might be tested to understand perpetrators of MSBP. In one effort Adshead and colleagues[16] attempted to evaluate attachment by scoring pieces of videotape obtained covertly from mothers who subsequently smothered their babies in the hospital. In a second project, Adshead and Bluglass[17] used an attachment measure to evaluate a mother and grandmother of a smothered child and speculated, "Theoretically, the insecurely attached maltreating parent has internalized a working model of dependency relationships characterized by hostility and fear."

Learning theory provides yet another theoretical model to explain psychological reasons for MSBP behavior. Rand and Feldman[18] present the most complete formulation. They hypothesize that perpetrators of MSBP behavior have powerful, dysphoric emotional drive states (intense anger or frustration) that they discharge through the abusive behavior to the child. The perpetrators need to avoid internal inhibitions that would ordinarily prevent a mother or other caretaker from acting out in this way, and neutralize external inhibitions at the same time. "We hypothesize that MBP behavior gains habit strength each time the perpetrator experiences the drive, overcomes internal and external inhibitions, experiences the sought after release, and successfully controls the responses of other people." While applying learning theory principles to MSBP behavior the authors also offer criticism for psychoanalytic formulations.

Libow,[19,20] writing independently from Schreier, has also used learning theory to describe how children come to participate in MSBP behavior.

Discussions of somatization often include references to learning illness behaviors from parents.[21]

Family systems theory is another model used to explain MSBP behavior.[22–25] In general, writers with a family systems perspective maintain that family units have an independent life of their own, and significant transactions have meaning for everyone within the family. Thus a recurrent behavior, such as falsifying information about the child's illness, affects everyone and is maintained by everyone within the family unit, whether overtly or covertly. A correlate of this theoretical perspective is that an intervention aimed at stopping the behavior is best made at the level of the family unit. Robins and Sesan[26] described the etiology of MSBP behavior from a family systems perspective but complemented this by adding feminist theory to try and explain why perpetrators are primarily female.

As we can see, there are a variety of theoretical points of view from which to choose if we seek to explain abusive parental behavior from a psychological perspective. As one would expect, there have been attempts to test hypotheses with clinical observations. These efforts have ranged from single case design studies to examinations of a series of perpetrators.

Sigal and colleagues,[27–29] in several papers about a man who injected gasoline under the skin of his wife and, later, his girlfriend, attempted, through psychiatric interviews and psychological testing, to discover why he would do such a thing. The gasoline injected under his wife's skin caused numerous atypical abscesses that eventually resulted in a painful death. The authors reported these actions as examples of MSBP where the victims were adults. A psychiatric interview conducted in prison showed no evidence of psychosis, anxiety, affective disturbance, or cognitive defects. Psychological testing confirmed that the perpetrator had no distortion of reality testing but did indicate a narcissistic personality disorder. When asked why he killed his wife he led his interviewers to understand that he "did not regard his behavior as criminal, but rather described it as an expression of 'love and caring.'"[27]

Another single case study attempting to understand the motivation of a murderer yielded a similar conclusion. Stanton and Simpson[30] interviewed a woman convicted of smothering to death 3 of her own children and attempting to murder 2 other youngsters in her care who, fortunately, survived. The investigators conducted long intense interviews with the woman while she was at home on leave from prison. She told them that she killed her first child because the child was suffering from apnea. She "described the killing of her much loved and wanted daughter as a 'mercy killing'—that is, where a child is killed to prevent them having to go through real suffering." The explanation she gave for the murders of her next 2 children was that she never really "bonded" with them.

Bools and colleagues[31] studied a group of 19 mothers evaluated for MSBP. Their work represents the best effort to date to gather systematic information about perpetrators of MSBP. They conducted a structured interview and administered psychological tests, sometimes years after the initial consideration for MSBP. The study indicated that the perpetrators had troubled childhoods including significant amounts of physical, sexual, and emotional abuse. Seventeen of the 19 mothers received a diagnosis of a personality disorder. None of the women was thought to be psychotic. However, 15 of 19 had a history of somatization disorder, most of which represented factitious illnesses in themselves.

This last characteristic, the propensity for communicating thoughts and feelings through somatic symptoms, appears to be the predominant difference between this group of medical abuse perpetrators and parents who committed other forms of child abuse. While not all abusive parents have abusive childhoods, and certainly not all parents who were abused as children abuse their children, parents who abuse their children often learn parenting from abusive parents.[32,33]

Sociological Theories—The Role of Illness Behavior

Others writing about MSBP have concluded that the answer to the question, "Why commit abuse in a medical environment?" lies not in examining the psychology of perpetrators but in studying illness behavior, or the "sick role." In fact, several authors[34-37] have referred to the classic reference by Talcot Parsons[38] written in the 1950s regarding the sociology of illness. Just as there exists a loosely understood concept of a "good mother," there is a similar understanding of what constitutes a "good patient." Good patients follow the rules of acceptable illness behavior. The following are some rules that define the sick role as adapted from Parsons:

- Patients are victims of the illness.

- The illness is outside oneself and one is not responsible for it.

- Sick people can put themselves in the hands of others (give over control).
- The sick person is exempted from work or school.
- The sick person is expected to cooperate with others trying to help and make a sincere effort to get well.

These rules represent how a patient should present himself or herself to the doctor and the community at large. Generally, if a parent is taking her child to the doctor the same rules apply. Children, and by extension their parents, are not responsible for the fact that they have contracted an illness. Children are excused from school and their parents can stay home from work to take care of them. In exchange for receiving the special treatment afforded a person in the sick role, the child and his or her parent agree to do everything in their power to get back to a normal state of health. Giving accurate information to the physician is part of the sick person using all efforts to get well.

Why Do People Lie?

In our description of medical child abuse we maintain that a parent who induces an illness directly in a child, for example, by feeding the child ipecac, is committing assault, or physical child abuse. It is the unnecessary and harmful or potentially harmful medical care administered by the physician that constitutes medical child abuse. We stipulate that to have medical care providers become the instrument of abuse in medical child abuse, parents need to provide doctors and nurses with false information. However, just as with many other behaviors, there can be many reasons why people do what they do.

Here are a few reasons why people might provide false information to their doctor and, by doing so, violate the rules for proper sick role behavior. The person providing the information might think it is correct. He or she might know that it is not true but not feel it is significant in the larger scheme of things. He might know the information is not accurate but pass it on with the understanding or intention that it will facilitate a good outcome ("a little white lie"). Or the provider of information might communicate untrue facts knowing that somebody acting on those facts will cause harm. How can we know which of these or one of the many other variations might be happening in the communication between a parent and a physician?

In this book, we will be extensively discussing one of our patients, a girl named Laura. She was admitted to the hospital as a 4-year-old to receive intravenous antibiotics because she was felt to suffer from "pansinusitis." She had received antibiotics in pill form several times for greenish-yellow drainage from her nose (by her mother's report) that was felt to be an indication for sinus infections. Laura's mother's insistence that she had recurrent sinus infections led to treatment in the hospital. While on the ward her attending physician asked for and received a consultation from the pediatric rehabilitation service. A senior medical student doing his rotation in rehabilitation medicine conducted a detailed interview of our patient's mother regarding the girl's medical history and documented what she told him. The medical student wrote in his consultation note in the chart that Laura suffered from "pancreatitis." She was in the hospital for 30 days. At no other time was there an indication in the hospital record that any of her attending physicians were concerned Laura might have pancreatitis. The discharge summary made no mention of pancreatitis but did record treatment for pansinusitis. Over the next several months specialists began commenting, in their evaluations of Laura, that she suffered from recurrent pancreatitis. In retrospect, we concluded that her mother tried to explain to the medical student why she was in the hospital, the medical student understood it incorrectly as pancreatitis, and communicated this diagnosis back to the mother. Laura's mother then transmitted a new illness for her child to the next 3 physicians she saw while repeating her medical history. We saw this child when she was 10 years old. By that time a dozen physicians, without any corroborating medical evidence, had reiterated that she suffered from recurrent pancreatitis and this information was used to justify treatment that she never needed.

Laura's mother obviously told a number of doctors, including us, that her daughter suffered from recurrent pancreatitis. Was she lying? She clearly passed on false information. There is no indication we can determine that she did this maliciously. But it did result in her daughter receiving unnecessary and harmful medical care. It does constitute behavior that led to harm and from which the child should have been protected. Once again, the determining factor of whether behavior constitutes medical child abuse resides in the harm experienced by the child and not in the motivation of the parent. We would agree with Jones,[39] who commented that he would rather describe the harm done to a child than give a medical label to someone for lying.

Chapter 6
So, Why *Do* They Do It?

There is one thing of which we can be certain. Everybody lies. Some people lie more than others. Some people lie with good intentions and others with malicious purpose. But at some time or another we all communicate falsely. We recently went to the promotion ceremony for a police officer friend. We were surprised to see his wife in attendance. We knew that she had asked for leave from work to see her husband receive his new rank and a well-earned citation. We also knew that she had been turned down. At the reception afterward we learned that she had called in sick. She lied to her employer. We agreed that she deserved to be with her husband for this important occasion and that the employer had been unreasonable in refusing her request. She could have informed her employer that she was taking the time without permission and received the expected reprimand. However, calling in sick was a behavior that we understood and that seemed appropriate given the circumstances.

If communicating things that are not true is commonplace we should not be surprised to see that it happens within the medical environment.[35] In fact, people lie so regularly about some things that physicians have routinely taken certain falsehoods into account. For example, 30 years ago in medical school we were told to assume when taking a history of alcohol use that our patients would admit to approximately half of what they actually consumed. If a man admitted to 1 drink before dinner we could be almost certain that he had 2. Today's medical students are being told the same thing. People lie to their dentist about whether they floss their teeth. Overweight people invariably eat like a bird. Some men claim much more sexual prowess than their wives would confirm.

People lie. People lie to their doctors. People lie to their doctors about their children's illnesses, and by doing so break the rules of expected illness behavior. Medical decisions made based on false information are almost invariably bad decisions. And as a result children receive unnecessary and harmful or potentially harmful medical care. We know that parents who abuse their children often have emotional problems of their own, and that parents who abuse their children medically often have a history of over-involvement with the medical community. It all seems fairly obvious. But still physicians ask the question, "So why *do* they do it?"

Even though we can explain that rules exist describing the social contract between doctors and patients, and parents sometimes break the rules with bad consequences for their children, it is still interesting to ask why doctors can't seem to get beyond the question. We began this discussion in the previous chapter and continue it now. We think the answer lies in looking at the *physician's response* to illness behavior in their patients and the parents of their patients. To examine this more closely we would like to look at some distortions of normal illness behavior and some physicians' responses.

Vulnerable Child Syndrome and Somatization Disorder

In 1964 Green and Solnit[40] described *vulnerable child syndrome*. This concept has had a long, productive life in child psychiatry and pediatrics as a description of a particular type of illness behavior exhibited by anxious parents. Curiously, unlike MSBP, vulnerable child syndrome has never taken on the trappings of an actual illness. Rather, it has remained a description of over-anxious parental behavior in the medical setting. Green and Solnit pointed out that circumstances surrounding birth could give rise to belief in some parents that their child was in danger of dying or being vulnerable to significant harm from a medical illness that may or may not have a basis in fact. An event in pregnancy, a difficult aspect of the delivery, a chance remark by a doctor that "we almost lost him," all of these could form the core of a belief that a child could die suddenly. This belief may result in parents taking their child for medical care unnecessarily.

Vulnerable child syndrome represents an example of how a parent's belief system can affect how and why the child goes to the doctor. In fact, it is fairly common. Levy[41] surveyed parents in outpatient pediatric clinic waiting rooms. She specifically asked if the parent thought her child was suffering from a serious, life-threatening illness. She then compared parents who had a belief in a life-threatening condition with medical records to see if there was evidence for the concern. She found that 27% of parents had the belief that their child was vulnerable to a serious illness, and for 40% of these, there was no clinical basis. Therefore, approximately 10% of all the parents in the waiting room believed their child to be seriously ill when it was not the case. What's more, these parents were identified as more frequent users of medical services, and were more frequently dissatisfied with care received than a comparable group of parents with realistic beliefs regarding their children's illness.

These vulnerable children are vulnerable in more ways than one. Their parents consider them potential victims of a serious illness. And in response to this belief subject them to doctor visits they may not need. Their perceived vulnerability actually makes them vulnerable to unnecessary medical care. But these children rarely turn out to be victims of medical child abuse. Usually they receive only treatment they do need. Doctors are usually able to identify the underlying issue before giving unnecessary care. These parents often respond to the question, "Is there something about your child that makes you feel that he or she might die?" with an open expression of their true concern. They express relief that a doctor would ask about their worst nightmares. With their anxieties manifest parents can begin to understand the actual nature of their child's medical condition and deal with their own fears. Occasionally, a parent cannot accept reassurance and continues with a fixed belief that puts a child at risk, and their behavior "crosses the line" resulting in the child needing protection. Once again, we can appreciate a continuum of behavior.

Somatization disorder is a description of illness behavior that has made the transition into a diagnosis in the *Diagnostic and Statistical Manual of Mental Disorders, Fourth Edition (DSM-IV)*.[42] Doctors identified more than 100 years ago that a group of patients, primarily women, repeatedly present themselves for treatment with symptoms that do not have an organic basis. The predecessor terms for somatization disorder include *hysteria* and *Briquet's syndrome*. People diagnosed with this disorder go to the doctor frequently with a wide variety of symptoms. In fact, in order to meet the *DSM-IV* criteria complaints have to refer to many different organ systems. The complaints are seldom associated with objective physical findings on examination or laboratory tests. As described in *DSM-IV*,[42] "These individuals commonly undergo numerous medical examinations, diagnostic procedures, surgeries, and hospitalizations, which expose the person to an increased risk of morbidity associated with these procedures."

Everyone has the occasional ache or pain that causes concern. We respond to signals from our bodies and make judgments about what should be considered serious enough to warrant medical attention. If the threshold is set particularly low a person can end up seeking medical treatment for bodily concerns that others would ignore. If this behavior is severe enough the conditions for somatization disorder can be met. A distinguishing feature of somatization disorder is that the person must actually believe the symptoms are, or might be, real. If the patient knows the symptoms are not real he or she would be diagnosed with a factitious illness or malingering.

Somatization disorder is a term that describes people for whom being sick is a way of life. It is understood that they fall on the far end of the continuum of health care–seeking behaviors. But they still play the medical game by the rules. They think they are sick. They seek medical treatment with the intent of becoming healthy again.

It has been suggested that MSBP might be understood as a form of somatization disorder by proxy.[43,44] Using this line of thinking, instead of or in addition to, taking oneself to the doctor as a way of life, some parents take their children to the doctor. Taking one's child to the doctor, even when he or she does not need it, is not a crime or an illness. However, once again, if the parent's behavior toward her child crosses a certain line then we must consider it to be child abuse. The salient fact is not the motivation of the parent, or whether the parent suffers from a somatization disorder, but whether or not the child is being harmed.

The Contribution of the Physician

In a much quoted paper written in 1992 Eminson and Postlethwaite[45] provided a schema to understand the health-seeking behavior of parents. They focused on the degree of agreement between the parent and her physician about whether to seek medical care. They suggested that most of the time parents and doctors are in general agreement. From the doctor's point of view parents could have a normal, appropriate response to the child's symptoms, have a slightly exaggerated or anxious view of the symptoms, or a somewhat lackadaisical view of the symptoms. All of these would be within a normal range. However, a parent might feel much more strongly about the need to seek care than a doctor feels is appropriate. Such a parent might exaggerate symptoms, invent symptoms, or induce symptoms in the child. On the other end of the spectrum, a parent's view about whether to seek treatment might also be significantly different from that of the average physician. These parents would neglect to give their child prescribed medications, would take unnecessary chances with their child's health, or might completely ignore symptoms. Outside the normal range of health-seeking behavior, to either extreme, either too much or too little, a child could be in danger. Health-seeking behaviors toward the exaggerated extreme represent what we call *medical child abuse*, while those at the other extreme represent *medical neglect*.

Eminson and Postlethwaite make an assumption that physicians understand when a parent should bring a child for medical care. Their schema describes parents who deviate to one extreme or the other from the physician's expected standard. However, physicians vary as well. Some are more inclined to do diagnostic tests than others. Some physicians are minimalists who feel that less treatment is better. In the case of Laura, the girl with the false diagnosis of "pancreatitis," her mother who exaggerated symptoms managed to find several physicians who gave exaggerated treatment. The result was a child getting very harmful medical care.

The doctor-patient relationship involves expectations of the doctor as well as of the patient. It is a complementary fit. Doctor and patient need one another. To be a healer a physician needs someone who requires healing. Typically, a patient asks for and receives care, and a physician offers and provides care. A patient is not obligated to request needed medical care. He or she can opt out of the treatment relationship at any time. Nor is a doctor obligated to provide unnecessary medical care. But once the doctor-patient relationship is established, expected rules of behavior generally dictate that care is requested and provided until the illness episode is over.

Eminson and Postlethwaite emphasize that a physician needs to have a "framework" within which to proceed with treatment. This framework includes generally accepted expectations on the part of both doctor and patient. A doctor doing his or her job can expect the patient to play his or her part. If the patient breaks the rules by, for example, giving false information and the doctor continues to play by the rules and provides treatment consistent with the information provided, the result is potentially harmful medical care. What is more, treatment given for a nonexistent illness is seldom successful. Because the false symptoms do not respond to unnecessary treatment the potential exists for the symptoms to be repeated and even augmented, resulting in more unnecessary treatment. This inappropriate use of the complementary relationship between patient and doctor leads to a situation where the framework is eventually broken. Either the doctor stops providing care (leaving the parent the option of seeking another doctor who *will* provide care), the mother stops making up new symptoms, or the child eventually experiences harm.

Physicians who realize that the rules of the relationship have been violated need to step out of their usual perspective and look at what they are doing from a new viewpoint. This is similar to what a physician needs to do when treating a patient with somatization disorder. The treatment is to give no medical treatment. The proper exercise of the doctor-patient relationship is to inform the patient that she does not have an illness that will respond to usual medical treatment.

But what if the patient is a child and the person distorting the doctor-patient relationship is the child's caretaker? Then, when the doctor steps out of the normal doctor-patient relationship, and takes an objective view of the treatment, he finds himself in a dual role. He needs to decide whether the behavior of the parent has possibly put the child in danger. Has the behavior crossed the line into the territory of child abuse?

A doctor reporting child abuse to the local child protection agency is stepping out of the primary doctor-patient relationship to serve as a representative of the community at large. Physician reporting laws dictate that not only is the physician required to make a report, but cannot be held responsible legally for violating his patient's confidentiality by the act of the reporting if that report is done in good faith. A new set of rules apply. The physician is required to balance his role as a healer and keeper of confidences with his role as a representative of society. The physician reporting an infectious disease to the local health department is acting in a similar dual role. Preventing a cholera epidemic that would harm many people supersedes the doctor's responsibility to the individual patient. Other examples of physicians with dual responsibilities include those who conduct forensic interviews and testify in court, and those who work for insurance companies, the military, or prisons. In each of these cases the doctor is responsible to the individual patient but with special considerations that are usually spelled out ahead of time.

Having roles ancillary to that of confidential healer has always been part of medicine. However, a doctor who has been deceived in the medical setting by a parent is likely to experience a role for which he or she is not prepared. Instead of, or in addition to, taking on the role of protector of children, the physician may feel more like a victim of the actions of the child's parent. People who feel violated experience a need to regain equilibrium however possible. A physician as victim can be expected to respond as victims do for any other type of assault. The natural response to victimization is to get angry and to push away the perpetrator. Then one might try to understand the situation, to make sense of something that at first seems senseless. This is what physicians have done when they become aware that they have been made complicit in harming a child through medical child abuse.

Victims of sexual abuse often ask a therapist, "Why did he do it?" and "Why did he choose me?" These are the same questions physicians ask when they find themselves victimized by the person who is medically abusing their child. More often than not, in the case of sexual abuse, the answers to the questions are, "Because he thought he could get away with it," and "Because you were available." These are often unsatisfying answers for the victim of sexual abuse. The abuse is experienced as highly significant to the victim and, in the victim's mind the reason for it should have just as high a significance. The victim of sexual abuse often feels not only that she is the only person in the world ever to experience such a thing, but that the perpetrator would not have ever violated anyone else. To a victim, a special event should have a special cause.

Over the years the medical community has come to accept that many different kinds of parents for many different reasons can commit physical or sexual abuse. But with medical child abuse the doubts, concerns, and speculation have never matured into commonplace awareness and acceptance that child abuse happens and sometimes there is no really good answer to the question, "So why *do* they do it?"

References

1. Eminson M, Jureidini J. Concerns about research and prevention strategies in Munchausen syndrome by proxy (MSBP) abuse. *Child Abuse Negl.* 2003;27(4):413-420
2. Bools C. *Fabricated or Induced Illness in a Child by a Carer: A Reader*. Oxford, UK: Radcliffe Publishing; 2007
3. Kempe CH, Silverman FW, Steele BF, Droegemueller W, Silver H. The battered child syndrome. *JAMA*. 1962;181:17-24
4. Pickel S, Anderson C, Holliday MA. Thirsting and hypernatremic dehydration— a form of child abuse. *Pediatrics*. 1970;45(1):54-59
5. Fleisher D, Ament ME. Diarrhea, red diapers, and child abuse: clinical alertess needed for recognition; clinical skill needed for success in management. *Clin Pediatr*. 1977;17:820-824

6. Souid AK, Keith DV, Cunningham AS. Munchausen syndrome by proxy. *Clin Pediatr (Phila).* 1998;37(8):497-503
7. Rosenberg DA. Web of deceit: a literature review of Munchausen syndrome by proxy. *Child Abuse Negl.* 1987;11(4):547-563
8. Mercer SO, Perdue JD. Munchausen syndrome by proxy: social work's role. *Soc Work.* 1993;38(1):74-81
9. Stern ES. The Medea complex: The mother's homicidal wishes to her child. *J Ment Sci.* 1948;94:321-331
10. Lesnik-Oberstein M. Munchausen syndrome by proxy. *Child Abuse Negl.* 1986;10(1):133
11. Schreier HA, Libow JA. *Hurting for Love: Munchausen by Proxy Syndrome.* New York, NY: The Guilford Press; 1993
12. Schreier HA. The perversion of mothering: Munchausen syndrome by proxy. *Bull Menninger Clin.* 1992;56(4):421-437
13. Schreier HA, Libow JA. Munchausen syndrome by proxy: diagnosis and prevalence. *Am J Orthopsychiatry.* 1993;63(2):318-321
14. Palmer AJ, Yoshimura GJ. Munchausen syndrome by proxy. *J Am Acad Child Psychiatry.* 1984;23(4):503-508
15. Szajnberg NM, Moilanen I, Kanerva A, Tolf B. Munchausen-by-proxy syndrome: countertransference as a diagnostic tool. *Bull Menninger Clin.* 1996;60(2):229-237
16. Adshead G, Brooke D, Samuels M, Jenner S, Southall D. Maternal behaviors associated with smothering: a preliminary descriptive study. *Child Abuse Negl.* 2000;24(9):1175-1183
17. Adshead G, Bluglass K. A vicious circle: transgenerational attachment representations in a case of factitious illness by proxy. *Attach Hum Dev.* 2001;3(1):77-95
18. Rand DC, Feldman MD. An explanatory model for Munchausen by proxy abuse. *Int J Psychiatry Med.* 2001;31(2):113-126
19. Libow JA. Child and adolescent illness falsification. *Pediatrics.* 2000;105(2):336-342
20. Libow JA. Beyond collusion: active illness falsification. *Child Abuse Negl.* 2002;26(5):525-536
21. Krener P. Factitious disorders and the psychosomatic continuum in children. *Curr Opin Pediatr.* 1994;6(4):418-422
22. Richtsmeier AJ Jr, Waters DB. Somatic symptoms as family myth. *Am J Dis Child.* 1984;138(9):855-857
23. Griffith JL. The family systems of Munchausen syndrome by proxy. *Fam Process.* 1988;27(4):423-437

24. Gray J, Bentovim A. Illness induction syndrome: paper I—a series of 41 children from 37 families identified at The Great Ormond Street Hospital for Children NHS Trust. *Child Abuse Negl.* 1996;20(8):655-673
25. von Hahn L, Harper G, McDaniel SH, Siegel DM, Feldman MD, Libow JA. A case of factitious disorder by proxy: the role of the health-care system, diagnostic dilemmas, and family dynamics. *Harv Rev Psychiatry.* 2001;9(3):124-135
26. Robins PM, Sesan R. Munchausen syndrome by proxy: another women's disorder? *Prof Psychol Res Pr.* 1991;22:285-290
27. Sigal MD, Altmark D, Carmel I. Munchausen syndrome by adult proxy: a perpetrator abusing two adults. *J Nerv Ment Dis.* 1986;174(11):696-698
28. Sigal M, Gelkopf M, Meadow RS. Munchausen by proxy syndrome: the triad of abuse, self-abuse, and deception. *Compr Psychiatry.* 1989;30(6):527-533
29. Sigal M, Gelkopf M, Levertov G. Medical and legal aspects of the Munchausen by proxy perpetrator. *Med Law.* 1990;9(1):739-749
30. Stanton J, Simpson A. Murder misdiagnosed as SIDS: a perpetrator's perspective. *Arch Dis Child.* 2001;85:454-459
31. Bools C, Neale B, Meadow R. Munchausen syndrome by proxy: a study of psychopathology. *Child Abuse Negl.* 1994;18(9):773-788
32. Kaufman J, Zigler E. Do abused children become abusive parents? *Am J Orthopsychiatry.* 1987;57(2):186-192
33. Anda RF, Felitti VJ, Chapman DP, et al. Abused boys, battered mothers, and male involvement in teen pregnancy. *Pediatrics.* 2001;107(2):E19
34. Lipsitt DR. Introduction. In: Feldman MD, Eisendrath SJ, eds. *The Spectrum of Factitious Disorders.* Washington, DC: American Psychiatric Press, Inc.; 1996:xix-xxviii
35. Sheridan MS. Munchausen syndrome by proxy in context I: deception in society. In: Levin AV, Sheridan MS, eds. *Munchausen Syndrome by Proxy: Issues in Diagnosis and Treatment.* New York, NY: Lexington Books; 1995:69-83
36. Feldman MD, Eisendrath SJ, eds. *The Spectrum of Factitious Disorders.* Washington, DC: American Psychiatric Press, Inc.; 1996
37. Ford CV. Illness has a lifestyle: the role of somatization in medical practice. *Spine.* 1992;17:S387-S342
38. Parsons T. *The Social System.* Glencoe, IL: Free Press; 1951
39. Jones DP. Commentary: Munchausen syndrome by proxy—is expansion justified? *Child Abuse Negl.* 1996;20(10):983-984
40. Green M, Solnit AJ. Reaction to the threatened loss of the child: a vulnerable child syndrome. *Pediatrics.* 1964;34:58-66
41. Levy JC. Vulnerable children: parents perspective and the use of medical care. *Pediatrics.* 1980;65:956-963

42. American Psychiatric Association. *Diagnostic and Statistical Manual of Mental Disorders, Fourth Edition*. Washington, DC: American Psychiatric Association; 1994
43. Livingston R. Maternal somatization disorder and Munchausen syndrome by proxy. *Psychosomatics*. 1987;28(4):213-214, 217
44. Donald T, Jureidini J. Munchausen syndrome by proxy. Child abuse in the medical system. *Arch Pediatr Adolesc Med*. 1996;150(7):753-758
45. Eminson DM, Postlethwaite RJ. Factitious illness: recognition and management. *Arch Dis Child*. 1992;67(12):1510-1516

Chapter 7

Description of 115 Cases Referred for Possible Munchausen Syndrome by Proxy

We propose that research energy would be more productively directed towards furthering our understanding of somatization and certain problematic aspects of modern pediatric practice.
— Eminson and Jureidini, 2003[1]

Introduction

In preparation for this book the authors reviewed their involvement with children suspected of having Munchausen syndrome by proxy (MSBP). We conducted a retrospective chart review of children we evaluated or treated during the past 12 years. During that time one of the authors (CJ), a pediatrician, directed a child protection program at a children's hospital, evaluating children referred for possible child abuse in all of its forms. The other author (TR), a child psychiatrist, directed a partial hospital treatment program for medically and psychiatrically ill children, including children suspected of having been abused in a medical context. Both continue to serve in those capacities. Children suspected of suffering from, or needing treatment for, MSBP have been referred to both programs.

We work in the State of Rhode Island, which has a population of approximately 1 million people. Working in a small New England state has its advantages. Nothing is very far away. The population is diverse and interesting. For the most part professionals know one another. *ChildSafe*, the child protection program at Hasbro Children's Hospital, is the only hospital-based child abuse program in the state. It works closely with the Rhode Island Department of Children, Youth and Families (DCYF) and is the state's primary resource for the medical evaluation of suspected child abuse and neglect. The program evaluates more than 1,800 children for abuse or neglect each year.

The Hasbro Children's Partial Hospital Program (HCPHP) is a pediatric/child psychiatric day treatment program recognized as a statewide resource for the evaluation and treatment of children with unusual medical conditions who also have psychological issues. The HCPHP treats approximately 175 children each year and has an average length of stay of 20 days. The HCPHP treats children between 6 and 18 years of age. In a small state combining the resources of the major child abuse evaluation unit and the principal treatment facility for children with combined medical and psychological problems results in broad coverage of the children for whom MSBP might be an issue. Because of these factors we feel it's fair to say that most (if not all) children in Rhode Island suspected of MSBP come to our attention.

How Were the Children Identified?

Despite this, we cannot claim that the 115 children described here are an epidemiologically representative sample of the children of Rhode Island. It remains a sample of convenience. How did we choose to include the children? We cast a wide net. Each of the programs maintains a log that allows children to be identified based on the reason for their referral. These resources were searched to find appropriate cases. The only inclusion criterion was that during the referral process someone identified a concern about MSBP. (More recently colleagues have begun to refer children for possible "medical child abuse" instead of MSBP and these cases have also been included.)

About 5 times per year the *ChildSafe* team (out of 1,800 referrals) is asked to evaluate a child for potential MSBP. Regardless of the outcome of that evaluation, those children are included in the sample. Similarly, when children are referred to the HCPHP for treatment of an illness, they sometimes come with a question by the referring doctor about whether this might be "Munchausen's." These children, too, are included in the data set. A third group of children in the sample of 115 were referred by child protection agencies in nearby states for second opinions regarding the question of MSBP.

We have commented previously on the difficulty that exists when drawing conclusions from extreme cases of MSBP. The availability heuristic limits what one can say in general terms about a condition that has a wide range of presentations if one only includes examples from one end of the spectrum.

It is much better to sample across the spectrum from mild to severe if one wants to make general statements about a phenomenon. By setting the bar for inclusion at "a possibility of MSBP," we almost certainly guaranteed that we would include mild cases and even some that would not meet the criteria for medical child abuse.

In many cases the concerns about MSBP were the primary reason to seek consultation. For other children, it was mentioned as a secondary issue. An example might be a primary care pediatrician referring a child with pseudo-seizures saying, "I think the mother might have Munchausen's." Once the issue was raised the child was included in our series. As we will see, the children surveyed here include those "tip of the iceberg" very dramatic cases, the type that usually find their way into published case histories and subsequently into review articles such as "Web of Deceit."[2] But it also includes the soft cases, children for whom a primary care pediatrician has a concern but does not know whether abuse has really taken place. As such, we feel our sample is more representative of the real world in pediatric and child psychiatric practice. More appropriately, however, the children surveyed could be considered to be representative of children who come to the attention of a specialty child abuse evaluation and treatment center.

Specifically, 13 children were seen exclusively by the *ChildSafe* program, and 68 children were treated exclusively in the HCPHP. A total of 16 children were evaluated in *ChildSafe* and also treated in the partial program. In addition to the children treated at the 2 programs at Hasbro Children's Hospital, the authors were consulted on 18 cases from other states.

Case Examples

We begin with a series of short case vignettes describing how some of the children in our series presented to us. We will refer to these cases by that name during the description of evaluation and treatment that follows.

Laura

Ten-year-old Laura was referred to HCPHP for evaluation of abdominal pain. It turned out she had many more things wrong with her as well. Her mother brought a paper shopping bag full of medications to the first visit. Laura was taking more than 30 different medications for a variety of ailments. Her list of symptoms included abdominal pain, constipation, headaches, easy fatigability, frequent fractures of major bones, seizures, immune deficiency, hypothyroidism, developmental delay, attention-deficit/hyperactivity disorder, depression, and enuresis. She had a gastric tube in place and was receiving hypoallergenic formula despite being significantly overweight. She had a central venous catheter through which she regularly received intravenous immunoglobulin (IVIG). She wore diapers at night and went to school only sporadically. In the past, several of Laura's treatment providers had entertained the idea of MSBP but their concerns were alleviated when she was given the diagnosis of presumed mitochondrial disorder.

June
June was a child we were asked to see when she was 2 months of age. She was hospitalized twice in the first 6 weeks of life for possible sepsis. In the hospital she did not show the signs of dehydration, fever, and listlessness claimed by her mother in frantic telephone calls to her pediatrician in the middle of the night. The third time June's mother took her child to the emergency department the house staff and attending pediatrician decided to admit the child to the hospital again, asking the question, "Is this MSBP?" The *ChildSafe* program was then consulted.

Nancy
Nancy was 10 years old when we first met her. She had a number of medical conditions among which were seizures, obsessive-compulsive disorder, and chronic diarrhea. Because of the diarrhea she had been taking oral antibiotics for more than 2 years. She had a half dozen specialty care providers, several of whom felt her mother exaggerated symptoms to a degree that real medical problems were obscured. She was admitted to HCPHP to "rule out MSBP."

Emilie
Fifteen-year-old Emilie was referred to the HCPHP by DCYF to be evaluated for possible MSBP. Emilie had missed most of the previous year in school and when she did attend she made frequent visits to the nurse's office. Her lack of school attendance led to a truant officer going to her home. The officer got into a verbal and physical altercation with Emilie's mother. The family practice physician who made the initial child abuse allegation to

social services felt that she had been lied to by both Emilie and her mother regarding medical symptoms. The physician asked for an evaluation of possible MSBP.

Pam
This youngster was 10 when we first met her. She was born with a significant cardiac anomaly and had surgery when she was a few months old. Her repair was excellent and she had no restrictions on her activity, but her parents treated her as if she was totally handicapped. They also feared that she had kidney disease, asthma, and psychiatric illness. But what concerned them the most was that she was spoiled. She was referred to us by a psychiatric facility where she was felt to be the victim of MSBP.

Janis
Janis was hospitalized with an infected mastoid and kept getting blood infections. She was 4 years old and was in the hospital for 8 weeks before the hospital staff determined that her mother was putting spit and feces in her intravenous line through which she was getting antibiotics.

Frank
Frank, an 11-year-old boy, was hospitalized repeatedly for severe asthma. The hospitalizations were precipitated by Frank refusing to take his asthma medications. When properly treated his asthma was under stable control. His treatment providers raised the issue of MSBP because of his non-adherence to treatment. As we began working with him we learned that his mother explained his asthma exacerbations by saying she believed he was severely allergic to eggs. She felt he was so allergic to eggs, in fact, that she did not allow anything in the house that might contain egg in any form. Both the mother and Frank were convinced that he would have a severe asthma attack if he touched the shell of an egg. After one of his inpatient admissions, he was referred to HCPHP for ongoing care.

Alice
Alice was an 8-year-old girl referred to HCPHP for treatment of Crohn's disease. She had not been to school for 2 years. For the past several years, Alice had been treated for immune deficiency with IVIG. An anonymous friend of the family had called DCYF saying she was afraid the child was a victim of MSBP.

Scott
Scott was an 11-year-old boy who was an only child living with his mother. She began taking him to his pediatrician and subsequently to specialist physicians for answers to why he had experienced a significant personality change. She described him as having periodic uncharacteristic episodes when he destroyed things in the home, and acted as if he could not hear what she was saying. By doing research on the Internet, his mother decided that his symptoms were consistent with porphyria. When his pediatrician completed a physical examination, did some general screening tests, and declared it unlikely that he had a serious metabolic problem, she ended treatment and asked for a referral to another pediatrician. Another round of tests led to a similar conclusion. She demanded he be admitted to the hospital to rule out serious medical illness. The chief pediatric resident raised the issue of MSBP, and he was transferred to the HCPHP.

Annie
Annie was only a few months old when her mother began bringing her to the emergency department saying she was vomiting and turning blue, precipitating multiple hospitalizations and extensive medical workups, all of which were normal. The baby only seemed to have difficulties when with her mother. Finally, an observer was placed in the hospital room and Annie did fine until one time when the hospital employee was called away for a few minutes. During that time Annie turned blue and the staff became concerned she was being smothered. Social services was called and Annie was taken from her mother's care.

Alex
Alex was referred to us at age 7 with mastoiditis that did not respond to antibiotic treatment. He had been hospitalized several times and received intravenous antibiotics only to have his infection reappear. While in treatment at the HCPHP he developed polymicrobial sepsis and was re-hospitalized.

Dan
Dan was referred to us several different times. In between his times with us he spent more than a year in a psychiatric hospital receiving treatment for uncontrolled psychogenic vomiting. He was 14 at the time of his last

admission to HCPHP. While he was in the psychiatric hospital he was adjudicated in family court to be the victim of MSBP. His mother was determined by the court to be such a noxious influence in his life that she caused him to vomit.

Molly

Molly was a 13-year-old eighth-grade girl whose primary care pediatrician reported suspected abuse to social services because of actions of her mother, saying the mother suffered from MSBP. Molly ate large amounts of food and vomited. She lied to her parents about how much food she ate. She completely denied that she was vomiting despite such evidence as hypokalemia (low blood potassium) and the smell of vomitus left behind in the bathroom. Her mother insisted that the primary care physician do an extensive workup for all possible illnesses that might result in nausea. When told that her daughter suffered from an eating disorder, the mother refused to accept the diagnosis and took her child to a gastrointestinal specialist in another city. That physician came to the same conclusion. Molly continued to deny eating disorder symptoms. Her mother chose to believe her and took her to yet another physician in another city for a third evaluation. She was eventually admitted to the HCPHP.

Brian

Brian was 7 years old when referred for treatment because he refused to eat. He was physically capable of eating but had been fed through a gastric tube since he was 6 months old and had never developed normal eating behaviors. He was taken from the custody of his parents when he was 4 years old and diagnosed with severe failure to thrive. He was the size of a 2-year-old, not talking or walking, and he vomited anything put in his mouth. Family court adjudicated him a victim of MSBP saying his problems resulted from his relationship with his mother.

Terri

Terri suffered from chronic fatigue syndrome. Her fatigue fluctuated and seemed to be most pronounced when she was asked to do something she did not want to do. Her mother had taken her to several experts before she was referred to us. Her primary care physician raised the issue of MSBP.

Richard

Richard was a 15-year-old boy referred for treatment of a debilitating neurologic condition. He and his mother maintained that his legs were paralyzed each morning when he awoke. He could feel sensation in his feet but he could not move his feet or legs. As the morning went on he gradually gained more control of his lower body and by early afternoon he felt completely normal. In fact, by 3 o'clock he was able to participate in his favorite sport, bicycle racing. He was so good at this that he won competitions all over New England. Unfortunately, his recurring early morning paralysis prevented him from attending school. His medical condition went away during the summer months when school was not in session. His mother and father were separated and argued frequently about the severity of Richard's condition, with his mother anxious to find a medical cause. He received numerous neurologic evaluations and diagnostic tests including several spinal taps, electromyelograms, and various imaging studies of his central nervous system. He was referred to the HCPHP by the pediatricians caring for him to "rule out MSBP."

Our Involvement With the Children in the Sample

As stated previously the children were included in the sample if a suspicion of MSBP was raised at the time of their referral. However, as the children came to us from a variety of sources, our involvement varied significantly. Some of the children were seen by the *ChildSafe* program in consultation to an inpatient service in the Children's Hospital, or as a referral from a primary care pediatrician in the community. These children and their parents were interviewed, the medical history was reviewed, and the case was discussed at the weekly child protection team meeting. This whole process might take a few hours to a few days. The medical records of these children might be only a few pages long or, in some cases, voluminous.

In contrast, the children referred for a second opinion by state child protection agencies usually required the review of thousands of pages of medical records. In some cases the child had previously been adjudicated as a victim of MSBP. There was occasionally a question about whether to reintegrate the child into a family previously deemed unsafe. In some of these cases we also interviewed the parents and evaluated the child. In others, we based our consultation solely on medical record review.

The largest group within our sample was children and their families with whom we had an extended treatment relationship that lasted from weeks to months. These children were admitted to the HCPHP, usually for treatment of a specific symptom or constellation of symptoms. The issue of MSBP was, at times, at the forefront of our concern, and at other times, only an ancillary aspect of treatment. Our treatment contract with the family centered on the symptoms, or illness, the child brought with him or her to the program. The treatment objective was to help the child be healthy and to promote a family environment where he or she could remain healthy. Sometimes this involved removing the child from the family. Other times the state child protection agency was not involved.

The children seen primarily by *ChildSafe* were evaluated as possible victims of child abuse. The children seen in the HCPHP were treated as children who had unusual illnesses with psychological factors, who might also be victims of child abuse. As noted earlier, 16 children were evaluated for possible child abuse by *ChildSafe*, and also treated in the HCPHP.

As we reviewed the charts of the medically abused children seen over the past dozen years, one question that we struggled with and determined not to be answerable from our available information was the issue of motivation of the perpetrator. We could not find an objective way to determine the perpetrator's incentive. Certainly, attempting to pass judgment consistently on a person's motivation from old medical records seemed difficult. It is not clear that the task would be easier if it were done in a prospective manner.

There are no psychological tests available to quantify motivation. Some widely used screening tests for personality, such as the Minnesota Multiphasic Personality Inventory employ "lie scales." However, such subscales only indicate inconsistencies in the person's reported answers to questions, not what the respondent specifically is lying about or the reason for the falsehood.

We did not think asking perpetrators to explain their motivation would give us reliable information. While we had long interviews with most of the parents, and in some cases spent weeks and even months in a treatment relationship, not one time did a parent reveal to us that she was harming her child to derive nurturance from the medical care environment. We had many examples of parents who described their behavior as exemplary, maintaining they should be held out as model parents. However, neither the denial of dependency on medical care providers, nor the self-description as a paragon of parenting, gave us sufficient information to clearly ascribe motivation to the parent for her behavior.

Neither did we feel we could rely on the opinions of doctors and nurses who worked with the mothers. Often they had strong views on the matter, but opinions frequently changed and often contradicted one another. One nurse might think one thing motivated the mother while a nurse on the next shift would advance a totally different opinion.

Determining motivation is a difficult task in any circumstance. Jury members asked to assess an alleged perpetrator's motivation might look for clues that imply intent. For example, to tell if a large corporation's chief executive officer (CEO) intended to deceive stockholders when giving optimistic reports about the company's prospects, jurors might look for evidence that the CEO was sending e-mails to colleagues saying what fools the stockholders were to believe him. This kind of evidence was hardly ever available in the medical records we reviewed or in our direct patient care contacts with children and their families. We could tell what was happening medically to the child, whether it was causing harm, and we could make judgments about whether the care was necessary, but we had no litmus test that would allow us to tell what was motivating the behavior of the parent in seeking medical care.

We know that for some of our colleagues who evaluate and write about MSBP the inability to ascribe motivation to the mother will be seen as a major shortfall of this retrospective series. We can only say that after examining all the possibilities there was no objective means of assessing motivation that we could apply in even a small percentage of the cases. We are left with the data we could confirm by direct observation.

There is another area in which this study will disappoint. We did not do formal psychiatric diagnostic interviews of parents or psychological testing on caregivers and, thus, cannot comment on psychiatric illness being present or absent in the potential perpetrators of medical child abuse.

The conclusions presented here are the result of a traditional, retrospective chart review process. We determined which variables we felt were salient and likely to be found in the medical record, constructed a data collection instrument, and reviewed medical records to access the appropriate data. Prior to surveying the records we obtained approval from the hospital human subjects review board to conduct the research. The data were entered into an SPSS database and analyzed using SPSS software.

Do the Children Meet Criteria for MSBP or FDP?

Before giving a detailed description of the children in the sample we wanted to see how they compare using definitions of medical child abuse, MSBP, and factitious disorder by proxy (FDP). In reviewing the case material to determine if the children met criteria for medical child abuse we asked 2 questions: Has the child experienced unnecessary and harmful or potentially harmful medical care at the instigation of a caretaker? Was the harm or potential harm to the child sufficient to warrant consideration for protection?

To answer the first question we looked at the medical care the child received, the supporting evidence that would indicate whether the care was necessary, and whether a caretaker initiated the care. We noted evidence for the caretaker exaggerating existing symptoms, fabricating symptoms, or inducing symptoms in the child. To answer the second question we used a commonsense approach frequently referred to as "what would a reasonable person conclude."

For example, if a mother called her pediatrician frequently with concerns that her child might have an ear infection, and that child received repeated courses of antibiotics prescribed over the phone, we might feel that this represented potentially harmful medical care but that it did not rise to the level that a reasonable person would feel the child needed to be protected from his mother. However, if a child received a yearlong course of intravenous antibiotics to treat undocumented Lyme disease, we would think a reasonable person would say this warrants an investigation for possible child abuse.

Obviously, making the determination that a child is the victim of medical child abuse and that the severity of the abuse might warrant protection of the child involves exercising medical judgment. Remember, however, we were able to make these decisions under optimal conditions. For all of these children we were specifically consulted to evaluate their medical situation. We were given access to all the medical records, permission to interview whomever we deemed appropriate, and in many cases shared weeks and months of an intense treatment relationship. It is hard to imagine being in a better position to make these judgments.

In doing this retrospective case analysis we noticed an interesting phenomenon. The answer to the second question (is the harm to the child sufficient to warrant consideration for protection) was essentially whether the child should be reported to a state agency for evaluation of potential child abuse. In theory all those we judged to have experienced medical child abuse should have been reported. However, we found that cases seen many years ago often went unreported while those seen more recently were much more likely to result in a child protection report. Over time we have lowered our "threshold" for reporting cases to child protective services.

Of the 115 children referred to us for evaluation of MSBP, 87 (75.7%) met the criteria for medical child abuse. Table 1 lists the type of unnecessary medical care received by medically abused children in our series.

How many of these children would meet criteria for MSBP as defined by Rosenberg's original criteria?[2] The first characteristic she lists specifies that the behavior produced by the parent must include fabrication or induction of illness. It does not allow for cases of extreme parental anxiety resulting in unnecessary medical treatment, or illness exaggeration, although in other writings Rosenberg has maintained that extreme illness exaggeration is the equivalent of fabrication.[3] The second necessary feature for MSBP according to Rosenberg is a parent presenting a child repeatedly for medical care. The third characteristic is denial of knowledge by the perpetrator regarding why the child is sick, and the last is evidence that the illness goes away when the child is separated from the perpetrator.

In the 87 children we diagnosed with "medical child abuse," illness was fabricated or induced in 78.2%. So about one-fifth of the "medically abused" children would *not* have met Rosenberg's first criterion. The second feature Rosenberg requires for a diagnosis of MSBP is that the child repeatedly receives medical assessment and care. There are children who go to the doctor frequently and receive multiple medical procedures for perfectly justifiable reasons. She does not specifically require that this medical attention be unnecessary, but we assume this must be what she means. All 87 of our children determined to be victims of medical child abuse received excessive, unnecessary medical care, and so they also would have met Rosenberg's second criterion. The third criterion, "denial of knowledge by the perpetrator as to the etiology of the child's illness," also presents difficulties in interpretation. It goes without saying that none of the parents we dealt with brought their child for treatment and volunteered that the symptoms were not real. No parent admitted that they themselves were the cause of the child's medical condition. From this standpoint literally all of the children in our sample meet this criterion. However, one could also interpret this as the parent giving a false answer when asked, "Do you know how your child got sick?" As this question was seldom asked in this way, we would be hard put to acknowledge parents as denying knowledge of the etiology of the child's illness. We did identify multiple examples of parents giving clearly false information to their treatment providers. As an example, Laura's mother stated that her daughter had experienced fractures on multiple occasions including a broken arm, a fractured spine, and several ankle fractures. The medical records documented that x-rays were taken but no fractures were ever seen. When confronted with this information she responded,

TABLE 1
Types of Unnecessary Medical Care Received by 87 Victims of Medical Child Abuse

Type of Unnecessary Medical Care	No.	%
Unnecessary physician visits and physical assessments	81	93.1
Unnecessary psychological/psychiatric evaluations	33	37.9
Unnecessary medications	74	85.1
Unnecessary noninvasive tests	80	92.0
Unnecessary minimally invasive tests	76	87.4
Unnecessary invasive tests	46	52.9
Unnecessary minor surgery	33	37.9
Unnecessary major surgery	21	24.1

Examples
Noninvasive tests—urinalysis, electrocardiogram
Minimally invasive tests—blood draw, radiograph
Invasive tests—computed tomography scan, fluoroscopy, endoscopy, spinal tap, bone marrow aspiration
Minor surgery—skin biopsy, removal of skin lesion, insertion of indwelling line
Major surgery—orthopedic procedure, neurosurgical procedure, intraabdominal or intrathoracic procedure

"The doctor put her in a cast every time so I thought it must be broken." In fact, casts were applied for each injury despite there being no documented fracture because of the mother's description of the extent of the child's pain. The plastic support provided for the possible spine injury was worn 1 day before it was discarded. Because this information is repeated numerous times in the medical record and gave the impression that Laura had weak bones when this was clearly not the case, we rated this as providing false information. We are not sure if this would meet the denial of knowledge criterion for Rosenberg. For the sake of this discussion we assume all the parents meet the third criterion.

Finally, regarding the fourth criterion, there were therapeutic separations from the parent in 31 (35.6%) of the 87 medically abused children. The children separated therapeutically all had improvement in their medical conditions and therefore would meet this factor. For the 56 children who did not experience therapeutic separations, we cannot confirm that they would have had improvement in symptoms.

If we assume that a diagnosis of MSBP requires all 4 of the sentinel criteria, we conclude that only 29 (33.3%) of our medically abused children actually meet all 4 of the conditions Rosenberg sets out to make the diagnosis.

We have also tried to analyze information using Rosenberg's criteria to see if they distinguish between those cases we feel meet criteria for medical child abuse and those that did not rise to that threshold. See Table 2. It is clear that the 4 criteria do not do a good job of separating the medically abused children from the non–medically abused children. While many medically abused children do not fulfill all 4 criteria, none of the non–medically abused children do so, although about half of the non-abused children would be positive for 2 criteria. Overall, of the children we found to be abused medically, only one-third meet all 4 criteria. Compared to our criteria for defining medical child abuse, the Rosenberg criteria were quite specific for making the diagnosis, but not very sensitive.

The picture is even less clear when trying to use criteria for FDP from the *Diagnostic and Statistical Manual of Mental Disorders, Fourth Edition*.[4] The first feature of FDP correlates strongly with the first feature of MSBP and includes finding examples of fabrication and induction of illness but not illness exaggeration. Hence, the number of children we documented having fabrication and induction (78.2% of the medically abused children) would

TABLE 2
Rosenberg's Criteria Compared to the Diagnosis of "Medical Child Abuse"

Rosenberg Criteria	Medically Abused Children	Children NOT Medically Abused
Fabrication or induction of illness	78.2%	0
Repeatedly presenting for medical care	100%	46.4%
Parent denies knowledge of why child is sick	100%	60.7%
Child improves when separated from parent	35.6%	0
Meets all 4 criteria	33.3%	0

meet the first criterion for FDP. The second and most significant feature for FDP involves determining that, "The motivation for the perpetrator's behavior is to assume the sick role by proxy." This we were not able to determine so none of our 115 children would meet formal criteria for FDP. In addition, the last criterion for FDP involves identifying another mental disorder in the perpetrator that would better account for the behavior. As we did not do structured psychiatric interviews on perpetrators, we cannot speak to this feature.

Evidence for a Spectrum of Presentations in Our Sample

We structured the inclusion criteria in hopes of having a broad range of cases available for study. The first evidence for this is that 28 children (24.3%) did not meet the threshold for inclusion in the group of children subjected to medical child abuse. Comparing the children in the 2 groups, those who were confirmed to have been medically abused with those who were not (Table 3), we see some significant similarities and differences. Children in both groups had similar frequencies of problems in infancy that might predispose them to be considered vulnerable children. The 2 groups had mothers employed in the medical profession in similar proportions. There was no significant difference between the 2 groups regarding the frequency of non-adherence to treatment. However, there was significant difference in frequency of illness exaggeration, illness fabrication, and illness induction. None of the children in the non-medical child abuse group had a parent who fabricated symptoms or test results or induced illness.

The children referred to us for suspected MSBP who we did *not* find to be victims of medical child abuse included many with significant illnesses. Almost half of the children in this cohort (12/28) had physicians who were seriously concerned about non-adherence to treatment and medical neglect. The doctors making the referral with a question of MSBP were frustrated that appropriate treatment recommendations were not being followed. School personnel were involved in referring 8 children with questions about MSBP because the children were not attending school and using illness as an excuse. Four non-medically abused children had physicians who complained that parents were persistently asking for unnecessary medical treatment. These children did not meet our criteria because their physicians actively refused to provide unnecessary medical care. As a result the children were not subjected to medical child abuse. Finally, the fathers of 2 children whose parents were involved in painful custody disputes made charges of MSBP against their ex-spouses. Neither of these cases met our criteria for medical child abuse.

In all of the non-medically abused children we could see no evidence a child received unnecessary and harmful or potentially harmful medical care. Some of them, however, were clearly the victims of medical neglect and were not receiving needed medical care due to actions by their caretakers.

Focusing more specifically on the children who *did* meet criteria for medical child abuse, we found that the cases were on a spectrum of severity of the caretakers' abusive behavior, from mild to severe. Table 3 lists the frequency of the parent behaviors documented in the record. The most common behavior of the parents leading to unnecessary medical care in the medically abused children was the exaggeration of existing symptoms. Less frequently we saw evidence for fabrication of symptoms of diseases that were not actually present, and least frequent was the actual induction of symptoms by a caretaker, where a person purposefully made the child ill.

Table 4 lists the types of unnecessary medical care received by the 115 children in our sample, comparing the medically abused children to those who were *not* medically abused. The most common form of abusive behavior was subjecting children to unnecessary medical examinations. The more intrusive and more dangerous the medical treatments/diagnostic procedures, the less frequently they occurred. The non-medically abused children received significantly less unnecessary care than the medically abused children.

TABLE 3
Comparison of Children Found to Be Victims of Medical Child Abuse to Those Who Were Not[a]

Criterion	Medically Abused Children (No. [%]) (N = 87)	Children NOT Medically Abused (No. [%]) (N = 28)	P Value
History of "vulnerable child" as an infant	31 (35.6)	5 (17.9)	NS
Male gender	38 (43.7)	10 (35.7)	NS
Minority[b]	13 (14.9)	2 (7.1)	NS
Suspected perpetrator in health care profession	16 (18.4)	5 (17.9)	NS
Caretaker was severely non-adherent to the child's prescribed medical care	42 (48.3)	12 (42.9)	NS
Caretaker exaggerated child's symptoms	78 (89.7)	17 (60.7)	0.001
Caretaker fabricated child's illness[b]	64 (73.6)	0 (0.0)	0.000
Caretaker fabricated child's test results[b]	7 (8.0)	0 (0.0)	NS
Caretaker induced illness in the child[b]	23 (26.4)	0 (0.0)	0.001

Abbreviation: NS, not significant ($P>0.05$).
[a] All children were referred as suspected victims of Munchausen syndrome by proxy. All P values were calculated with Pearson's chi-square test unless otherwise noted.
[b] Fisher's exact test.

We were able to document a total of 37 children who received surgery they did not need (4 received major surgery, 16 received minor surgery, and 17 received both major and minor surgeries). The most common unnecessary surgery was the placement of gastric tubes (10) in the face of no or minimal evidence of growth failure. Four children received Nissan fundoplication surgery with minimal documented signs and symptoms of gastroesophageal reflux disease. Three children received unnecessary colostomies or cecostomies, and 2 toddlers had sinus antrum procedures for nonexistent recurrent

TABLE 4
Types of Unnecessary Medical Care Given to Medically Abused and Non-Medically Abused Children[a]

Criterion	Medically Abused Children (No. [%]) (N = 87)	Children NOT Medically Abused (No. [%]) (N = 28)	P value
Unnecessary medical visits and examinations[b]	81 (93.1)	5 (17.9)	0.000
Unnecessary psychiatric/psychological evaluations and/or treatment	33 (37.9)	2 (7.1%)	0.002
Unnecessary medications[b]	74 (85.1)	10 (35.7)	0.000
Unnecessary noninvasive tests	80 (92.0)	4 (14.3)	0.000
Unnecessary minimally invasive tests	76 (87.4)	4 (14.3)	0.000
Unnecessary invasive tests	46 (52.9)	0	0.000
Unnecessary minor surgery	33 (37.9)	0	0.000
Unnecessary major surgery	21 (24.1)	0	0.002

[a] All P values were calculated using Fisher's exact test unless otherwise noted.
[b] Pearson's chi-square test.
Examples
Noninvasive tests—urinalysis, electrocardiogram
Minimally invasive tests—blood draw, radiograph
Invasive tests—computed tomography scan, fluoroscopy, endoscopy, spinal tap, bone marrow aspiration
Minor surgery—skin biopsy, removal of skin lesion, insertion of indwelling line
Major surgery—orthopedic procedure, neurosurgical procedure, intraabdominal or intrathoracic procedure

sinus infections. There were 3 children in our sample who had central venous access catheters placed in their chests to receive IVIG with no documented laboratory evidence of immunodeficiency. One child received IVIG for 6 years despite 3 different negative evaluations.

Illness Presentations in the Medical Child Abuse Group

While many authors[5] have documented that almost any illness in a child can be part of a medical child abuse case, it is useful to keep in mind that certain illnesses occur more frequently in medically abused children and can increase the index of suspicion. We categorized by organ system illnesses treated in the children who met criteria for abuse. We then looked at the illnesses to see if there was evidence indicating a need for treatment. We rated each illness presentation as having enough medical evidence to confirm the need for treatment, having evidence that partially confirmed the need for treatment, and having no evidence that the illness required treatment. Figure 1 presents this information in graphic form.

We hypothesized that we would see illnesses more frequently in medically abused children when the diagnosis depended on parent report. The most common body systems where illnesses were *not* supported by any medical data were gastrointestinal diseases, neurologic disorders, respiratory diseases, infectious diseases, and allergies. A high number of children also had psychiatric diseases, but more of those conditions were actually "real" diagnoses, supported by objective data. This may be because 60% of the children in our series were treated in the HCPHP. All children who enter the program have both medical and psychological problems.

There were 18 of the medically abused children (18/87, 21%) who received medical treatment but for whom *no* illnesses were confirmed. An additional 5 children had no verifiable physical illness but did have symptoms consistent with psychological illness. If we add these 5 children to the others, we see that 26% of our medical child abuse sample received treatment for medical illnesses when there was absolutely no confirmatory evidence that they were ill in any way. The other side of this coin is equally important. Seventy-four percent of the medically abused children had actual illness but also received harmful medical care that was not required. These children who had documented illness received excessive medical care that was *not* appropriate given the objective data about the children's illnesses.

Interestingly, when we went back and looked at the children who did not meet criteria for medical child abuse, only 1 of the 28 children had no confirmatory signs or symptoms of a physical illness. That child did have a confirmed psychiatric illness. Children who did not meet criteria for medical child abuse were demonstrably *more* ill than children in the medical child abuse group.

FIGURE 1
Systems Involved in Cases of Medical Child Abuse

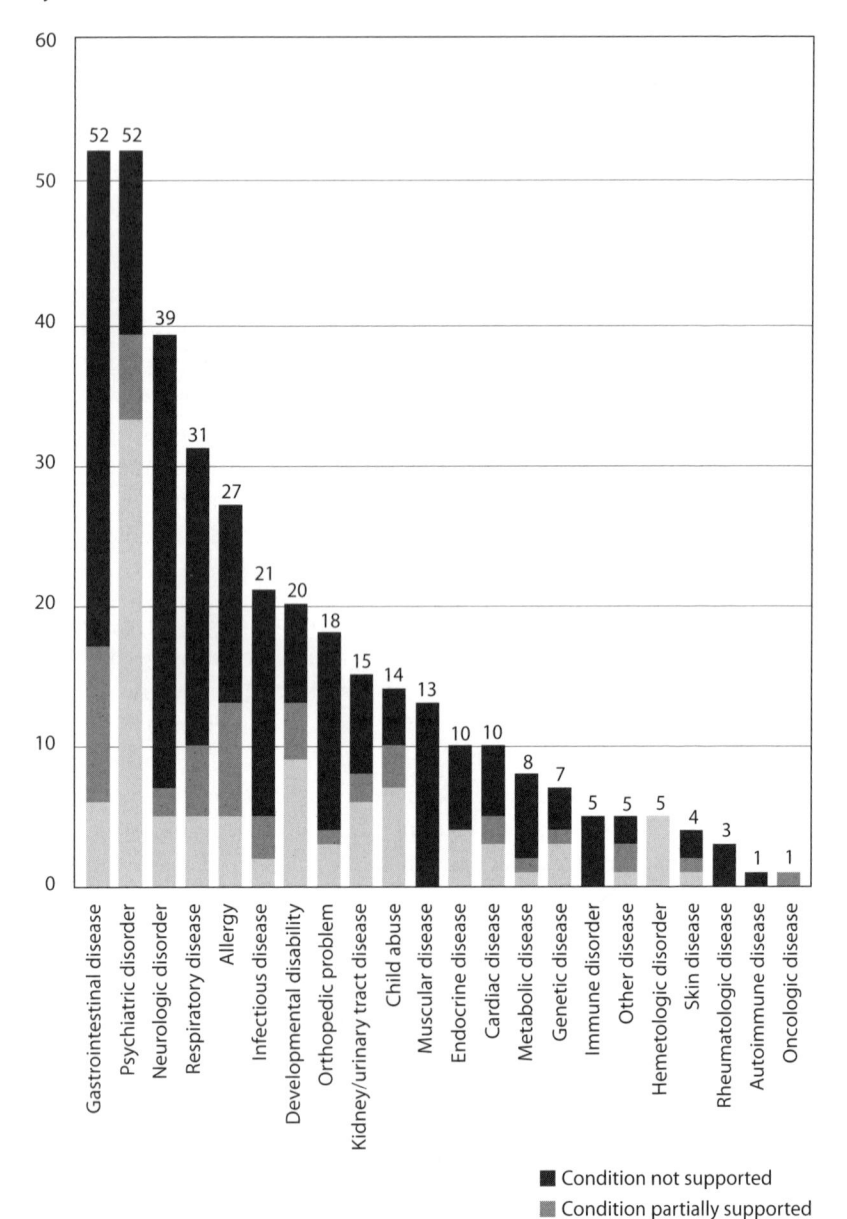

System	Total
Gastrointestinal disease	52
Psychiatric disorder	52
Neurologic disorder	39
Respiratory disease	31
Allergy	27
Infectious disease	21
Developmental disability	20
Orthopedic problem	18
Kidney/urinary tract disease	15
Child abuse	14
Muscular disease	13
Endocrine disease	10
Cardiac disease	10
Metabolic disease	8
Genetic disease	7
Immune disorder	5
Other disease	5
Hemetologic disorder	5
Skin disease	4
Rheumatologic disease	3
Autoimmune disease	1
Oncologic disease	1

■ Condition not supported
■ Condition partially supported
□ Condition supported

Treatments Experienced by Children Judged to Have Experienced Medical Child Abuse

For most of the children in the medical child abuse group seen in the HCPHP, treatment was similar to that received by other, non-medically abused children who are routinely treated in the program. They received appropriate medical care that was reevaluated daily; individual, group, and family psychotherapy; and exposure to a number of other families who were struggling with complex medical issues and trying to make healthy choices.

Table 5 lists the types of interventions that medically abused children received. In some cases, even when medical child abuse was clearly established, and particularly in the early years of the study, no mention of child abuse was made to the family. As previously stated this has happened much less frequently in the last few years. There were 2 main reasons why some of the confirmed cases were not referred to child protective services. In some cases, the family responded to treatment, and excessive medical care was stopped with treatment in the HCPHP. Another reason was that the primary physician caring for the child disagreed with the diagnosis of medical child abuse and insisted the child was getting appropriate medical care, even in the face of obvious evidence to the contrary.

One question that intrigued us was the difference between the children we actually saw at the children's hospital (at either *ChildSafe* or HCPHP) and the cases that were referred for second opinions from other states. The second opinion cases were, on the whole, much more dramatic and severe than the cases we diagnosed and treated clinically. Table 6 points out some of these differences.

Obviously, the second opinion cases congregate on the more severe end of the spectrum. Were we to exclude them from the sample there would only be one child removed permanently from the parent's home, no criminal prosecutions, and no deaths. Someone writing about MSBP having available only a sample of second opinion cases would have a very different perspective on the seriousness of the condition than we have seen in our clinical experience. From that perspective one could understand making statements advocating for every child diagnosed with MSBP to be removed from the home, and prohibiting any visitation from the perpetrating parent.

TABLE 5
Interventions in Cases of Medical Child Abuse

	Number (%)
Children staffed at a multidisciplinary team meeting	40 (46.5)
Children reported to child protective services	36 (41.4)
Cases where children or parent was removed from home[a]	29 (34.1)
Cases where parental rights were terminated for the perpetrator	5 (5.7)
Cases where the patient died	2 (2.3)
Cases where perpetrator was convicted of a crime	1 (0.9)
Cases where perpetrator was incarcerated	1 (0.9)

[a] Child and parents were separated in 29 of 85 cases where the child survived the abuse.

In contrast, our patient sample allowed us to be much more flexible in our treatment efforts. In many cases we worked with the family to help them establish an appropriate level of concern given the severity (or absence) of illness. In later chapters in this book we go into considerable detail about the treatment process.

A total of 29 of the 85 surviving medically abused children were removed therapeutically from their home environment by social service agencies. Of those almost all returned home. The most common placement option was with a parent either divorced or separated from the perpetrator. Criminal action was taken against only one parent (one of the second opinion cases). This was a mother with a history of 2 previous children dying in suspicious circumstances who was discovered by a hospital nurse placing a plastic bag over her toddler's head, attempting to suffocate him. Retrospectively, it was determined that her 2 previous children died due to illness induction. The perpetrator was tried and convicted only for the third incident. Hence, although 2 children died, in only one case was the perpetrator tried and convicted.

Conclusion

We come away from this survey of 12 years' experience seeing children suspected of MSBP with some general thoughts. First of all we feel confident

TABLE 6
Characteristics of Second Opinion Cases From Social Services Agencies Compared to Children Evaluated and Treated at HCH[a]

Characteristic	HCH Cases	Second Opinion Cases	P Value
Number of cases of MCA confirmed out of all cases evaluated	71/97 (73.2%)	16/18 (88.9%)	NS
Number of MCA cases where patient died	0/71 (0.0%)	2/16 (12.5%)	0.046
Number of survivors of MCA referred to child protective services[b]	25/71 (35.2%)	14/14 (100%)	0.021
Number of medically abused children removed from the perpetrators' care[b]	19/71 (26.8%)	10/14 (71.4%)	0.004
Number of criminal prosecutions	0/71 (0.0%)	1/16 (5.6%)	NS
Medically abused child permanently removed from parent's care[b]	1/71 (1.4%)	4/14 (28.6%)	0.005

Abbreviations: HCH, Hasbro Children's Hospital; MCA, medical child abuse; NS, not significant ($P>0.05$).
[a] By Fisher's exact test.
[b] Two of the 16 MCA cases in the "second opinion" group died before the diagnosis of medical child abuse was made.

that by carefully reviewing the medical care received by children, we can distinguish which children have been subjected to medical child abuse and which have not. This ability to distinguish abused from non-abused children is fundamental. In our next chapter we focus specifically on how to identify children who may have been medically abused, the first step in the child protection process.

We were able to confirm that having a suspicion that a child might be harmed in the medical environment does not necessarily mean that harm has actually taken place. Asking the question does not make it true. This is an important point because we advocate maintaining a healthy suspicion that abuse might be taking place as part of the practice of quality medicine. As a result of this healthy suspicion we were able to discriminate between children who had been medically abused and others experiencing serious medical neglect and to get help for both.

When we did make the determination of medical child abuse, we saw evidence for a spectrum of presentations ranging from mild to severe. We were able to show that mild presentations may not require protection and may respond to customary medical interventions. The diagnosis of medical child abuse does not necessarily require a child to be removed from his or her parent's home. A child might be subjected to medical examinations too frequently, might receive too many diagnostic tests, and because of this meet criteria for medical child abuse. It would be appropriate to report this child to social services just as one would report a child who presents in the office with a slap mark across the face. However, in neither example would one expect the child to be immediately removed from home.

We also saw extremely serious and life-threatening situations where immediate intervention by child protection services was essential to save the child's life.

As mentioned previously we were curious to see that our ability to decide when a child needs protection has been improving. We have felt much more comfortable in recent years in invoking child protective services, and more successful when we do make the call in receiving the kind of help that keeps a child safe from future harm.

References

1. Eminson M, Jureidini J. Concerns about research and prevention strategies in Munchausen syndrome by proxy (MSBP) abuse. *Child Abuse Negl.* 2003;27(4):413-420
2. Rosenberg DA. Web of deceit: a literature review of Munchausen syndrome by proxy. *Child Abuse Negl.* 1987;11(4):547-563
3. Rosenberg DA. From lying to homicide: the spectrum of Munchausen syndrome by proxy. In: Levin AV, Sheridan MS, eds. *Munchausen Syndrome by Proxy: Issues in Diagnosis and Treatment.* New York, NY: Lexington Books; 1995:13-37
4. American Psychiatric Association. *Diagnostic and Statistical Manual of Mental Disorders, Fourth Edition.* Washington, DC: American Psychiatric Association; 1994
5. Rosenberg DA. Munchausen syndrome by proxy. In: Reece RM, Ludwig S, eds. *Child Abuse: Medical Diagnosis and Management.* 2nd ed. Philadelphia, PA: Lippincott Williams and Wilkins; 2001:363-383

Chapter 8

Introduction to Treatment

When it was proved, or extremely probable, that the epilepsy was false, it was usual for the child to be protected in the same ways as for other forms of child abuse: the social services department was notified, a case conference convened, and very often a court order imposed for the safety of the child. —Meadow, 1984[1]

In the first chapter we commented that some experts have written that treatment of Munchausen syndrome by proxy (MSBP) is extremely difficult or impossible, while others say that treatment can be quite successful. Two early papers epitomize the contrasting positions. Waller[2] wrote "Obstacles to the Treatment of Munchausen by Proxy Syndrome," a pessimistic view of treatability. Two years later, Nicol and Eccles[3] contributed "Psychotherapy for Munchausen Syndrome by Proxy" expressing the opposite view.

Waller began his paper with a case report of a 2-year-old boy whose mother added her own blood to his urine. The boy had been hospitalized several times with various symptoms, none of which was explained by thorough medical evaluations. During the hospitalization when the mother's behavior was uncovered, he was said to be suffering from easy bruising, coughing up blood, hematuria, and bloody stools. The hematologist who evaluated the child for a possible bleeding disorder noted that none of his symptoms seemed to occur out of the presence of his mother, and suggested that the blood found in the child's urine might come from her. This was established quickly through blood typing.

The mother was confronted with this information. She agreed to a follow-up appointment but did not appear for the meeting because she was in another hospital being evaluated for severe abdominal pain. Despite having a normal white blood cell count and no elevated temperature, presumably on the basis of her self-reported pain, she received an appendectomy. The appendix was normal. While recovering from her surgery, she hired an attorney who arranged with the court to have her child put in the custody of his grandmother and, in addition, to send the mother for psychotherapy. However, the agreement negotiated by her attorney also prohibited the mother's therapist from participating in any discussions about the welfare of the child, as this would be a violation of confidentiality.

Once the child was removed from his mother's care it was assumed that everything would go smoothly. Instead, the mother began explaining to people why the blood in the child's urine was discovered to be identical with her blood by telling a lie, namely that her child had received a blood transfusion from her. Child welfare personnel caring for the child initiated a new evaluation to find out "what was really wrong with the child medically." Instead of there being a legal settlement that protected the child, he was exposed to a new round of unnecessary medical evaluation and treatment.

This paper was written in 1983 just as the field was beginning to shift from considering these cases "uncommon manifestations of child abuse" to MSBP. The author argued that MSBP shared many similarities with non-accidental poisoning. He accumulated examples from the literature where parents both fabricated and induced illness in their child. He wrote that a parent fabricating an illness could easily progress to doing direct physical harm. Because of this, "A primary goal of legal intervention must be to ensure that the child's health status is monitored, and that any subsequent medical treatment is appropriate." He maintained that the management of MSBP should include the involvement of the physicians who diagnosed the condition. He stated that the consulting psychiatrist should develop and keep an alliance with all of the professionals influencing the child's environment. In conclusion he said that we needed to provide for the long-term safety of the child by periodic involvement by social services or other responsible parties.

Waller also noted that getting the cooperation of the legal system and other medical professionals offered some of the biggest obstacles to protecting the child. As an example he made reference to another case in which the perpetrator was able to bring forward 5 medical doctors who would testify on her behalf. His comments are generally considered to be evidence of the difficulty in providing effective treatment and are an example of the frustration of professionals who try to intervene.

Many of the concerns he raised are repeated in other articles regarding management of MSBP. For example, McGuire and Feldman,[4] who focused primarily on the potentially dismal long-term psychological outcome of children abused in this particular way, cited Waller while saying, "...both parents' level of denial and their psychiatric diagnoses often mitigate against successful psychotherapy." They went on to say that in the cases they had seen, "...treatment had been attempted for significant periods of time and appeared to have had little effect on either the behavior of the mother or on the development of insight into her condition. We have yet to see a case, and know of only one in the medical literature, in which treatment of the mother was successful."

The one case in the medical literature to which they referred was reported by Nicol and Eccles.[13] They, too, began their discussion with a case study. The child spent almost half the first year of life in the hospital being treated for a variety of medical symptoms including apathy, dehydration, diarrhea, vomiting, peripheral edema, and unexplained nocturnal hypothermia. It was only after 12 admissions, despite continuing suspicions, that her physician was able to confirm the mother was adding salt to the child's diet. Both mother and father were confronted with the information regarding the cause of the child's illness. After the confrontation, but before the determination the child would be removed from the family, a child psychiatrist interviewed the mother and listened to her deny any involvement. In her own defense she continued to hold tightly to descriptions of illnesses with which the child had been diagnosed previously. Once it became clear the child would be placed in foster care, the mother confessed to poisoning her with salt. Out of the mother's presence the child quickly regained health, gained weight, and made significant advances in motor development.

Subsequent to the mother acknowledging responsibility for her actions the authorities agreed to have the child remain in her custody with close supervision. The mother agreed to get psychotherapy as a condition to keeping her child at home. One therapist met with her weekly for 6 months and then "fortnightly" for an additional 6 months. He began with supportive treatment but quickly moved to insight-oriented psychotherapy. He described in some detail the patient's struggle with the knowledge of the harm she had done to her child and the possible consequences. She explored with her therapist the organization of her family of origin in which everyone had been victimized by her father's bullying. An escape from the corrosive atmosphere in the home was provided by a withdrawal "into anxiety and overconcern with health." The perpetrator, as a young child, made frequent visits to the doctor with her mother. She discussed the comfort she felt as an adult seeking care for her own child, at being in a medical environment, and also her pleasure in fooling the medical professionals she worked with and admired so much.

Nichol and Eccles noted that an inherent difficulty in treating a condition that includes significant deception is the need to find collateral evidence for everything the patient offers. To this end they attempted to confirm that their treatment was successful by looking at observable changes in the family, the health-seeking behavior of the mother, and in her functioning in other aspects of her life. They concluded that they saw objective evidence of significant change in the mother and her family. They offered that, for most treatment of child abuse, stopping the abusive behavior and providing general support is indicated, and may be all that is possible. "Individual interpretive psychotherapy may have a place in this minority of cases, and where the patient is reasonably well motivated in trying to confront his or her difficulties, is of average intelligence, and not beset with family and social problems." They stated that their observations applied, in addition to MSBP, also to sexual, emotional, and even physical abuse.

The cases offered by these 2 papers are quite similar. They were written in an environment where professionals were just coming to understand this type of child abuse. The treatment conceptualized by the authors shares many common features. One case had an unfortunate outcome while the other was successful. Based on these 2 early experiences should we conclude that treatment is relatively straightforward or nearly impossible?

Themes introduced by these 2 papers include:

1. The importance of physicians maintaining an index of suspicion of possible abuse.
2. The necessity to search objectively for evidence to confirm signs and symptoms reported by parents.
3. When parents are informed that deception has been discovered, it is reasonable to expect they will deny involvement as long as possible.

4. Past behavior predicts future behavior. One can expect that a parent who has been abusive in the past will continue to be abusive until stopped.

5. The primary goal of treatment is maintaining safety for the child.

6. For the child to be safe it is important to have open communication between all adults, including caretakers and treatment providers, affecting the child's environment.

7. Conversely, if the various caretakers and professionals do not communicate effectively with one another it is quite likely that abuse will reoccur and the child will suffer.

8. Uninformed doctors and legal professionals can undo attempts to protect children.

9. Treatment of a psychiatric illness in an abusive parent is a related but separate matter from the management of the abuse of the child.

10. Children removed from abusive situations can recover significantly.

11. When an abusive parent refuses to take responsibility for her actions, and the child remains in her custody, it is reasonable to expect the child will be abused again.

12. For psychotherapy of an abusive parent to be successful that person must acknowledge some responsibility for her actions and enter into a genuine treatment relationship.

13. When the child's safety can be guaranteed in no other way, it is necessary to remove the child from an abusive family.

These 2 papers written 25 years ago include most of the ideas important in the treatment of medical child abuse. Ironically, one is cited as proof that MSBP is untreatable and the other offers evidence for successful treatment. Yet the authors did not contradict one another. They both approached their task as describing treatment for child abuse, and both offered cogent descriptions of the difficulties facing the treatment team. They both maintained that providing for the child's safety was the first priority. They both addressed the importance of establishing a workable treatment alliance with the people taking care of the child. They both discussed the difficulty dealing with ancillary medical (and legal) personnel. And they both discussed the need of the perpetrator to accept responsibility for her actions before treatment can proceed successfully.

Reading these 2 papers today it seems apparent that the confusion comes from not specifying what it is we mean by "treatment." If the reader means individual psychotherapy of an individual who has caused harm to her child and is refusing to acknowledge any responsibility, then treatment will be difficult. If, by treatment, we mean discovering if and how a child is being harmed, stopping it, and preventing it from occurring in the future, then treatment is not only possible but necessary.

Once again, we are reiterating concepts put forth by our colleagues many years ago. For example, Donald and Jureidini[5] wrote, "We know of no empirical evidence that indicates that the application of standard child abuse management principles hamper's the management of Munchausen syndrome by proxy." And Meadow[6] commented referring to perpetrators of MSBP, "I don't think the principles are a lot different from other forms of child abuse. If a person can recognize what they're doing and have some insight into it, I believe they can be helped."

We propose that treatment of medical child abuse follows the general concepts involved in treatment of all child abuse. The first step is to recognize that it is occurring. The second step involves stopping the abuse. Next we must provide for the ongoing safety for the child. Following this, we want to treat the damage, both physical and psychological, caused by the abuse. Finally, we want to accomplish these goals while helping the child's family maintain its integrity as much as possible. This last goal, preserving the family, involves helping the perpetrator deal with the results of her actions, and the reasons she came to harm her child. To do this it is often important, but not always necessary, to ascertain the motivation of the caretaker for exposing her child to harm.

There is one difference between treatment of medical child abuse and that of other forms of child maltreatment. Before treatment can begin, those responsible for treatment (ie, the medical community) must recognize that the largely unspoken medical treatment contract is not working. The agreement the doctor has with the family is not functioning in the interest of the child and must be re-examined. For treatment to proceed there must be a renegotiation of the primary contract.

Chapter 8
Introduction to Treatment

In responding to all forms of child maltreatment a necessary step includes calling a halt to the abuse. There is a time when the community says, "This is not right. This needs to stop." But the behavior that is halted, the sexual abuse, emotional torment, or neglect, is embedded in the life of the family taking care of the child. Those who act to protect the children step in from the outside. The protectors have no prior involvement in the abuse itself. With medical child abuse the maltreatment is a direct result of medical treatment being applied by doctors and nurses, albeit under false pretenses. The abuse occurs when the medical contract is broken. The physician cannot carry out the medical contract alone. It is the caretaker's responsibility to help the physician make sure that this oath is honored.

Apart from the special role of medical child abuse occurring in a medical setting, the treatment paradigm applies equally to all types of child abuse and neglect. Sexual abuse provides a comparable example. The first and sometimes most difficult task is recognizing that it is occurring. Some children are abused sexually in their families for as long as 10 years before the abuse is discovered or the child discloses what he or she has been experiencing. Treatment cannot begin until after the disclosure. The first action taken in the treatment process is to stop the abuse. To do this perpetrators are required to have no contact with the child, to leave the home or, if necessary, to be incarcerated. It is not enough to stop the abuse for 1 week or 1 month. Controls must be in place to prevent indefinitely the child from being exposed to further sexual abuse. In the case of intrafamilial abuse, it is important to evaluate whether the non-offending spouse supports protection of the child or sides with the perpetrator against the child. The child disclosing sexual abuse is not always believed or supported by family members. The professionals involved in the treatment process need to assess if the child can be maintained safely in the family of origin even if the perpetrator has been extruded.

As soon as the safety of the child can be ensured therapy can begin to assess and treat the physical and psychological consequences of the abuse. These consequences can be mild or devastating. Treatment is tailored to the needs of the individual child.

And finally, once abuse has been identified and stopped, and controls are in place to prevent it from reoccurring and remediation efforts have begun, then the role of the perpetrator in the child's life can be evaluated. If the perpetrator can admit responsibility for his actions, and seek treatment, perhaps eventually he can be reintegrated into the family. On the other hand, he may deny responsibility, refuse treatment, and effectively exclude himself from the child's life. Successful treatment is defined by the success of each step in the treatment sequence. Identifying the abuse and stopping it constitutes success. Accomplishing this and maintaining the integrity of the core family unit (absent the perpetrator) is further grounds for declaring victory. And if the perpetrator can be rehabilitated and reintegrated successfully into the family without sacrificing the safety of the child or the siblings, all the better.

As those of us who have spent time evaluating and treating child sexual abuse will attest, treatment can be difficult, often frustrating, but can also be extremely rewarding. Treatment of medical child abuse is no different. Fortunately, a child protection system exists in this country that has been working for more than 30 years to evaluate and treat child sexual and physical abuse. The specific issues in medical child abuse are different but the treatment strategies are very similar. We can take advantage of the child protection apparatus available in most communities simply by defining medical child abuse clearly as abuse.

Each of the next few chapters will focus on a specific element of the treatment process. For example, the next chapter will deal with identifying medical child abuse. We will look at the task confronting the primary care physician who suspects medical child abuse in the outpatient setting. Then we will look at identifying medical child abuse from the viewpoint of the specialist in the hospital setting. And finally we will outline the role of a child abuse expert asked to evaluate suspected medical child abuse.

While the MSBP literature contains relatively little specific information regarding treatment, it is clear that many of our colleagues over the years have come to a conclusion similar to what we present here.[7-19] In general, recommendations for treatment specify putting the welfare of the child first, taking action to make sure the abuse stops and is not begun again, and dealing with the perpetrator. In addition, almost everyone who writes about treatment identifies the need to have a multidisciplinary team to support the treatment effort. Most professionals working in the area of child abuse concur that attempting to identify and treat child abuse as a sole practitioner is extremely difficult if not impossible. Child abuse is a multifaceted problem and requires a multifaceted solution. As with other forms of child abuse treatment, intervening in medical child abuse should only be attempted with the help of a team of professionals working together for the benefit of the child and the child's family.

References

1. Meadow R. Fictitious epilepsy. *Lancet.* 1984;2:25–28
2. Waller DA. Obstacles to the treatment of Munchausen by proxy syndrome. *J Am Acad Child Psychiatry.* 1983;22(1):80-85
3. Nicol AR, Eccles M. Psychotherapy for Munchausen syndrome by proxy. *Arch Dis Child.* 1985;60(4):344-348
4. McGuire TL, Feldman KW. Psychologic morbidity of children subjected to Munchausen syndrome by proxy. *Pediatrics.* 1989;83(2):289-292
5. Donald T, Jureidini J. Munchausen syndrome by proxy. Child abuse in the medical system. *Arch Pediatr Adolesc Med.* 1996;150(7):753-758
6. Meadow SR. Munchausen syndrome by proxy. *Med Leg J.* 1995;63(Pt 3):89-104
7. Lansky LL. An unusual case of childhood chloral hydrate poisoning. *Am J Dis Child.* 1974;127(2):275-276
8. Meadow R. Munchausen syndrome by proxy and pseudo-epilepsy. *Arch Dis Child.* 1982;57(10):811-812
9. Meadow R. Munchausen syndrome by proxy. *Arch Dis Child.* 1982;57(2):92-98
10. Black D. The extended Munchausen syndrome: a family case. *Br J Psychiatry.* 1981;138:466-469
11. Meadow R. Management of Munchausen syndrome by proxy. *Arch Dis Child.* 1985;60(4):385-393
12. Masterson J, Dunworth R, Williams N. Extreme illness exaggeration in pediatric patients: a variant of Munchausen's by proxy? *Am J Orthopsychiatry.* 1988;58(2):188-195
13. Masterson J, Wilson J. Factitious illness in children: the social worker's role in identification and management. *Soc Work Health Care.* 1987;12(4):21-30
14. Senner A, Ott MJ. Munchausen syndrome by proxy. *Issues Compr Pediatr Nurs.* 1989;12(5):345-357
15. Kravitz RM, Wilmott RW. Munchausen syndrome by proxy presenting as factitious apnea. *Clin Pediatr (Phila).* 1990;29(10):587-592
16. Leonard KF, Farrell PA. Munchausen's syndrome by proxy. A little-known type of abuse. *Postgrad Med.* 1992;91(5):197-204
17. Fisher GC. Etiological speculations. In: Levin AV, Sheridan MS, eds. *Munchausen Syndrome by Proxy: Issues in Diagnosis and Treatment.* New York, NY: Lexington Books; 1995:39-57

18. Eminson DM, Postlethwaite RJ. Factitious illness: recognition and management. *Arch Dis Child.* 1992;67(12):1510-1516
19. Bools C. *Fabricated or Induced Illness in a Child by a Carer: A Reader.* Oxford, UK: Radcliffe Publishing; 2007

Chapter 9
Identifying Medical Child Abuse

Training in pediatrics and child health does not encourage us to doubt the veracity of parents' histories. Clinical practice is based on an assumption of truthfulness and a shared interest in the welfare of the child. We also naturally enjoy the admiration and approval of our patients and are reluctant to offend them. We may therefore be poorly prepared to deal with those motivated to deceive in this way. —Morley, 1995[1]

Introduction

Before we can undertake the central task of reconstituting the medical contract with the patient and his or her family, we need to identify that the contract has been broken. We need to establish that the child is being maltreated in the medical environment.

The first and single most important step in identifying medical child abuse is to think that it might be occurring. One of the most frequently asked questions we hear is, "Why did you ever think that the mother might not be telling the truth?" Our answer is that having medical abuse in the differential diagnosis is part of good medical practice.

In the medical community *practice good medicine* is a mantra that means many things in many different circumstances. It might mean knowing which test to order, or when not to order a test. It could mean knowing when to refer to a subspecialist. On the other hand, it could mean feeling comfortable treating the patient or condition oneself. To practice good medicine it is necessary to listen to the patient, or the parent of a patient. But sometimes, to practice good medicine one must know when to listen critically. *Practicing good medicine* means that 99% of the time the doctor should believe what the parent says. But 1% of the time a good physician will take what the parent says with a large grain of salt.

More and more, practicing good medicine has come to mean providing medical care based on scientific medical evidence. There has long been a subtle, and sometimes not so subtle, tension between "the art of medicine" and "the science of medicine." Gradually, it has become more acceptable to base treatment on observable, reproducible scientific evidence rather than anecdotal experience. Evidence-based medicine dictates that treatments adhere to principles established through controlled clinical trials. There are no controlled clinical trials for the treatment of medical child abuse. There are, however, principles accepted in evidence-based medicine that apply. First and foremost is the expectation that treatments will be based on observable clinical evidence, and not just on information gleaned from interviewing parents.

We will illustrate this point with a more detailed description of the patient described in Chapter 7 as "June." June's mother took her to the primary care pediatrician's office at 2 weeks of age. Her mother was extremely anxious and gave an elaborate account of her baby's high fever, listlessness, inability to feed, vigorous vomiting, and lack of urination. At this age, these are serious symptoms and could represent life-threatening sepsis. Based solely on the symptoms reported by the mother her physician hospitalized the infant. June received a spinal tap, and blood cultures were done to determine whether she had a systemic infection. She was begun on intravenous antibiotics. While in the hospital the baby showed no symptoms. She had no more than the usual amount of fussiness. She urinated regularly and took the bottle with no problem. Forty-eight hours later, when her blood cultures showed no evidence of infection, her pediatrician stopped the antibiotics and offered the mother reassurance that her daughter was doing fine.

A week later, in the middle of the night, the pediatrician's partner received a phone call from the same mother repeating a similar story in concerned anxious tones. June's mother was advised to take the infant to the emergency department immediately. Once again the infant was worked up for possible sepsis and received yet another spinal tap. Once again she had no symptoms in the hospital. When her cultures were negative for infection, she was sent home. After the third frantic telephone call the pediatrician decided to admit June for observation but not start aggressive treatment. He chose not to listen to the mother. Instead he consulted the hospital child abuse team to evaluate whether this behavior on the part of the mother represented medical child abuse. At this point the child was only 2 months old and had already experienced 3 unnecessary hospitalizations, 2 spinal taps, 2 courses of intravenous antibiotics, and numerous arterial and venous blood draws.

Chapter 9 **167**
Identifying Medical Child Abuse

If unnecessary, each of these medical procedures represented an act of child abuse. Her doctors were correct in listening to the mother the first 2 times. They practiced good medicine by treating the child for presumed sepsis. They also practiced good medicine by not listening on the third occasion and observing her without treatment. After 2 unnecessary treatment episodes, the proper treatment was to initiate an evaluation for medical child abuse.

The pediatrician thought about potential child abuse. He recognized that June was receiving significant medical care that was appropriate given the symptoms related by her mother. But it was not appropriate if the accounts given by the mother were not true. He was not sure what was motivating the mother to report dramatic symptoms. But it was clear that something needed to be done differently to avoid exposing June to more medical trauma.

For a patient to be abused in a medical care environment, he or she needs to receive medical care that is unnecessary and harmful or potentially harmful. And that medical care must be the result of actions on the part of the caretaker. When this happens the caretaker is violating the rules that govern the doctor-patient relationship. By giving distorted information or false information, or causing there to be false information in the system, for example, by falsifying test results, the parent or caretaker leads the physician to prescribe the wrong treatment. Practicing good medicine means listening to the parent, but also getting information from other sources that confirms what the parent says.

We cannot stress this enough. For medical child abuse to occur there needs to be a violation of the doctor-patient relationship, the rules of engagement between doctors and those they treat. To be eligible for the special treatment accorded to people who are sick, a person must adhere to the unwritten agreement that one should do everything possible to get well again. This applies equally as much to parents of toddlers or children who cannot speak for themselves as it would for adults seeking their own care. Working together with the doctor to get well involves an exchange of accurate information. The evaluation of medical child abuse requires a physician to practice the kind of good medicine that keeps in mind that not all patients play by the rules.

The same characteristics that make for a good doctor may render him or her vulnerable to being made an unwitting participant in medical child abuse.[2] The attributes of a good pediatrician include a willingness to work closely with parents, a desire to go the extra mile to find out what is wrong with children, and sensitivity to the emotional needs of parents as well as children. Good pediatricians are usually caring, trusting, and sympathetic. These traits of model physicians are exactly the features that render them vulnerable to being deceived by parents offering false information.

In Chapter 3 we discussed the report by Guandolo[3] written in 1985. The author introduced the phrase *the medical game* and specifically discussed how he felt the mother of his patient was not playing by the rules. After many years of attempting to treat nonexistent illnesses the author relates how the mother one day dropped in the conversation that she might be using her new law degree to pursue her interest in "negligence law." At that point the primary care pediatrician decided to get corroborating evidence for some of the statements made by the mother. He called her husband and the entire story unraveled.

It is not our intention to suggest that physicians give up traits such as empathy, sensitivity, and a trusting nature. Rather, we think it is appropriate to follow the adage, "Trust but verify." Specifically, we want to encourage the medical community to consider medical child abuse consistently. If doctors think about the quality of information they are getting from caretakers, they can prevent medical child abuse. Children can avoid the types of harm they experience when an abusive situation is allowed to continue over months and years. In this chapter we want to set the stage for early identification, even before the situation raises to the level requiring intervention by child protection authorities. More than anything else, we want to encourage our colleagues to *practice good medicine*.

As we described previously, to identify medical child abuse, the physician making that determination must distance himself from the treatment role to some degree and look at what is happening objectively within the doctor-patient relationship. The doctor must question what he or she is doing even while it seems appropriate given the information available at the time. It is much easier to see what someone else is doing than to observe one's own actions. We liken this process to becoming "meta" to ongoing treatment; to the dancer stepping out of the dance to watch it taking place.

While obtaining an accurate history of signs and symptoms is essential in all medical practice, in the treatment of small children information gained from the caretaker is more important than any test one can do. As Meadow[4] says, "I teach my medical students 'Listen to the mother. She will tell you the diagnosis, not tests and examinations'. You get it from the story, and unless you listen and believe the carer when you are dealing with children, you're an absolutely rotten doctor. You won't get any rapport with the family and you won't help them, and you won't make the right diagnosis." This lesson has been ingrained in most of us at some time in our training. If listening to parents is such an important part of pediatrics, how are we to know when to listen and when not to listen?

In fact, there are no hard and fast rules. If there were a rule, it would be always to have in the differential diagnosis the possibility that information received from the parent *might* be erroneous. The number of illnesses that might generate a particular set of symptoms can be quite extensive and take us in many different directions. Having the account of the symptoms be untrue might be the 10th item on a complicated differential diagnosis. But even having it far down the list is better than not thinking about it at all. If medical abuse is on the list of possible diagnoses and is ruled out there is no harm done. However, if it is not considered at all, the consequences can be life-threatening. In fact, the sooner it is considered and ruled out the better for all concerned.

Identifying Abuse in Primary and Specialty Care Practices

Primary care pediatricians, pediatric subspecialists, and child abuse pediatricians all have advantages and liabilities in making the diagnosis. Primary care physicians and specialty care physicians enter into slightly different contracts with their patients. The role of a primary care physician is to create a close partnership with parents and work together toward the overall medical health of the child over an extended period. A specialty care pediatrician is more likely to be focused on a specific disease entity or organ system while still maintaining the perspective of the child's overall health. Because of this difference in perspective we think the primary care pediatrician has the more difficult task in identifying medical child abuse.

A primary care pediatrician is likely to have a long-standing relationship with a parent. While this means that the physician has a lot of experience listening to a particular parent, the relationship actually can make it more difficult to consider medical child abuse. It is asking much of a primary care pediatrician to stop one day and ask if the care being provided might be unnecessary and the direct result of inaccurate information. On the other side of the coin, a primary care pediatrician who has been working with a mother for a number of years comes to understand the parent's threshold for asking for help. Some parents respond very quickly to the slightest symptoms while others wait too long to bring the child to the doctor. A good pediatrician comes to understand this and compensates for it.

We recently were asked to advise a pediatrician who had worked with a mother for 6 years regarding illnesses in her twins. The mother had complained of symptoms in her children on multiple occasions, and for the most part the doctor was able to avoid unnecessary treatment. However, the mother was now requesting a referral for a cardiac evaluation for her 6-year-old son, as she was convinced he had developed a serious heart condition. The pediatrician doubted this but could not bring herself to refuse to order the consultation on medical grounds for fear that she would alienate the mother.

In fact, she had already called a cardiology colleague and scheduled an appointment for the boy but felt it was the wrong thing to do. She was convinced that arranging a subspecialty appointment for a nonexistent illness would only make the situation worse in the long run. She asked if we had other ideas about how to handle the situation. Specifically, she wanted to know if this was Munchausen syndrome by proxy (MSBP) and should she report this to her local child abuse agency.

We asked if she felt the child had experienced any harmful or unnecessary medical care. She responded that up to this point she did not think that was the case. Instead of suggesting she make a report of child abuse when no abuse had yet taken place, we recommended she schedule an hour-long appointment with the mother and specifically include the child's father who had been an infrequent visitor to the pediatrician's office. We suggested that she discuss her concerns with both parents and slowly and carefully give her reasons for not wanting to ask for an unnecessary consultation and potential round of diagnostic tests that were unlikely to discover an underlying illness.

The pediatrician followed our advice, canceled the cardiology consultation, and scheduled an appointment at the end of the day for the mother and her husband. The meeting stretched to 2 hours. At the end of the visit both parents thanked the pediatrician for her honesty and concern and agreed with a plan not to pursue an aggressive medical diagnostic workup when there was no real reason to do so. As anticipated, the presence of the husband was invaluable in this meeting. The pediatrician called to report the outcome of her intervention. Even though she could not charge a fee that would adequately compensate for the time spent, she felt very positive about sparing the child needless medical care and perhaps setting a bad precedent for the future. She had practiced good medicine.

We find that many primary care pediatricians have 5 to 10 parents in their practice who require considerable time on the telephone or during office visits. They acknowledge that one of their functions is helping these parents deal with their own anxiety about their children's health or their tendency to exaggerate symptoms. Each doctor has his or her own way of approaching these patients. We evaluated one family for possible medical child abuse and found extensive comments in the original pediatrician's office records about this issue. There was a standing order that no treatment would ever be prescribed over the telephone. The mother was to bring the child for an office visit because, "You can never trust what she says." Symptoms were only treated if they could be validated by direct observation in the office. Unfortunately, the family moved to another city and the next several doctors were not as vigilant. We found documentation of the child receiving treatment many times based on telephone reports of symptoms, referrals to subspecialists that were not necessary, and other evidence of inappropriate medical care resulting from the mother's communication of false information.

Primary care physicians generally engage in long-term medical relationships with families of the children they treat. The suspicion that a parent is exaggerating symptoms or lying about symptoms might occur at the beginning of that relationship or well along, even years after the initial visit with the child. The awareness that things may not be what they seem might grow slowly or come on suddenly. There might be a long series of nagging doubts that finally crystallize in the doctor's awareness of a new understanding of the child's illnesses. Or there might be one event that is so far out of the ordinary that it calls for a new hypothesis. The feature in common is the doctor reaching a tipping point in his or her relationship with the parent that involves switching from a primarily trusting stance to a questioning one. Doctors can find this shift in perspective easy to do or almost impossible, or they may fall anywhere in between. Some physicians are born suspicious while others can hardly do anything but trust.

Imagine a mother bringing her 5-year-old son to the doctor and saying, "I took his temperature and it was 107 degrees!" You look at the child and see that he is walking, talking, and smiling. Immediately, you think that the extremely elevated temperature and clinical presentation do not match and your suspicion that the mother has exaggerated or simply misread the thermometer is present from the first instant you receive this history. A temperature taken by your office nurse is read as 99.2°F. From that point on your relationship with the mother is marked by an understanding that symptom reports might not be accurate. Now imagine a mother who calls saying her child's temperature is 104°F. By the time he gets to the office, however, his rectal temperature is 99°F and the child looks well. The mother says she gave her son Tylenol an hour before bringing the child to the doctor's office. It seems perfectly reasonable that the child may have experienced an elevated temperature at home that responded to medication. But what if this scenario is repeated month after month? After the sixth or seventh such incident, while scratching his head to think of a disease that would explain repeated bouts of essentially asymptomatic fever, the physician might consider not trusting the mother's story. A primary care pediatrician at this point, with an element of doubt in his mind, might ask the mother to bring the child to the office without giving medication so that he can be evaluated while experiencing the full set of symptoms. The mother's response to this request provides new data that are useful in finding out what is really going on.

For example, a mother could say, "That's a great idea! I was beginning to think you might not believe me when I said my child was having a fever. Maybe this will help us find out what's really happening." Or instead, a mother could say, "I can't possibly do that! Johnny suffers so much when he has a fever and I will not put him through the experience of waiting for two hours to get to the office." The response given by the parent allows the physician to recalibrate his understanding of the doctor-patient relationship using new information.

It is appropriate at this point to remember that the medical contract between child, parent, and physician is always subject to reexamination and renegotiation. We know that it usually goes unspoken. When a pediatrician makes an appointment with a new mother he or she does not have that mother sign a piece of paper saying she will tell the truth, the whole truth, and nothing but the truth. The medical contract is embedded in the culture and it is understood that everyone agrees to it without question. The fact that it is usually assumed to be functioning in all cases and at all times does not make it any less real. Nor does this assumption absolve the physician from keeping in mind the possibility that the contract may not, in fact, be operating as expected.

If the primary care pediatrician's job is the hardest, what about a subspecialist called to evaluate children in consultation? A subspecialist has the opportunity to take a fresh look at the situation. By definition, the subspecialist is hired to look at all the facts from a new perspective; exactly what is necessary to diagnose medical child abuse. A consultant usually has a variety of powerful diagnostic tools at his disposal. Of course, these tools can be assets or liabilities. One function of the pediatric subspecialist is to rule out significant illness in the child. A diagnostic test that can definitively exclude the possibility that a child has an illness can be of great help to the referring physician. It can give the referring doctor the ability to reassure a parent that she need not worry about a serious illness.

However, the special diagnostic tools come with a price. They can induce anxiety by their mere use, cause pain and discomfort, possibly provide false-positive results, lead to further tests, and sometimes carry potentially lethal risk to the patient. In many cases a specialty physician does not have the advantage of a long-term relationship with the mother. He or she cannot as easily judge when the mother is exaggerating or minimizing symptoms. In the absence of a well-established therapeutic relationship, a subspecialist might come to rely more and more on diagnostic procedures.

Imagine the position of a gastroenterologist evaluating a child for abdominal pain. Many things can cause abdominal pain. Some of them can be ruled out by tests such as x-rays, computerized tomography (CT) scans, ultrasound, endoscopy, biopsies, motility studies, and more esoteric examinations like hydrogen breath testing for lactose intolerance. Imagine that 1 or 2 tests show equivocal findings and the doctor suggests taking a "wait and see," conservative course. He schedules a follow-up appointment in 1 month expecting that symptoms may resolve spontaneously. However, when the mother returns she maintains that the symptoms have worsened and at times are totally debilitating even though today her child is feeling well. What can the subspecialist do? Repeat the tests? Order different tests? Send the child to another subspecialist? Tell the mother he doesn't believe her?

We said at the beginning of this chapter that the primary ingredient in making the diagnosis of medical child abuse is practicing good medicine. What constitutes good medical practice for a subspecialist who is getting a clear message from a mother that her child is experiencing significant symptoms that cannot be seen in the office on the day of the examination? Many illnesses, particularly chronic remitting illnesses, do not exhibit symptoms every day. It is perfectly understandable that a child could be suffering from abdominal pain but not be in pain at the time of the examination in the office. For a subspecialist, sometimes the only evidence he has available to aid in making a diagnosis is the history given by the parent. Obviously, the primary care pediatrician has the advantage of being able to schedule a patient on consecutive days if needed to afford a better chance of seeing the full clinical picture.

One option available to the subspecialist is to call the referring physician and coordinate the treatment. The consultant not seeing symptoms in the office could call the primary care doctor and get confirmatory evidence. Rather than take the word of the parent, the primary and consulting physicians can confer about the existence of objective evidence of illness. Close coordination between physicians treating the same child, however, does not guarantee that a child can avoid medical child abuse. Laura had 7 active subspecialists involved in her care. They were all competent clinicians and they communicated with each other with good referral letters. They generally felt comfortable working with one another. In this case, noting the complexity of the medical presentation, the family had been assigned to a specific primary care pediatrician with a particular interest in monitoring complex medical conditions. However, even the presence of a special primary care doctor specifically designated to coordinate the efforts of all the subspecialists did not result in Laura avoiding harmful medical care.

If a primary care physician's long-term relationship with the parent makes it difficult to diagnosis medical child abuse, the subspecialty pediatrician does not have this problem. But he or she does have special concerns. Foremost among these is the need to dig deeper and deeper into medical situations to justify the medical specialist status. It is said that to a man with a hammer in his hand everything begins to look like a nail. A specialist with a diagnostic tool is likely to use it and when this happens, positive or partial results are certain to show up every so often, even in the absence of an underlying illness. Some experts go so far as to attribute the current prevalence of medical child abuse to the existence of subspecialty medicine.[5]

Dr Leland Fan, a pediatric pulmonologist at National Jewish Hospital in Denver, CO, first diagnosed the case cited in the introduction to this book that led us to a major reconceptualization of MSBP. When Dr Fan assumed care as the attending physician, the child was several months into a terrible series of apparent life-threatening events (ALTEs). He looked at the patient, talked to some of us who had been involved in treating the child, and then sat down to review the hospital record. Many hours later he emerged with several pages of notes and said he was certain that the mother had induced the child's illnesses. He had the facts to prove it. He revealed that our care of the child, all the diagnostic tests and special procedures we used in search of ever more esoteric illnesses, occurred because of the mother's actions. He demonstrated that all of the 22 ALTEs the boy experienced in the hospital occurred in the mother's sole presence, and not one happened when she was not there. After we escorted the mother from the hospital and stopped any further diagnostic testing, we watched as the child slowly recovered from the repeated bouts of aspiration pneumonia caused by his mother. Dr Fan's analysis of the record quickly convinced the medical team and, subsequently a judge, that the child needed protection.

What about child abuse pediatricians? Is it easier for someone with specific interest and training in child abuse to make the diagnosis of medical child abuse or is the opposite true? Occasionally a child is referred specifically to a child abuse pediatrician or other child abuse professional to make a diagnosis of medical child abuse. This represents a huge advantage for the consultant. It means that other physicians or professionals involved in the welfare of the child have already considered the diagnosis and are asking for its confirmation. A child abuse specialist (whether a pediatrician, social worker, psychologist, or psychiatrist) has the easiest job of all when it comes to determining medical abuse. A child abuse specialist does not need to step out of an ongoing treatment role to see that the treatment might be harmful. Because this is a major part of the battle, child abuse professionals begin the diagnostic process well ahead of others. However, some child abuse professionals suffer from another liability.

We have been involved in the evaluation of several situations where children and their parents had been referred previously for a specialty evaluation for possible MSBP. After numerous hours of interview, 2 different child abuse experts concluded that there was no evidence of MSBP because they could not establish that the mother was subjecting her children to medical treatment to meet her own dependency needs from medical care providers. One even maintained in her written report that MSBP could only be diagnosed when a mother was observed on videotape causing harm to her child.

In one of these families, 3 children between them had been treated for symptoms of seizure disorder, attention-deficit/hyperactivity disorder, psychosis, immune deficiency, asthma, developmental delay, gastroesophageal reflux, brain tumor, and need for a permanent wheelchair. For none of these conditions was there any biological basis demonstrated on physical examinations or diagnostic tests. The question of MSBP was first raised 10 years before our involvement. Five years before we were asked to consult, the family was sent specifically to a mental health evaluation and treatment center for an MSBP evaluation. The report written by a child psychiatrist described the mother representing herself as a "major advocate for her children." The expert accepted this characterization and noted that he could find no specific dependency on the medical profession on the part of the mother. Obviously, he was asking the wrong question. The expert made no assessment about whether the children received unnecessary medical care. On the basis of this report, the child abuse investigation was closed. A by-product of the attention focused on the mother's possible contribution to excessive care was a significant decrease in the number of doctor visits for all 3 children for the next several years before the mother began abusing her children anew by initiating unnecessary medical treatments. At that point we were contacted.

Usually when a child abuse expert is consulted, it is in a complicated case like the one just described. Unnecessary treatments have been taking place for many years. There may be multiple children involved, multiple prior illness events, and many hospitalizations or surgeries. A specialty care pediatrician often is asked to review symptoms involving a specific organ system (eg, the gastrointestinal system). The child abuse professional may have less of a challenge in making the diagnosis but may have to work much harder. He or she usually gets sent the complicated, extensive, and very distressing cases. These are also the cases that get presented in the literature as "interesting case reports."

A primary care pediatrician considering medical child abuse must review objectively his own medical practice with a child and decide if medical care was given inappropriately because the caretaker provided inaccurate information. A specialist is usually asked to consider a specific set of symptoms and determine if the symptoms constitute a treatable illness. The task of the child abuse professional is to review the entire treatment history of the child and the child's family to look for patterns of inappropriate medical behavior. Hopefully, if the primary care pediatrician and subspecialty physician practice good medicine there will be no or minimal inappropriate medical care, and the situation will not develop that would require a child abuse pediatrician to do an extensive evaluation for medical abuse. Practicing good evidence-based medicine represents primary prevention for medical abuse.

The Child Abuse Expert's Evaluation

Procedures for conducting a thorough subspecialty evaluation for medical child abuse are well-established.[6] For example, Sanders and Bursch[7] give an excellent review of how to approach a major case. They emphasize that the primary approach to making the diagnosis of medical child abuse in a complex case is to review the medical records looking for harm. These authors participated in the American Professional Society on the Abuse of Children's task force redefining MSBP and use the language agreed on in its report. "Similar to the assessment of other forms of child abuse, such as physical or sexual abuse, the determination of whether abusive illness falsification has taken place is typically based on circumstantial rather than direct evidence because it is rare that someone directly observes an abusive act. The question of illness falsification can often be answered by conducting a thorough medical record review."

The medical record review is the central feature of the evaluation. It is a complicated process, made more difficult by the large number of records usually involved, by the complexity of the medical issues, and by the possibility that many accounts cited in the records might be erroneous. Our most intricate case required the review of a stack of 7 feet of medical records.

Contradictions in the medical record might represent misunderstandings between physicians and caretaker, misunderstandings between physicians, or frankly erroneous information provided by the caretaker. Lies can be subtle or gross. A mother might say, "I think she had an ultrasound and I think I remember it showed kidney stones." When the medical record is consulted it might reveal an ultrasound report that documents no evidence of kidney stones, or no sign of an ultrasound being conducted or even considered. As an example of a not so subtle prevarication, a patient once told us that her *brother* had had surgery to treat cervical cancer. Not surprisingly, the medical record offered no proof of this claim.

Sanders and Bursch[7] give an example of a table used to compile medical record information. Most experts, including us, have found useful similar methods of organizing records. Basically, we begin with the birth records of the child and record on a table every medical event in the child's life. A typical child might, at age 5, have 10 to 15 medical visits documented in the pediatrician's record. A child with a more significant history of illness might have several dozen. A typical case of suspected medical abuse evaluated by a child abuse specialist could have several hundred medical visits. We were consulted about one child who had seen a physician on average every 2½ days of his life. This meant reviewing more than 400 medical visits.

On the table recording the child's medical history, we record the date and location of treatment, the chief complaint, supporting medical information, the treatment given, and specific comments. For example, we might document an outpatient visit made when the child was 3 years old with the chief complaint of "pulling on ears." The doctor's physical examination showed no evidence for otitis media, but a prescription for amoxicillin was given. Under the comment column we might write, "This is the 7th time antibiotics were prescribed for symptoms claimed but not supported by direct visualization of abnormal tympanic membranes."

We want to emphasize that the above entry does not alone constitute medical abuse. It is simply documentation of a pattern of medical behavior. Many such entries describing the treatment of a single child could add up to medical abuse. At a certain point a threshold is reached and we must consider whether the child needs protection from ongoing unnecessary medical care. Table 1 is a typical example of a chart that might be constructed in a medical child abuse case.

The reviewer is looking for a number of indicators of potential medical abuse. Occasionally there will be evidence for illness induction; direct physical harm committed against the child by her parent. In our survey of 115 possible cases of MSBP we found evidence of illness induction in 23. Typical of how illness induction is identified is the child with 22 ALTEs.

TABLE 1
Example of a Chart Used to Review Medical Records in Cases of Suspected Medical Child Abuse[a]

Date	Provider	Complaint	Comments
2-05-07	Jones, ENT	Recurrent OM	Mom says audiogram at Kerman Hosp. shows conductive hearing loss. He snores and mouth breathes. He has had 12 ear infections. *Audiogram report says it's normal. He has had 3 documented ear infections.* Mother says child has eosinophilic granulama. *Not true.* Child is allergic to Keflex, penicillin, and erythromycin. *No evidence of drug reactions in medical record.* MD says based on history, child needs T & A and PE tubes inserted.
2-17-07	Marshal Hosp. Jones, ENT	Recurrent OM	**SURGERY.** T & A, PE tubes. No fluid noted behind ear drums. No unusual tonsilar or adenoidal pathology.
2-24-07	Jones, ENT	Postop visit	Tubes in place. Doing well.
3-11-07	Marshall Hosp. ED	Tube fell out of ear	Mom was cleaning child's ear with a water pik. PE tube came out of ear. Ref. to Dr. Jones.
3-15-07	Wilson, Pediatric cross cover	Ear pain and fever	Telephone call from mom. Fever and ear pain. Child allergic to penicillin and erythromycin. Rx: Ceclor.
3-17-97	Jones, ENT	Evaluate lost PE tube	Missed appointment.

[a] Reviewer's comments are in italics.

The mother gave her toddler something to drink and then held his nose and mouth until, gasping for air, he inhaled the liquid. She was never directly observed doing this. It was inferred from the medical documentation available to us. Even though no one ever caught her in the act, when confronted with our suspicions she admitted what she was doing. We considered this an assault on a child and that was the charge to which the mother eventually pled guilty. The medical child abuse the child experienced ceased immediately when his mother was prevented from physically assaulting him.

Sometimes a third party observes a parent doing something to the child that causes the child to be ill. This is rare. In many more instances illness induction is never observed. Of course, the lack of a witness to the abuse is something medical abuse shares with almost every other kind of child maltreatment.

Once the table of all medical events has been completed, the next step is to begin looking for patterns. The table will tell you if medical appointments ceased for a significant time or became more frequent. It will tell you if several different medical providers are treating the child for the same condition. And it will reveal the caretaker's role in the child receiving unnecessary medical care. On one such table we found adjacent entries documenting medical events in 2 different doctors' offices on the same day. The first entry was from an orthopedic surgeon. The note read, "Problem has resolved, examination normal, no need for further orthopedic care." The next entry in the table documents a telephone call made an hour later to the primary care pediatrician from the mother of the child. The pediatrician's note stated, "Mom just back from Dr J's office, surgeon recommending above the knee amputation." This kind of disparity, which jumps off the pages of a medical record table, calls for immediate efforts to protect the child. Reading the records from just one provider often will not reveal the parent's behavior. It is the ability to see the consolidated medical timeline that reveals the diagnosis.

Information provided by the parent to various medical personnel as reflected in the medical record becomes the basis of determining whether the parent initiated unnecessary or harmful treatment. For example, a child was admitted to our hospital because she had multiple episodes of vomiting blood. The next day, her mother called the principal of her daughter's school and told him that the child was in the hospital awaiting dialysis for kidney failure. He relayed this information to the treatment team in the hospital. The girl had no kidney disease and when the mother was asked the next day in the hospital if she had ever made such a statement she said, "Of course not!" It was determined that the blood in the child's vomitus was from the mother, not the child. Once again, one falsehood does not constitute abuse. However, a number of such statements that lead directly to improper medical care may call for protection.

To document every medical event in a child's life it is necessary to have all of his or her medical records. Several factors militate against accumulating the complete set of records. Remarkably, getting permission to view the records is usually not the most difficult part. While there is an occasional parent who is wary about giving permission to view medical records, most give permission quite readily. Signing permission to obtain medical records is a routine part of seeing a new physician. Parents are asked to do this all the time. Parents being evaluated for medical child abuse are often comfortable in doctors' offices, having spent a great deal of time in them, and in some cases are even rather proud of their medical accomplishments. A mother once told us, "Wait until you read all those records! If we had all the money spent on medical care on that boy we would never have to work again." The more difficult task surrounding getting access to all medical records involves knowing which records to request. Parents forget the names of doctors they've seen, or hospitalizations that took place years ago. Often one begins a medical record review and finds references to hospitalizations or emergency department visits that had not been previously mentioned by the parent.

It is important when asking for medical records that the reviewer specify a complete copy of the records. Many hospitals believe a doctor requesting records is only interested in discharge summaries, laboratory tests, and consultation notes. However, the most interesting and valuable information is often retrieved from nursing notes and daily progress report comments. Sometimes a hospital will send records for a specific hospitalization and neglect to include information about 25 emergency department visits. In a complicated case it is often necessary to request medical records for the index patient, the siblings, and the parents or caretaker suspected of abusing the child.

We were once requested to offer an opinion about whether a mother should regain custody of her children. One of her children had died from a purported accidental overdose of chloral hydrate. Her other children had been placed in protective custody with relatives. The mother was suing the doctor who prescribed the chloral hydrate for malpractice. This was a military family and medical records existed in several states because the family had moved frequently. In addition, there were records stored in the military central records depository. The most important information we reviewed was the accused mother's records. There we found a persistent pattern of lying to physicians about important medical events dating back to her teen years. Because of this and other information gathered in the review, we recommended the children not be returned. Although we were unable to say with certainty from the available data whether the mother purposefully overdosed her child with chloral hydrate, we suspected this to be the case. Years later we learned she eventually confessed to poisoning the child.[8]

We cannot stress enough the need to review all appropriate medical records. There are situations where the child's life might be in danger. Sometimes it is necessary to ask for an order from a court or a subpoena from a child protection agency to access all the records that might shed light on the risk of danger.

Many authors[9] have commented on the futility of a psychiatric interview to determine if a parent is perpetrating or suffering from MSBP. However, the interview of a parent can be a very important part of an evaluation of child abuse. The interview allows the evaluator to hear the parent's point of view regarding medical treatment. It is just as important in the evaluation of medical child abuse as it is to the evaluation of other types of child abuse. As with physical or sexual abuse, it is important to find out whether the history provided by the caretaker fits the circumstances of the child's situation.

Distinguishing Between Parental Anxiety, Illness Exaggeration, Illness Fabrication, and Illness Induction

For the physician, the process to recognize medical child abuse is similar to that used in identifying other forms of child maltreatment. The doctor is asked to determine if there is enough evidence of abuse that the child might need protection. The physician provides information regarding medical symptoms, interview details, and evidence from a clinical examination to the civil authorities who make the determination whether the child is sufficiently in harm's way to require the state to step in. The response by the agency can take many forms from deciding no action is indicated, to providing support to the family, to removing the child.

Certainly the most common cause of a parent overreporting symptoms in her child is anxiety. A parent might have very real, or imagined, reasons to anticipate her child to be ill even in the absence of observable signs or symptoms. It may be that the parent is anxious about most things in her life. Or her anxiety may focus specifically on the child. The anxiety might be part of a diagnosable anxiety disorder in the mother such as obsessive-compulsive disorder, or might be just a pattern of overreacting to the world. A primary care physician can usually detect rather quickly whether a mother is prone to oversensitivity and screen the reports given by her accordingly. A special form of parental anxiety we referred to earlier in the discussion of vulnerable child syndrome focuses specifically on the parents' fear that their child might be prone to death or serious illness.

The best way we have found to determine if the parent is overreacting to the child's symptoms because of a belief in vulnerability is to take an extremely thorough history of the child's birth. Most doctors ask a few questions about the pregnancy and birth of the child as part of the medical history. We recommend, when vulnerable child syndrome is a concern, sitting with the parents in a comfortable setting and slowly reviewing the events of the pregnancy, birth, and perinatal period with a particular emphasis on real or imagined loss. Questions such as, "Was there ever a time when you thought he might die?" or "Were you afraid, and are you still afraid, your child might not be normal?" Given an opportunity, a parent sometimes reveals long-standing, deep-seated fears never shared before, even with her spouse. For example, a parent might have the experience of another child in the family dying from sudden infant death syndrome (SIDS) and fear that this child might also die. Expressing the fear out loud, exposing it to the light of day, and talking sensibly with the physician about the risk of SIDS might be enough to defuse the anxiety. Parents might be hesitant at first to admit to fears and concerns, but once revealed these thoughts can rapidly lose their potency. As a result their child is the beneficiary of a more benign parental belief system.

Severe illness exaggeration is further along the spectrum that begins with parental anxiety and ends with parents causing direct harm to their child. Many parents at some time in the life of a child might find themselves exaggerating medical events. For example, take the parent who says to her neighbor, "You can't believe how sick Johnny was last week; I thought he was going to die!" To constitute medical abuse illness exaggeration needs to be demonstrated to be part of a persistent pattern that results in the child getting unnecessary medical care. In our experience, illness exaggeration was the most common parental behavior that resulted in children being harmed in the medical environment. The more persistent and severe the exaggeration, the more likely the child is to receive harmful medical care.

To establish whether a child is the victim of medical abuse, the medical community is asked to determine if medical care was unnecessary and potentially harmful, and in what way the caretaker promoted the unneeded medical care. Determining if care is necessary requires medical judgment. Laura, first introduced in Chapter 6, had frequent infections when she was 4 years old. Her mother told her pediatrician that she had greenish nasal discharge and headaches. He prescribed oral antibiotics to treat a presumed sinus infection. Her mother reported continued symptoms and the oral antibiotic treatment was reinstituted. She underwent x-rays and a CT scan of her sinuses that showed no signs of sinus infection. Her mother continued to complain of greenish-yellow discharge, and Laura was admitted to the hospital to receive intravenous antibiotics for "pansinusitus." After she went home from the hospital, her mother repeated that the nasal discharge was copious and green and wondered if something else could be done for her daughter's sinuses. Laura ended up receiving sinus antrum surgery, a procedure that is rarely required in children this young. The ear, nose, and throat surgeon sent sinus contents to be cultured for evidence of infection, but no organisms consistent with sinusitis were found.

At some point in this narrative it was possible to say that Laura was receiving harmful medical care resulting from her mother's account of her symptoms. This determination alone should be sufficient to bring a halt to the ongoing medical intervention. Her medical team could have decided that 4-year-olds contract numerous viral infections and seldom need antibiotics for nasal discharge. Or her doctors could have tried oral antibiotics 1 or 2 times and then reevaluated treatment based on closer direct observation of symptoms.

Another step in the process would have been to try oral antibiotics, then intravenous antibiotics, but then say that 4-year-olds are unlikely to need surgery on their sinuses and opt to observe her over time to see if she improves. These are all steps in medical judgment expected from the medical team. But present all along the sequence was the persistent and, presumably, persuasive account by Laura's mother regarding how much the child was suffering from nasal and sinus congestion.

In determining that the child is being maltreated in the medical care environment the doctor is appropriately required to provide an explanation of how that can happen. What was the nature of the parent's participation that resulted in harmful medical care? What was the extent of the parent's behavior? It is useful to characterize this behavior on a spectrum ranging from mildly inappropriate misuse of the doctor-patient relationship due to parental anxiety or some other need of the parent, to exaggeration of existing symptoms, to falsification of information including lying about symptoms or fabrication of test results, to actual induction of illness in the child requiring treatment. Keep in mind that the central question is, "Does the child need protection?"

This is the same question we would ask about a child who has been *sexually* abused, that is, where on the spectrum of perpetrator behavior does this case fall? The child protection agency will often ask, "What did the perpetrator do?" Has the child told the physician the perpetrator talked to her in a lewd way? Exposed himself to her? Fondled her? Raped her violently? They will also want to know if these allegations are supported by clinical evidence. In sexual and physical abuse, perpetrator behavior falls on a spectrum from mild to severe, just as it does in medical child abuse.

Clearly, it is easier to make the case for protecting a child who has been intentionally poisoned or suffocated by his parent. It is easier to convince the system to protect a child whose parent is caught obviously falsifying test results. However, our experience has been that most children for whom MSBP is suspected actually have existing illnesses, and their parents exaggerate symptoms of their illnesses. Induction of an illness or fabrication with tests results is much less common. Hence, an essential element in identifying medical child abuse is an ability to characterize what contribution the parent is making that results in harmful medical care.

In the anecdote regarding Laura, there is no suggestion in the medical record that her mother caused her to have sinus infections. Nor is there concern that she fabricated laboratory tests or even made up accounts of Laura having copious nasal discharge. It is easy to understand that Laura, as is frequently the case in toddlers, had recurring viral infections with nasal discharge. Given her mother's tendency to exaggerate all illness that we observed while treating Laura, we concluded that years before we met her, her doctors were subjected to a continuous barrage of embellished descriptions of the child's illness. The child received intravenous antibiotics and unnecessary surgery because her doctors did not appreciate that they were receiving grossly exaggerated information.

The following is another example demonstrating the complexity of interpreting mothers' accounts of illness. Nancy's mother told us her child was having diarrhea every night. She had been telling doctors this for a number of years and as a result her child had been treated for *Clostridium difficile* infection with daily (and very expensive) antibiotics for more than 2 years. The 10-year-old child was in diapers and we asked the mother to bring the diapers to the hospital for us to inspect so we could evaluate her stooling pattern. Day after day we received diapers with soft or semi-formed stool consistent with the child's largely liquid diet. Each day we examined the diapers with the mother and informed her that her child did not have diarrhea. Laboratory tests conducted on the stool looking for causes of diarrhea were completely negative. She continued to begin each day's visit with a comment on her child's diarrhea. With the permission of her gastroenterologist, we stopped the antibiotic with no significant change in her symptoms.

In an attempt to determine the contribution of the parent, one must always keep in mind that the *interaction* between doctor and patient is part of the problem. A number of parents have been accused of MSBP because a previously workable relationship between the doctor and the family deteriorated. For example, a community physician reported a 15-year-old she suspected was a victim of MSBP (Emilie) to the state child protection agency. The local agency was unable to determine if Emilie was suffering from MSBP and arranged for the child and the child's mother to be court ordered to participate in our treatment program. Both the mother and teen were aware that an investigation was underway regarding MSBP.

Emilie gave a vague and inconsistent history of abdominal pain, sore feet, and headaches. She and her mother were extremely close. They lived alone together and were constant companions. Emilie's mother was disabled by her own multiple medical problems and visited doctors frequently. The mother's last significant full-time employment was as a nurse's aide.

To evaluate Emilie and her mother we pursued 2 paths simultaneously. We requested all of Emilie's medical records and did a thorough review. While reviewing Emilie's records, we required daily attendance in our day treatment program and we monitored her symptoms on an hour-by-hour basis. We noted that she was able to take part in all the normal activities within the therapeutic milieu, including attending and participating in community meetings, group therapy, individual and family therapy, school, mealtimes, and afternoon activities such as playing softball, doing art projects, and watching movies. She did complain of discomfort on occasion, but this did not interfere with her functioning to any significant degree.

In individual therapy Emilie admitted that despite the closeness between her and her mother, she had managed to acquire a boyfriend and become sexually active. She stated that her mother had no knowledge of this involvement and that she had no intention of telling her. In fact, an admission and later denial of sexual activity had led to charges and countercharges of lying between Emilie, her mother, and the primary care physician. Also, in her medical record was a reference to an inadequately treated sexually transmitted infection. We felt that her abdominal complaints might be the result of lingering pelvic inflammatory disease. She agreed to be tested once again to see if her infection had persisted. Cultures were positive and she reluctantly agreed to a course of treatment, stating that she had not liked the taste of the medication prescribed previously.

The review of the medical records showed a pattern of numerous missed appointments. However, each time Emilie did appear in her doctor's office there were physical signs and symptoms consistent with her complaints. In other words, she was not going to her doctor's office for unnecessary medical care. In fact, the frequency of visits turned out to be less than one might expect considering her mother's pattern of using medical services frequently. In addition, there was no indication from the medical record that Emilie's mother was encouraging her to make extra doctor visits.

Through her participation in our day hospital program Emilie demonstrated she was capable of regular attendance in a structured environment such as school, and was able to function despite complaints of abdominal pain or headache. In addition, with adequate treatment for her pelvic inflammatory disease her abdominal complaints decreased. We wrote a report to social services indicating there was no evidence for medical child abuse, but that Emilie and her mother needed significant help in negotiating normal adolescent differentiation. We recommended that the court continue to mandate family therapy and to make her mother responsible for Emilie attending school on a regular basis.

Emilie's family physician was frustrated by her inability to get adequate medical care for her patient, and felt that Emilie's mother was getting in the way of this process. Her report to social services with concerns regarding MSBP was reasonable. There were numerous red flags that medical child abuse might be an issue. We had evidence that the family used signs and symptoms of illness as a means of communicating with one another. Emilie's mother had experience as a nurse's aide. There were frequent missed appointments and disappointments with treatments resulting in the changing of providers. But when all was said and done, the problem facing this family had more to do with adolescent acting out behavior than it did with misuse of the medical care system. However, the family's lack of cooperation with the family physician, and subsequently the police and juvenile court system, precipitated a concern for MSBP.

The fact that Emilie had a true infection is important, but not a deciding factor in determining whether she was a victim of medical abuse. Children evaluated for medical child abuse often have intercurrent illnesses. This is important to remember, as there is a tendency when evaluating medical abuse to believe that the child was never sick. In fact, we are more often faced with determining which illness or which part of the illness is in fact medically justified. We treated a 9-year old boy with documented electrical seizure activity who had a history of seizure treatment dating back to early childhood. However, his treating physician became concerned about possible MSBP when the boy began having seizures many times a day, seemingly occurring when he did not get his way. He had video electroencephalogram test results that documented a mixture of rare, well-controlled electrical events and many more nonelectrical seizures. His mother, while an educated woman, seemed incapable of grasping the notion of nonelectrical or pseudoseizures and responded to all of his outbursts as if they were uncontrollable seizures. The result was that he was unable to attend school, had many medical evaluations, and was on a list to receive a surgical treatment for uncontrolled seizures. Our task was to determine when he was having "real" seizures and to bring his mother along with us to respond appropriately.

Detecting Illness Fabrication

The medical literature is replete with ingenious examples of doctors discovering the source of fabricated laboratory findings. The first such example, of course, is contained in Meadow's[10] original publication. To test his theory that the child's mother was manipulating urine specimens, adding blood products and other foreign materials to make it seem as if the child had a serious urinary tract problem, he instituted an elaborate urine collection system involving the hospital nursing staff. Specifically, he ordered that some urine samples be collected in a way that the mother had access to them while only nurses and specific hospital staff, from collection to laboratory evaluation, handled the others. The staff kept notes on which samples were handled by the mother and which were not. They also gave the girl xylose that later showed up in both the clean and contaminated samples, evidence that mother was adding her urine to that of the child. Finally, blood testing gave added proof that some of the mother's blood was turning up in the child's urine. The evidence for fabrication was overwhelming.

Kurlansky and his colleagues[11] were faced with trying to understand how an infant got blood on his face. They marked his blood with a radioactive isotope and discovered that the blood on his face did not contain any radioactivity. Subsequently they did blood typing and confronted the parents with the knowledge that the blood on the child's face did not come from the child. Clark and colleagues[12] suspected a mother of fabricating a bleeding disorder in her child by injecting the child with heparin. They covered blood draw sites with electrocardiogram leads. They then found new puncture sites on the child caused by the mother's hypodermic needle.

Our own experience suggests that less creative methods work just as well. We are more likely to ask a mother to bring in diapers soiled with "diarrhea" so we can see for ourselves how serious the child's illness might be. We have, on occasion, encouraged parents to allow us to test purported food allergies with double-blind, placebo-controlled food challenges. Basically, any reasonable noninvasive medical test that can clarify the clinical situation and does not put the child at risk is appropriate to test for severe illness exaggeration issues as well as possible illness fabrication or test fabrication.

Therapeutic Separation

We need to consider a special case in the evaluation for medical child abuse—the separation of the child from the parent in a hospital setting. Many authors have suggested hospitalization as a therapeutic test to see if symptoms continue once contact with a parent is regulated.[13] Rosenberg[14] made it a criterion for diagnosing MSBP. Because we see the behavior involved in medical child abuse as existing along a continuum from mild to severe, we have long since abandoned the notion that every child suspected of being a victim of medical child abuse be hospitalized apart from the parent. Having said this, we have offered several examples of situations in which a parent having access to a child can be dangerous. As a diagnostic tool, separation of the parent by putting a child in the hospital or restricting access to the child by the parent through some medical means, such as admitting the child to the intensive care unit where he will be constantly observed, has some utility but is not specific for determining medical abuse. Having symptoms disappear suddenly after a child is separated from his or her parent offers supportive evidence but is not diagnostic. In the final analysis we are looking for evidence the child has been harmed or could be harmed by medical care.

In fact, one of the early factors distinguishing medical child abuse from other serious child abuse was that harm often continued while the child was in a hospital. A child hospitalized for repeated trauma inflicted by a parent usually did not get revictimized while in the hospital, but this has been noted in many cases of medical child abuse. Because of this, hospitalization alone is not enough. If hospitalization is to be used as a diagnostic strategy, proper constraints need to be specified, such as constant observation of the patient by staff, visitation of parents only in the presence of staff, or duplicate medical charts to prevent a parent from changing notation in the record.

Preliminary Interventions as Diagnostic Tools

We have found several interviewing strategies useful in delineating between parental anxiety, vulnerable child syndrome, and illness exaggeration. For example, it is sometimes quite helpful to simply ask the parent if she is an anxious person. "Do people (eg, your husband, your mother, your pediatrician) consider you to be a worrywart?" We have had numerous responses to this question, each of which can lead to a different diagnostic conclusion. A parent might answer, "Oh yes, I worry all the time, especially about the children." The follow-up question in this case might be, "So how much of your concern about Johnny's diarrhea comes from your worry (anxiety) versus how much do you think it is really a bad medical problem?" A mother who answers this question by saying it's probably 90% her own anxiety falls in a totally different category than someone who says she truly believes her child is sick and her feelings have nothing to do with the symptoms.

Parents' belief systems can be extremely powerful determinants of not only their children's behavior, but also of their children's health, and of the response of community members and physicians involved in their lives. As a not so trivial example we cite a study of parents in Britain.[15] Parents were queried about whether they felt their child was allergic or sensitive to any particular food. Parents who answered in the affirmative had children who were, on average, 1 cm shorter, even after compensating statistically for other possible causes for decreased growth such as objective evidence of allergy. The conclusion of the study was that the children of parents who believe their children were sensitive to foods ate less well-balanced diets and ended up shorter.

This is an example of a parental belief system manifested in a physical health consequence. Just because it has a consequence that can be measured does not mean that it constitutes abuse. We cannot imagine calling for the protection of a child merely because a parent believes (without clear medical justification) he or she is sensitive to foods and therefore withholds them from his diet. But we have reported a series of children with severe dietary restrictions caused by parental belief in food allergy that resulted in profound growth retardation.[16] In a situation like this a child might easily need protection from medical abuse. Once again, the common denominator is whether the child has or could experience significant harm.

Many times we have used a similar strategy to that described above for anxiety to evaluate the significance of exaggeration behaviors of parents. The diagnostic intervention involves the interviewer holding up his hands 3 feet apart and telling the parent that all parents fall between the right hand and the left hand regarding how much concern they may have for their child's health. A mother might fall close to the left hand if she really didn't pay much attention to her child's health, let her child be exposed to all kinds of harm, and never took him to the doctor even if he were really sick. She might fall close to the right hand if she watched her child like a hawk, took her child to the doctor for every little thing that might be wrong, and tended to make a mountain out of a molehill. Of course, parents might fall somewhere in between. The mother is then asked to place herself somewhere along the spectrum between the left hand and the right hand.

Usually, parents with a tendency to exaggerate symptoms cooperate by acknowledging they fall on the over-involved end of the spectrum. This is an excellent prognostic sign and offers hope that health-seeking behavior might be modifiable. An illness exaggerating mother who places herself directly in the middle of the spectrum between over-involved and under-involved causes considerable concern. And the parent who describes herself as tending toward under-involved when that is far from the case is potentially dangerous.

Pam was born with a severe cardiac anomaly successfully treated surgically in the first year of life. Her mother spent most of her waking moments attending to the girl, asking her if she was getting sick, and going to school to pick her up when Pam complained of stomachaches, dizziness, or headaches. The child had been treated for numerous illnesses for which there was little or no objective medical evidence. When asked to place herself on the spectrum between the interviewer's hands, Pam's mother replied, "You have to move your right hand a lot farther out there to get to where I am." Almost immediately she continued, "Do you think I'm the problem, the reason why she's getting sick all the time?" Over the next year after a combination of individual therapy for the mother, and family therapy, Pam turned into a normally functioning fourth grader with only the usual number of childhood illnesses, and her mother returned to work at a job she really enjoyed.

Identifying that medical child abuse is occurring is the first step. It is the acknowledgment that the medical contract has been broken. At this point we still do not know whether it can be fixed. Everything we have discussed thus far in this chapter has implications for what happens next. If the evaluation indicates that a parent has been inducing illness in a child, causing the child to be sick, then our next step is to make sure that this behavior does not continue. If it is determined that a child has experienced harm, or could experience harm, from medical care, then the next step is to stop the harm. The behaviors we are discussing fall along the continuum from mild to severe. A child might have a parent with mild anxiety that resulted in mildly overusing medical treatment. There may be a moderate degree of illness exaggeration that results in a moderate degree of harm to the child. There might be a severe degree of illness exaggeration resulting in the child experiencing a potentially lethal surgical procedure. An evaluation for potential medical abuse should take all of these things into consideration.

Not every evaluation for possible medical abuse will result in a report of suspected child abuse to the local child protection agency. The fact that the physician included the possibility in the differential diagnosis, evaluated it, and determined its likelihood does not mean the family faces automatic reporting. In fact, this is what happens in offices on a day-to-day basis. If a parent were to bring in a child with extremely poor hygiene for an evaluation, the doctor may comment on this fact in his record and may speak to the parent about the child's hygiene, but he does not necessarily report to the local child protection agency. However, if this neglect persists, and the doctor becomes progressively concerned about the child's welfare, at a certain point a threshold is reached and a report is indicated. Many times a pediatrician might consider the plight of a young girl being seen in the office and speculate about the possibility of sexual abuse in the child's life. She might offer the child an opportunity to talk about possible abuse but in the absence of more evidence a report is not indicated. A consideration of possible child abuse does not always constitute a reportable event. But it might sensitize the doctor to look for evidence that could be essential in protecting the child.

With medical child abuse, it is possible we have set the bar too high. McClure[17] comments that physicians in England delay reporting until they are almost certain the child's life is in danger. There are obvious reasons for this. It takes a major effort to step outside the dance and declare treatment previously given as health-promoting to be potentially life-threatening. Beyond the doctor's own issues, we have witnessed the confusion currently present in the medical, the child protection, and the legal communities about what constitutes medical child abuse. We can only hope that it will get easier to take the next step after identification and develop the means of stopping medical abuse.

Covert Video Surveillance

Before proceeding to discuss issues in stopping the abuse we want to consider one other issue in identifying medical child abuse. No issue in the field has generated more controversy then the use of covert video surveillance (CVS) as a diagnostic tool. Curiously, one of the early case reports invoking the MSBP construct involved a child who was videotaped being maltreated by her mother. Epstein[18] reported that a mother was videotaped giving a laxative to her child in the hospital. That same year Southall and colleagues[19] published the first 2 accounts of the use of covert video surveillance of mothers suspected of smothering their infants. Almost immediately[20,21] the debate began in the British medical literature that has persisted for many years regarding the ethical underpinnings of videotaping a mother with her child without her knowledge.

Southall and colleagues[22] went on to develop a detailed protocol for videotaping parents suspected of smothering their children. They published several other accounts including the influential report in *Pediatrics*[23] describing 39 cases in which 33 parents or caregivers were directly observed harming their children via a covert system including videotape recordings, many of which were subsequently used in legal proceedings. The videotape recordings themselves were powerful evidence that the children were at risk for further harm from their parents if allowed to go home with them.

However, from the very beginning, discordant voices were raised about whether such observation was ethical or moral. Over the years a number of arguments have been put forth. For example, Evans[24–26] argued that CVS is an experimental procedure, a research protocol, and anyone wanting to use CVS should therefore ask the appropriate institutional review board for permission to proceed, and develop a procedure for informed consent of all those participating. Of course, having a parent give informed consent to be videotaped eliminates the possibility that they could be videotaped without knowing it. Southall and Samuels[27] responded to this line of reasoning by saying that they presented their protocol to the appropriate hospital ethics committee and institutional review process and were reassured that the procedures were both ethical and not considered research. The authors went on to explain that CVS was a diagnostic test, in the best interests of the child, and had been well established as a standard part of medical practice.

Others[28] maintained that CVS violates the privacy of the parent. The counterargument to this stance is that parents visiting or taking care of their children in a hospital setting do not have an inherent right to privacy because they are participating in an effort to help their child get well and have given implicit and written permission to the hospital to do what is necessary for that to happen.[29]

A third argument against CVS involves issues regarding entrapment. Those using this approach state that once a medical team has determined there may be a suspicion of abusive behavior, creating a situation that would allow such behavior to be videotaped is, at best, unethical in its own right and, at worst, somehow encouraging parents to commit illegal acts.

Dozens of authors have entered into this discussion from both sides of the debate. The central issue seems to be around whose rights are most important. Is there a significant right of a parent not to be observed in a hospital setting in a way that would allow them later to be arrested and charged with a crime? Are doctors and hospital staff guilty of falsely representing themselves to parents as helping their children while in fact they are promoting a situation that could be harmful to the parent? Or is the child's right to be protected from harm more important than the rights of the parent? What if the only sure way to obtain the irrefutable evidence needed to protect the child is through the use of CVS?

There is no getting around the fact that a videotape showing a parent putting a pillow over a child's mouth until the child turns blue makes the task of decisively protecting the child much more straightforward. We have commented previously that child maltreatment in most of its forms is seldom observed by a third party, and having a witness to the abuse is rare. Covert video surveillance allows there to be a witness.

Conceptualizing MSBP as medical child abuse clarifies the issue about whose rights are more important. We are more concerned about the rights of the child than we are for the rights of a potentially abusing adult.[30] While the rights of an accused individual are important, and we must always guard individual liberties, over and over again society has made a determination that protecting children who, by definition, cannot protect themselves takes precedence over the right to privacy of an adult caring for that child.

Having said this, in no other form of child maltreatment would we consider placing the child in harm's way to make sure of our diagnosis. The child we suspect has been shaken violently by a parent is not sent home with that parent with a video camera hidden in the closet. If we think a child is being sexually abused we do not send her to the abuser's apartment with a tape recorder in her pocket. We take what steps we deem necessary given the information available. It is reasonable to conclude that the same general principles should apply to situations where recurrent suffocation is suspected.

There are other things to consider before entering into a program of CVS. It is difficult to do it right. In the early days Southall and his team had a policeman sit in an adjoining room watching the child's crib and the mother in attendance. This sometimes required several days of around-the-clock observation by a police officer. Subsequently, the police officer was replaced by nurses who were prepared to intervene at a moment's notice if they saw potentially harmful behavior in the next room. Installing a hidden camera and attaching it to a video recorder that is unsupervised is clearly unethical. The abuse observed when the videotape is replayed 2 hours later has already occurred and, at that time, it might be too late to protect the child. Hence, anyone entertaining CVS must be prepared for 24-hour monitoring and have procedures in place for immediate intervention. Despite suggestion by Hall et al[31] that every tertiary care children's hospital be prepared to conduct CVS, the commitment is a major one and not within the means of many institutions. This leaves everyone who does not do CVS at a significant disadvantage, as a defense attorney can easily argue that the hospital did not videotape the abuse so it must not have happened. The opposite can also be argued. If physicians suspect a mother is medically abusing her child and set up CVS to observe her, what if no episodes of abuse are recorded? Does this mean the physicians should then abandon their efforts to protect the child?

While we defend CVS as ethical and moral as a diagnostic procedure, the idea that medical child abuse can only be diagnosed in the presence of videotaped evidence is completely unsupportable. For this reason we maintain that identifying child abuse in all its forms is basically the same; it is based on good medical practice and procedures, using the best evidence available. When a reasonable suspicion that child maltreatment is occurring is reached, the medical community is charged and expected to do its part in seeing that it is stopped.

References

1. Morley CJ. Practical concerns about the diagnosis of Munchausen syndrome by proxy. *Arch Dis Child*. 1995;72(6):528-529; discussion 529-530
2. Jenny C, Roesler TA, Barron CE. *Munchausen Syndrome by Proxy* [audiotape, Pediatric Update Series]. Elk Gove Village, IL: American Academy of Pediatrics; 2002
3. Guandolo VL. Munchausen syndrome by proxy: an outpatient challenge. *Pediatrics*. 1985;75(3):526-530
4. Meadow SR. Munchausen syndrome by proxy. *Med Leg J*. 1995;63(Pt 3):89-104
5. Meadow SR. Who's to blame—mothers, Munchausen or medicine? *J R Coll Physicians Lond*. 1994;28(4):332-337
6. Eminson DM, Postlethwaite RJ. *Munchausen Syndrome by Proxy Abuse: A Practical Approach*. London, UK: Arnold; 2001
7. Sanders MJ, Bursch B. Forensic assessment of illness falsification, Munchausen by proxy, and factitious disorders, NOS. *Child Maltreat*. 2002;7(2):112-124
8. Guarnero RA. A case of Munchausen syndrome by proxy presenting as a medical negligence action. *J Healthc Risk Manag*. 1999;19(2):33-39
9. Meadow R. Management of Munchausen syndrome by proxy. *Arch Dis Child*. 1985;60(4):385-393
10. Meadow R. Munchausen syndrome by proxy. The hinterland of child abuse. *Lancet*. 1977;2(8033):343-345
11. Kurlandsky L, Lukoff JY, Zinkham WH, Brody JP, Kessler RW. Munchausen syndrome by proxy: definition of factitious bleeding in an infant by 51Cr labeling of erythrocytes. *Pediatrics*. 1979;63(2):228-231
12. Clark GD, Key JD, Rutherford P, Bithoney WG. Munchausen's syndrome by proxy (child abuse) presenting as apparent autoerythrocyte sensitization syndrome: an unusual presentation of Polle syndrome. *Pediatrics*. 1984;74(6):1100-1102
13. Sullivan CA, Francis GL, Bain MW, Hartz J. Munchausen syndrome by proxy: 1990. A portent for problems? *Clin Pediatr (Phila)*. 1991;30(2):112-116
14. Rosenberg DA. Web of deceit: a literature review of Munchausen syndrome by proxy. *Child Abuse Negl*. 1987;11(4):547-563
15. Price CE, Rona RJ, Chinn S. Height of primary school children and parents' perceptions of food intolerance. *Br Med J (Clin Res Ed)*. 1988;296(6638):1696-1699
16. Roesler TA, Barry PC, Bock SA. Factitious food allergy and failure to thrive. *Arch Pediatr Adolesc Med*. 1994;148(11):1150-1155
17. McClure RJ, Davis PM, Meadow SR, Sibert JR. Epidemiology of Munchausen syndrome by proxy, non-accidental poisoning, and non-accidental suffocation. *Arch Dis Child*. 1996;75(1):57-61

18. Epstein MA, Markowitz RL, Gallo DM, Holmes JW, Gryboski JD. Munchausen syndrome by proxy: considerations in diagnosis and confirmation by video surveillance. *Pediatrics*. 1987;80(2):220-224
19. Southall DP, Stebbens VA, Rees SV, Lang MH, Warner JO, Shinebourne EA. Apnoeic episodes induced by smothering: two cases identified by covert video surveillance. *Br Med J (Clin Res Ed)*. 1987;294(6588):1637-1641
20. Zitelli BJ, Seltman MF, Shannon RM. Munchausen's syndrome by proxy and its professional participants. *Am J Dis Child*. 1987;141(10):1099-1102
21. Frost JD Jr, Glaze DG, Rosen CL. Munchausen's syndrome by proxy and video surveillance. *Am J Dis Child*. 1988;142(9):917-918
22. Southall DP, Samuels MP. Guidelines for the multi-agency management of patients suspected or at risk of suffering from life-threatening abuse resulting in cyanotic-apnoeic episodes. North Staffordshire Hospital Trust, Staffordshire Social Services and Staffordshire Police. *J Med Ethics*. 1996;22(1):16-21
23. Southall DP, Plunkett MC, Banks MW, Falkov AF, Samuels MP. Covert video recordings of life-threatening child abuse: lessons for child protection. *Pediatrics*. 1997;100(5):735-760
24. Evans D. Covert video surveillance in Munchausen's syndrome by proxy. *BMJ*. 1994;308(6924):341-342
25. Evans D. The investigation of life-threatening child abuse and Munchausen syndrome by proxy. *J Med Ethics*. 1995;21(1):9-13
26. Evans D. Covert video surveillance—a response to Professor Southall and Dr. Samuels. *J Med Ethics*. 1996;22(1):29-31
27. Southall DP, Samuels MP. Reply to Dr. Evans re covert video surveillance. *J Med Ethics*. 1996;22(1):32
28. Morgan B. Spying on mothers. *Lancet*. 1994;344(8915):132
29. Yorker BC. Covert video surveillance of Munchausen syndrome by proxy: the exigent circumstances exception. *Health Matrix Clevel*. 1995;5(2):325-346
30. Gillon R. Covert surveillance by doctors for life-threatening Munchausen's syndrome by proxy. *J Med Ethics*. 1995;21(3):131-132
31. Hall DE, Eubanks L, Meyyazhagan LS, Kenney RD, Johnson SC. Evaluation of covert video surveillance in the diagnosis of munchausen syndrome by proxy: lessons from 41 cases. *Pediatrics*. 2000;105(6):1305-1312.

Chapter 10

Stopping the Abuse

Medical treatment of the child is the first priority and often is only possible on separation from the parent. The second task is to create an umbrella of protection, including the mobilization and coordination of pediatric, psychiatric, social and legal services. —Palmer and Yoshimura, 1984[1]

Introduction

Stopping the abuse means ending harmful medical treatment. This can happen only when people administering the treatment realize that it is based on false information and decide to undo any damage that may have occurred. Needless to say, this is easier said than done. We have talked about the tipping point where the relationship between doctor and patient undergoes scrutiny and open trust is replaced with healthy skepticism. This is a cognitive process, a rational step that is essential for good medical practice, but it is also emotionally wrenching. Remember, it is usually not just one individual medical practitioner who needs to make this shift, but sometimes an entire medical team or institution. How does one go from providing medical care previously assumed to be appropriate, health giving, and in some cases lifesaving, to not giving medical care for exactly the same reasons? This is the first task facing medical care professionals once they have identified medical child abuse.

Building a Consensus

Reevaluating a child's care usually starts with one person on the medical team raising concerns. It might be a nurse, a resident physician, a new attending, or even a ward clerk who introduces the first element of doubt. Needless to say, if the team has been practicing primary prevention and including the possibility of a broken medical contract in the differential diagnosis, much harmful care can be avoided. But once care based on false information has begun it can continue for a long time. In all cases the direction of treatment must be brought to a halt before it can be reversed. The comments of one person introducing doubt may be insufficient to begin the reversal. Even in a primary care physician's office medical care delivery is a group endeavor. A primary care physician has office staff, nurses, partners, and covering physicians who take part in the ongoing care of her patients. One person on the team, even the pediatrician herself, can be "out voted" by the rest and the needed change in treatment can go by the wayside.

The doubt introduced into the medical care system should be given careful scrutiny, discussed, and considered by all members of the team. Many times the doubt is short-lived as new information becomes available that supports prior treatment. Usually the treatment contract with the child and his or her family is not really broken. However, sometimes the doubt is justified but then gets put aside without thoughtful examination. The opinion of a nurse with extensive experience with a particular case can be disregarded when someone else on the team says, "I've known this mother for years and she would never do such a thing." The tipping point is never reached. One of the authors (CJ) has had just such an experience. In the case of the boy who was abused by his mother multiple times in the hospital when she caused him to aspirate soft drinks, a nurse contacted Dr Jenny, who was head of the child protection team at a treating hospital. The nurse said she was very concerned that the mother was hurting the child. Dr Jenny approached the attending physician in the intensive care unit with these concerns and asked if he wanted help. The attending responded briskly that the child had a serious, chronic lung disease and that the child protection team was not welcome to come to the intensive care unit (ICU) to review the case. The medical abuse of the child then continued for several weeks until Dr Leland Fan became the attending and made the correct diagnosis.

The more people that are involved, the more difficult it is to bring a halt to harmful practices. This was noted as early as 1986 when Waller[2] wrote his paper regarding the difficulties in treatment of Munchausen syndrome by proxy (MSBP). He commented that a mother he was treating was able to invoke 5 other physicians who would dispute his claim that the treatment was unnecessary.

For the abuse to stop, the entire treatment team, or a substantial portion of it, must come to the same general conclusion about the necessity for change. If the team is split with some parties arguing for a reevaluation of whether to trust the information provided, while others are content to continue to treat the child based on that information, it is almost impossible to bring the abuse to a halt.

Understandably, leadership is required for the medical care delivery team to take a fundamentally new direction. It is unreasonable to assume that a perceptive ward clerk calling attention to troublesome behaviors can change the direction of an entire treatment team. The primary care physician can assume this leadership role, or a respected consulting physician or a primary nurse in charge of a child's care. But the person who is organizing the new way of thinking must have the respect of the team and the authority to motivate people to reconsider the information used to dictate treatment.

The most difficult situation arises when there are multiple attending physicians, all of whom have strong opinions. We were recently asked to consult with a hospital team struggling with the care of a young child. The child had spent many months in the hospital for a variety of medical conditions. Eventually, a staff member made an anonymous child abuse report to the local child protection agency. When the agency's investigator went to the hospital he found the team in complete disagreement about whether the child was receiving appropriate or abusive care. Some of the involved attending physicians were ready to entertain the idea of medical abuse but others were just as adamant that even considering abuse constituted a "witch hunt." The primary care pediatrician and state agency together requested an outside consultation. Our review revealed that while the child had real underlying medical illness, the insistence on more aggressive care by his mother had resulted in numerous procedures and treatments that were completely unnecessary. In fact, some of the care given was life-threatening. Over the years the hospital staff had developed a close relationship with this family, and while attending physicians, house staff, and nursing staff all had issues with the care-seeking behaviors of the parents, they were unable to conceive that these behaviors were putting the child at risk. As outside consultants we met with the hospital staff on several occasions and provided the documentation from their own medical records that convinced a significant majority of the medical team to begin reconsidering the child's care.

It is not easy to cause a group of people thinking in one direction to change their perspective. Doctors like to think they are rational. Most physicians embrace at least the idea of evidence-based medicine. However, many pediatricians and family physicians always consider information gathered from parents as reliable evidence when, on occasion, this may not always be the case. Bringing a halt to abusive treatment requires questioning the very sources of information traditionally used to make treatment decisions. In a reasonable world, doctors would have constant permission to reevaluate their sources. Peers and patients alike would reward them for maintaining an open attitude regarding data sources and for being willing to reexamine the medical contract. In everyday practice, as much as physicians might want to consider themselves to be rational, emotions can get in the way. Questioning the medical contract and suspecting that parents might not be playing by the rules can be experienced as threatening. Emotionally, raising the question opens the door to feelings of betrayal. Indeed, even *asking* the question implies that the previous level of trust is no longer operational. In an earlier chapter we discussed how the emotional response to feeling betrayed leads to focusing on the perpetrator rather than on practicing good medicine on behalf of the child.

One can change the beliefs of a group of people by offering them a new set of facts that are inconsistent with their previous beliefs. However, introducing a new emotional element can also change beliefs. This has been one of the functions of the MSBP concept. If the medical care team has been trusting, supportive, and accepting of a parent, labeling the parent with MSBP may allow the group to exchange their positive feelings for negative ones, to be unsupportive and unaccepting. The emotional stance of the group shifts from acceptance to rejection and the unnecessary care can be brought to a halt. If the parent previously considered saintly is now characterized as a scheming liar, then the treatment team can find a quick justification for changing direction. Sometimes what cannot be accomplished using reason can come to pass based on pure emotion.

The last thing we want to do is to engage in "witch hunts." What we really want to accomplish is to practice good medicine and to institute an empathic but rational approach to the child's care. It is not necessary to have a scapegoat, a negative object, to bring harmful care to an end and to begin appropriate medical care. Nevertheless, the temptation to respond emotionally is difficult to overcome. It is the responsibility of the leaders of the team to make sure that good medical practice comes first.

In the previous chapter we discussed how abuse in the medical setting can only be identified if someone is able to think that it might be occurring. For the abuse to come to a halt the medical team needs to arrive at a consensus that harmful medical care is indeed taking place. Without the entire team or a significant portion of the team agreeing, the next step in the process cannot and should not be attempted. Bringing a treatment process to a halt is not an easy thing to do. Many people may be invested in one aspect of the treatment or another. It is a much more complicated process than, for example, starting a different antibiotic. Different members of the team will be at different stages in their awareness of the problem. Physicians accustomed to directing treatment may take umbrage to having that treatment questioned. So, even if one physician decides to end abusive medical care, nothing will have changed unless the entire treatment team acts in concert.

The conversion from the old treatment strategy to the new one is a particularly vulnerable time for everyone. Facts are reexamined. Beliefs are challenged. Both medical care givers and recipients can feel rejected or dismissed. In this chapter we offer suggestions about how to negotiate the necessary reevaluation process.

The first step is to bring the team together to consider a new treatment strategy, and to develop a plan to stop the harmful care. The next step is to communicate with the child and the child's family the new course of treatment. The family needs to be brought around to accept the new approach, and encouraged to join the team in its new direction.

Recently we followed these steps to protect a young child who had several unexplained bacterial infections in her bloodstream over a 6-week period. Janis was a 4-year-old with pressure equalization (PE) tubes in her eardrums. The tubes had been placed to treat her recurrent inner ear infections. She developed an external ear infection. She was treated with antibiotics topically, then orally, and when this was unsuccessful, she was admitted to a community hospital to receive intravenous antibiotics. Janis would seem to get better for a few days and then, once again, would have an exacerbation of her illness with pus draining from her ears. Her otolaryngologist operated on her mastoid, thinking that an underlying mastoid infection was causing the persistent drainage from her ears. He was surprised to find little pathology in her mastoid. She then received a central venous line to provide access for her continuing intravenous antibiotics.

After several weeks in the outlying hospital she was transferred to our facility. At first she was treated on a general medical floor. However, she became quite ill with a bloodstream infection (sepsis) and was transferred to the ICU. While in the ICU she made a rapid recovery. After transferring back to the general medical service she developed another bloodstream infection.

Her mother was with her constantly. Janis's mother commented on several occasions that she had not left the hospital even to take a shower for weeks at a time. At the 5-week mark of her hospitalization, including the time spent in the previous hospital, the infectious diseases specialist raised the issue that the multiple episodes of sepsis might be a product of contamination of her intravenous access port. This doctor was not convinced that the child's mother was inducing illness despite the curious pattern of infections with multiple organisms for which she had been treated over the course of the 6 weeks. But he put the question to the medical team involved in the child's care. The primary care physician had known the family for years. She said that she had never suspected Janis's mother of causing her children to have unnecessary care but was willing to entertain the idea and asked for a child protection team consult.

By this time a number of physicians including interns and residents had been involved in the child's care. Several nurses had developed a close relationship with the mother. The child protection physician interviewed staff, spoke to the mother, and reviewed medical records. The most prominent feature of the record review was the almost complete recovery of the child while in the glass bowl environment of the ICU where she was continually observed by nurses. However, another significant factor involved Janis's older brother. He had a history of bowel disease dating back to 6 weeks of age. He was being treated by a specialist in a nearby city who had scheduled him for a cecostomy operation. When we contacted the gastrointestinal specialist he confirmed that he had been puzzled for several years about the lack of response to treatment by this young man. He felt that, given the lack of response, surgery was his only option.

At this point everyone involved in the treatment of this child knew about the suspicions of abuse. The child protection team organized a meeting of all the medical personnel to discuss the medical evidence. At the meeting there was cautious concern but no immediate consensus. None of the nurses had specific evidence that would point to contamination of the central line. The infectious diseases experts confirmed that Janis should have responded to antibiotics any of a number of times and should no longer be in the hospital. The consensus was building but was not yet at a point where the medical team could take a unified stance. The plan that everyone could agree on was to introduce an observer to sit in the room with the patient and her mother 24 hours a day. The mother was told that the observer's job was to make sure the child's central line was adequately cared for.

The day the 24-hour observer was instituted our young patient began to improve. Her temperature returned to normal within 12 hours and the recurrent infections came to a halt. After 3 days the treatment team concluded there was sufficient evidence to indicate the mother had induced illness in the child. By then, Janis was totally normal and was ready to go home. The medical treatment team, including the primary care pediatrician, had reached a consensus that she was in significant danger if she were left with her mother. We took the evidence to our hospital child protection team meeting. That meeting was attended by representatives from the Attorney General's office and the state child protective services agency. As a result of that meeting, the child was determined to be "at imminent risk of harm," and was placed in the custody of the state so she would not be removed from the hospital by her parents. In retrospect, it became obvious that the child's persistent external ear infections that caused her initial hospitalization were most likely due to her mother putting a foreign substance in her ear, which traveled through the PE tube in the ear drum into the middle ear.

From the initial concern by the infectious diseases specialist, to the growing consensus of the hospital medical staff, to the formal consultation with the child protection physicians, to the deliberation of the child protection team and state agencies, there remained one more step. We had to inform the mother and father of our new knowledge about what was causing the child to be ill and what needed to happen for her to be safe.

The Informing Session

The event in the treatment process when the medical care team communicates to the family the change in treatment strategy is referred to as the *informing session*. Given the continuum of presentations of medical child abuse there is no one formula for such a session; there are, instead, as many different ways of doing this as there are patients and families. As one progresses up the spectrum of seriousness of harm to children, the specific issues change but the fundamental process is the same. It is necessary for the doctor and treatment team to communicate clearly what they think constitutes reasonable treatment given the new facts available. It is then the job of the family to respond to this information in a way that confirms that a treatment contract is in place, and that everyone is in basic agreement about what needs to happen. Usually, when one goes to the doctor, this negotiation happens more or less automatically. The doctor examines the patient, makes a diagnosis, suggests a treatment, and the patient says, "OK." While treatment contracting can be done almost instinctively, it can also be made into a deliberate act.

Early on, clinicians discussed "confronting" mothers accused of MSBP. Quickly, professionals recognized the need to generate a positive treatment relationship with parents and that confrontation was more likely to alienate families than to lead to accepting a new healthy approach to the child's medical care. For example, Meadow[3] stated, "Subsequently the aim is not so much to get the family to look back on what was really happening but to look forward to the future and feel good about the positive steps they're taking."

Prior to the informing session, the treatment team has to speak with one voice. If the treatment team has come to a clear realization of the need to take a new direction, the task of communicating this to the family is much easier. Take a common situation where a parent advocates for excessive treatment for her child. An example might be a mother insisting that her daughter with a sprained ankle be prescribed a wheelchair to go to school, when crutches or a soft supportive boot would be sufficient. With a particularly insistent parent the course of least resistance might be to order a wheelchair "only for a few days" with the understanding that most people get tired of being in wheelchairs quite quickly and revert to walking upright. However, if the team has determined that this mother overreacts to symptoms to a degree that her child is suffering significant negative consequences, then it is necessary to take special care to spell out the treatment contract to the parent and ask for her agreement with the plan.

One could imagine the following conversation.

Doctor: "Good news. The x-rays are negative. Even though she is in pain, it's a sprain not a break."

Mother: "When my aunt sprained her ankle she was in a wheelchair for three months! Mary is so sensitive to pain. How long do you think she will need a wheelchair?"

Doctor: "Actually, I discussed this with my orthopedic colleague and we are in complete agreement that Mary will heal faster without the wheelchair."

Mother: "Are you sure?"

Doctor: "Absolutely. Promise me you will give her Tylenol in the morning as you send her off to school in her soft boot with crutches"

Mother: "OK."

Communicating clearly what is in the best medical interest of the child may be all that is necessary to avoid harmful medical care. In a more complicated situation, conducting a specific diagnostic test and communicating that we are seriously listening to the concerns of parents can lead to family acceptance of a new course of treatment. Frank was an 11-year-old boy with asthma who was hospitalized on numerous occasions. His primary difficulty was failing to adhere to usual and customary treatment for his asthma. However, his mother was convinced that his hospitalizations resulted from exposure to eggs. Her misplaced belief resulted in her son not getting the treatment he really needed.

In fact, her conviction regarding allergy to eggs was so strong that she had not allowed them into her house in any form for 10 years. She checked every label of every product in the store to make she brought home nothing containing egg. She was convinced that if he touched an egg in its shell that he would have an asthma attack. She agreed to allow us to test this premise after we assured her that we had the ability to respond to a catastrophic allergic reaction. In fact, we opened the emergency crash cart and prepared several epinephrine syringes should he have a severe reaction to contact with eggs. We cut 2 wrist-sized holes in a sheet of cardboard and asked him to put his hands through the holes. By doing this he was shielded from seeing what we were doing to his hands. We brushed Elmer's glue on the back of one hand and egg white on the other. He said that he felt the hand with Elmer's glue begin to itch but in fact, there was no visible local or systemic reaction to either substance. We went on to test him for allergy to egg white taken by mouth using a double-blind placebo-controlled food challenge protocol. He eventually ate the equivalent of 2 eggs with no reaction of any kind. Immediately afterward he called his mother at work to report on the experiment. "Really," she said, "it wasn't supposed to come out that way. I guess you are not allergic to eggs." We were able to build on this success to motivate his mother to work with us to get Frank to adhere to his prescribed treatment. We redefined the treatment contract with Frank and his mother so we could work on something we could actually change, namely his cooperation with standard treatment.

There are clearly times, however, when the parent needs more than gentle, or even not so gentle, encouragement to see her child's medical symptoms in a new light and to begin participating cooperatively in a new course of treatment. Usually the medical team undergoing its own reevaluation will have an opportunity to discuss the case together and then predict a parent's possible response to significant new changes in treatment. The case of Alice is an example of a classic informing session.

Alice was 8 years old and had been treated for immunodeficiency, ulcerative colitis, attention-deficit/hyperactivity disorder, and seizures. She had received intravenous immunoglobulin treatments for her immunodeficiency and "frequent infections," but at the time we saw her she had been tested again and was found to have a normal immune system. By reviewing her records, we determined that she had had no more than the usual number of childhood illnesses. We observed her in our treatment program for several weeks, gathering baseline information about her level of functioning. She had occasional complaints of abdominal pain but nothing that affected her ability to participate normally in all activities. She was socially immature and could not tie her shoes, cut her food with a knife, or zip up her jacket. We concluded that her inability to do these normal 8-year-old tasks was the result of her mother not encouraging her to do them for herself. With gentle coaxing from our staff she quickly gained all of these skills.

We reviewed her medical records, consulted her past and present medical providers, and concluded that she had received potentially harmful medical care due to her mother fabricating symptoms. For example, there never was any evidence of immunodeficiency. Our experience with the family supplemented by information from the medical team led us to believe that Alice's mother would not easily be able to modify her belief in her daughter's illness. We involved the hospital child protection team and discovered that several months previously a family member had made a child abuse report anonymously because he or she thought the child was receiving too much medical care. The state child protection agency had done a brief investigation but the case had been declared unfounded. We called a meeting of the relevant medical professionals, our hospital child protection team, and a representative of the state child protection agency to discuss our options. The consensus of the team was that, contingent on the mother's response to our recommendation of significant changes in Alice's medical care, Alice might need protection from her mother. As a team, we decided to meet with Alice's mother, father, and maternal grandmother, along with the state child protection worker who had visited the family to investigate the anonymous report.

We introduced the family meeting by explaining that we wanted to review all the medical findings regarding Alice and to inform the family of our recommendations for further treatment. We said that we had very good news. We explained that in consultation with all of her past medical care providers, and based on our observations and diagnostic tests, she did not have ulcerative colitis, did not have immunodeficiency, did not have a seizure disorder, and in fact was basically a healthy child. We informed the family that she was socially immature, and behind her peers in academic functioning because of her significant absences from school. Once again, we emphasized how pleased we were to be able to give such good results. We explained that we would like the family's help in getting Alice to see herself as a healthy child and to reintegrate her into normal classroom activities. We went on to say that, now that we had a good understanding of Alice's medical condition, taking her to doctors for any of these conditions would be harmful to her and we were prepared to make sure that it did not happen. Her father beamed in appreciation, and the grandmother nodded knowingly. Alice's mother, however, sat quietly for a minute and then made a not so veiled threat to kill herself by saying, "I guess I'm not needed around here anymore."

Everyone present agreed that Alice's mother was not in a position to participate cooperatively in Alice's new treatment regimen. We sent the mother for an immediate psychiatric evaluation that resulted in her hospitalization for suicidal ideation. Alice went home in the custody of her father, and although she missed her mother, quickly began seeing herself as healthy, announcing to children at school that she was not sick anymore, and continuing to make rapid strides in socialization. The mother hired an attorney to help her regain custody of her children. The court denied her request and she was prohibited from having unsupervised contact with any of her children.

We had a follow-up meeting with the father and grandmother and asked if they were surprised at the mother's response to learning that her child was basically healthy. The grandmother said that she had been telling her daughter for years that the child was getting too much medical care. She had also tried to tell her granddaughter's doctors that the mother was not telling them the truth. She said she was not at all surprised at the reaction. Alice's father gave a similar response. He said he had been told many times by his wife to go to work and leave taking care of the children to her. He said he had long suspected that Alice was not as sick as her mother claimed but was unable to do anything about it. Shortly thereafter he filed for divorce and was awarded continued custody of the children.

In this example we see the team going through the process of suspecting abuse, reevaluating the medical facts, organizing a comprehensive approach that includes all significant treatment providers, and deciding to include social services after considering what the mother's reaction might be. After all these steps have been taken, an attempt is then made to frame the *new* approach to the child's illness in a positive way. This new approach is then presented to the family, while recognizing that the mother might not be able to accept it. If this is the case, the team should be prepared to respond to a possible negative outcome. Underlying the entire effort is the need to ensure that the child will be safe and that the abuse will be stopped.

In the case of Janis (the child with the life-threatening bloodstream infections), the informing session with the family occurred after the child had already been placed in protective custody. We felt the situation was too dangerous to risk the family leaving the hospital with the child. The child protection physician, the primary care pediatrician, and a favorite nurse met first with the father and then with both parents together. The decision to meet with the father was based on the need to assess his willingness and ability to protect his children. During this meeting, medical information was presented in a calm and thoughtful manner. The staff expressly emphasized that all of the physicians involved in treating his daughter agreed with the conclusion. The doctors explained to Janis's father that there was only one reasonable explanation for the long illness. He was told that his daughter had almost died on several occasions because his wife had purposely put spit and feces into the central line. His reaction to the information was curious. He did not become passionately defensive of his wife. In a calm, hesitant voice, he said that she had always been totally committed to the children and that he could not imagine her doing them any harm. But he said this in a way that made us feel he could be trusted to protect the children from her.

Next we invited Janis's mother to join the session. We repeated the information for her using almost exactly the same language. Her response was also curious. She said, "I never tried to hurt my daughter." She defended her actions and denied any involvement but did so without any conviction in her voice. She was told that she was not to have any contact with her children unless it was supervised by child protective services. Janis and her siblings were sent home in the custody of the father and his parents.

What You Can Expect

When the treatment team "informs" the child and his or her family that treatment will now be moving in a new direction, they are, of course, hopeful that the family will accept the plan and engage cooperatively in the new treatment process. In our experience most families are able to make this transition fairly easily. Yet some cannot do so. In the literature we find reference to all manner of responses to this fundamental change in expectation and treatment. Rosenberg[4] concluded that this was an extremely dangerous time in the life of the family. Meadow[5] responded some years later that he felt most families were able to tolerate the new information without significant danger. Authors come down on both sides of the issue. Some experts say the parents are able to accept the new information and take responsibility.[6–8] And others say that parents routinely reject the implication that false information is driving inappropriate medical treatments.[9]

Our conclusion is that many factors impact what the response will be when the medical treatment team communicates its intention to stop the medical abuse. When the abuse is caught early with only minimal harm to the child, there may be only a slight adjustment necessary in the treatment relationship between medical care providers and care receivers. When the abuse has been going on for years or even decades, there is much more at stake both for the perpetrator of the abuse, and also for the medical care providers who have been unknowingly colluding with the abuse.

One thing is certain. The manner in which the medical care team presents the shift in treatment has a great deal of impact on how the message is received. When the change is presented calmly in an empathic and rational way with well-documented supporting evidence, it is much more likely to be received positively. The presentation should be factual and non-judgmental. Likewise, when the message is given without any ambiguity, and with no split in the treatment team, there is a much greater likelihood that it will be accepted. If the informing session is done in an accusatory, blaming tone, the parents' reaction to the message is most likely to be defensive and angry in return.

Involving Social Services

In our sample only 41% of those children who met the criteria for medical child abuse became involved in the child protection system. Some may ask why this percentage is so low. Do not most laws governing child abuse in the United States use language that requires reporting any reasonable suspicion of child abuse to the authorities? The answer to this question is "yes." But in practice, mandatory reporters of child abuse always have a certain degree of discretion. Not every child who goes to school in winter without a warm coat is reported to social services as a victim of neglect. If every child with poor hygiene seen in pediatric outpatient clinics became the subject of a child neglect investigation, the system would be completely overwhelmed. When a teenager tells his teacher that his mother slapped him across the face, the disclosure sometimes justifies reporting, but sometimes not. The same is true in medical child abuse.

Having said this, there are other reasons why reporting to social services is less common in medical child abuse than in other forms of child maltreatment. We find that most medical caregivers who discover they have been the instruments of abuse would like the opportunity to reverse that process themselves. After having been unknowingly involved in harming a child, they want to do whatever they can to give the child appropriate medical care. This is consistent with putting the child's welfare first. It is in the best interest of the child to receive the appropriate medical care and to have a workable relationship between parents and care providers.

The other primary reason why more reports of medical abuse are not made is that most jurisdictions in this country are not adequately prepared to evaluate medical child abuse. Charges of neglect are far and away the most common reports investigated by protective services. Physical abuse is next most frequent, with sexual abuse representing approximately 10% of all reports to social services. While we do not have accurate information regarding the prevalence of medical abuse, it is safe to say that reports of this form of maltreatment are unusual compared to other forms of child maltreatment. As a result, there is little preparation by the child protection supervisory or line staff about how to approach these cases. In addition, the judicial system is equally unprepared to understand how a child can be harmed in this particular way and what steps need to be taken to prevent it from happening.

Understandably, physicians and other medical care personnel who suspect a child is being harmed medically by parents or caretakers have reservations about exposing the family and their own medical involvement to a system that may not be able to give appropriate consideration to the complexity of the situation. Because of this only the most extreme cases ever come to the attention of the child protection community. We cited previously a survey[10] of pediatricians in Great Britain finding that they "…do not make this diagnosis on tenuous evidence but do so only when they feel there is a very high probability of abuse." This is a much greater degree of certainty than would be appropriate in responding to most mandatory reporting statutes in the United States.

As our understanding of other forms of child maltreatment matured, as we became familiar with the characteristics of physical abuse and sexual abuse, the comfort in reporting became greater and the partnership with social services on behalf of children grew commensurately. Previously we noted that our own experience is moving in this direction. We are reporting medical abuse more frequently and receiving more useful support from state agencies. We assume a similar process will take place nationally as medical child abuse becomes better understood.

But we are talking about child abuse. Child maltreatment is the responsibility of the entire community and not just the medical establishment. There are clearly situations that require a response by the child protection community. We have been discussing how to stop the abuse. The process begins with our own medical judgment, the appreciation of the appropriateness of prior care given, and the need for new medical care treatment plans. It continues with the development of a new treatment contract with the family that takes into account the new medical information and the change in treatment strategy. When it is clear, or highly likely, that the family is unable to enter into a revised, appropriate, doctor-patient relationship, and we suspect the child will continue to be harmed by medical care, a report to child protective services is absolutely necessary.

Many communities and hospitals have a functioning child protection team (CPT). A CPT is a group of people who meet regularly to communicate across disciplines about children in need of protection. The typical team has representatives from nursing, medicine, social work, social service agencies, and police or prosecutors. This is the natural place to bring concerns regarding medical child abuse. Addressing a concern about a particular child to a CPT is not the same thing as making a formal child abuse report. The CPT allows for discussion from many points of view both prior to and after a formal report. The discussion at the CPT meeting may well result in a child abuse report being made. The advantage of the CPT is that complex situations such as those present in medical child abuse cases can be discussed by a group of people who regularly communicate with one another. The result is that one's concerns can get an objective hearing and a plan for ongoing action can be outlined.

Someone taking a concern about medical child abuse to the CPT should be prepared to discuss the situation in a clear, objective manner with specific evidence of medical care given that was not required, and how the mother or caretaker instigated the harmful care. The first few times a discussion of medical child abuse occurs at the CPT meeting someone will undoubtedly ask if this is MSBP. We routinely say that we find it more helpful to talk about the child abuse that is taking place and then discuss specifically the harm being done to the child. While a discussion of the motivation of the caretaker to commit abuse is always appropriate, we are more interested in what the CPT feels about the need to protect the specific child.

It is much more likely that a CPT will understand the complexity of a medical child abuse case compared to a single caseworker at the state agency who investigates many cases of neglect or physical abuse each week. Nevertheless, members of the CPT are charged with the responsibility to look at each child's situation from as many points of view as possible. It is important for the team to raise questions. The CPT process sets the stage for the involvement of the child protection agency in the case. It is probable that a representative from the state child protection agency will be a member of the CPT and can be the liaison to his or her colleagues in the agency.

When involving child protection in a medical child abuse case, we have the same goal in mind as with any other form of child maltreatment. Our first objective is to stop the abuse. If that can happen without state involvement, all the better. If there is any significant doubt, however, that the abuse will stop, having the backing of the state legal establishment can ensure the child avoids further harm.

One of the first decisions to be made, similar to that involving other serious forms of child abuse, is whether the parent should be prevented from having contact with the child. If the child is in the hospital, in many states a physician can invoke a temporary legal status where the parent is not allowed to visit the child. In our state this is referred to as "putting a hold" on the child. It is a legally sanctioned process that stops the parent from removing the child from the hospital against medical advice, and must be reconsidered by the family court within 72 hours. The doctor makes a medical decision that having the child be exposed to the parent would be unhealthy. In other jurisdictions, the doctor does not have the authority to put the child in the temporary custody of the state. There, a judge makes the decision with advice from physicians and child protection workers.

Once a decision is made that a protection order must be filed to guard the child, the function of the physician and the medical community becomes one of providing information, support, and medical advice to the larger child protection network. It is possible that a physician who involves the child protection services of the community to stop medical child abuse can no longer maintain a therapeutic relationship with the child and the child's family and care must be transferred to someone else. While this does not happen frequently, it is the price that sometimes must be paid to ensure that the child is no longer harmed in the medical setting. Once again, this can happen when making any report of child maltreatment. The best interests of the child come first.

Need for a Family Systems Response—A Team Effort

We think stopping child maltreatment is a family matter. It's the family's responsibility to keep children safe. If a family does not have the ability, the resources, or the will to provide for the safety of its children, it is unacceptable to allow the children to go without the safety they require. So the next step is to make the family bigger and add resources until safety can be guaranteed. We have seen evidence of this in the discussion of how to stop medical child abuse. The question is not whether child abuse should be stopped, but what resources need to be brought to bear for that to happen.

Fortunately, most families do a good job providing for the safety of their children. For some families there may be a temporary period when they need more support from extended family members, friends, or community or professional resources. Most health issues of children can be addressed without ever seeing a doctor. Most children are basically healthy and require only well-child care, vaccinations, and a few medical visits to get treatment for minor illnesses. When a family decides that special medical care is needed to provide for the health of a child, it enters into a partnership with a medical care provider. Within that partnership a child receives the care it needs and then returns to the family until some future time when the partnership is called on once again.

Medical child abuse occurs when the partnership becomes flawed. In these unusual instances, the child receives medical care that he or she does not need. It is the responsibility of the medical care provider to recognize this fact, and to renegotiate the partnership with the family. This is how physicians help families provide for the medical safety of their children. If, as medical care providers, we find ourselves unable to perform this function, unable to generate and maintain a stable partnership with the family, then we need to bring in more resources. We need to make the group taking responsibility for the care of the child larger and more effective. In this chapter we have given examples of progressively larger groups enjoined to help protect the child.

An individual practitioner who is unable to enter into an effective medical partnership can bring in his colleagues, his office staff, the answering service, or anyone else involved in the treatment of the child as well as the family to reestablish a working relationship. We think of this as creating a safety net, a human interactive matrix of people willing to cooperate with one another for a common goal. In this case the goal is the medical safety of the child. To guarantee the child does not experience harm in a medical setting, we want to make the safety net as large as required to operate effectively. If this can happen within the primary care setting, all well and good. It might be necessary to extend the safety net to an inpatient or partial hospital environment to make the child safe, while recognizing that the more people who are involved, the more possibilities exist for disagreements between caregivers. Lack of cooperation among providers leads to tears in the safety net and results in an inability to keep the child safe.

When this occurs the first response needs to be repairing the net, reassessing the common goals, and finding ways for everyone on the team to work together in support of those goals. If the medical team is working well together and the child is still not protected from medical harm, the answer is to make the net larger by including the hospital CPT and possibly the child protection agency in the community.

Protecting children is the responsibility of the family. If the child is not safe, we need to make the family bigger and more effective.

References

1. Palmer AJ, Yoshimura GJ. Munchausen syndrome by proxy. *J Am Acad Child Psychiatry.* 1984;23(4):503-508
2. Waller DA. Obstacles to the treatment of Munchausen by proxy syndrome. *J Am Acad Child Psychiatry.* 1983;22(1):80-85
3. Meadow R. Management of Munchausen syndrome by proxy. *Arch Dis Child.* 1985;60(4):385-393
4. Rosenberg DA. Web of deceit: a literature review of Munchausen syndrome by proxy. *Child Abuse Negl.* 1987;11(4):547-563
5. Meadow R. Letter to the editor. *Child Abuse Negl.* 1990;14:289
6. Clayton PT, Counahan R, Chantler C. Munchausen syndrome by proxy. *Lancet.* 1978;1(8055):102-103
7. Griffith JL, Slovik LS. Munchausen syndrome by proxy and sleep disorders medicine. *Sleep.* 1989;12(2):178-183

8. Goldfarb J. A physician's perspective on dealing with cases of Munchausen by proxy. *Clin Pediatr (Phila).* 1998;37(3):187-189
9. Feldman MD. Spying on mothers. *Lancet.* 1994;344(8915):132
10. McClure RJ, Davis PM, Meadow SR, Sibert JR. Epidemiology of Munchausen syndrome by proxy, non-accidental poisoning, and non-accidental suffocation. *Arch Dis Child.* 1996;75(1):57-61

Chapter 11
Providing for Ongoing Safety

The long-term therapeutic aim is to stop the abuse and protect the child and secondly to get the mother to understand the consequences of her actions, and to try and achieve motivation for continued treatment and help. —Meadow, 1985[1]

Introduction

Identifying abuse and stopping it are the first goals of treatment. Next, we want to make sure that the child remains safe once the abuse has been brought to a halt. Then we can begin treating the physical and psychological effects of the abuse on the child. And finally, it is always a treatment goal whenever possible to preserve the family unit. These are the goals for treatment: identify it, stop it, provide for ongoing safety, treat the psychological and physical effects of the abuse, and preserve the family if at all possible.

Although we usually work on these goals sequentially, one can easily appreciate that working on one goal can help in accomplishing another. Yet not surprisingly, attempting to reach one of these goals can negatively affect our ability to achieve a different one. For example, the best way to guarantee that a child remains safe from abuse is to remove him or her permanently from an abusive environment. This, however, directly impacts the preservation of the family unit. Moreover, guaranteeing physical safety by removing a child can have the effect of magnifying the psychological harm done by the abuse. Thus we find ourselves working on multiple goals at the same time, and needing to balance progress in one area with progress or lack of movement in another.

Once again we find parallels between the treatment of medical child abuse and other types of child maltreatment. The same steps are involved. The differences are specific to the situation of each individual child and family. The child who appears in the emergency department with welts left from a beating requires the same treatment approach as the child who has experienced severe abusive head trauma needing medical life support, although the initial medical response to the case will vary. Likewise, the child fondled through her clothing deserves the same treatment strategy as the victim of serial rape. In all cases the abuse must be identified, stopped, and then addressed within its context to determine if there is a chance for reoccurrence. The effects of the abuse need to be evaluated and treated, all the while considering the integrity of the family.

Ayoub and colleagues[2] correctly identified Munchausen syndrome by proxy (MSBP) as an "interactional disorder" requiring a child victim and an adult perpetrator. Needless to say, this situation exists in all forms of child maltreatment. Still, a significant difference between medical child abuse and other forms of child maltreatment is that the same professionals asked to identify medical abuse and conduct treatment may have been previously the instrument of the abuse by the caretaker.

Make Sure the Child Remains Safe

Most experts agree that the safety of the child should be the first concern whenever dealing with suspected MSBP. If safety were our *only* concern we should consider that removal of the child from an abusive environment is the only way to guarantee safety.

So, should all children suspected of being abused medically be removed from their homes? There are many examples in the literature of children suffering significant disability due to medical child abuse. At the extreme end of the spectrum, medical abuse is a lethal form of child maltreatment. Indeed, of the 87 children in our series who met criteria for medical child abuse, 17 (19.5%) experienced potentially life-threatening events, and 2 died. In view of this it is easy to understand those who advocate for immediate and permanent removal of a child from the abusive environment. Removal of the child not only stops the abuse but also offers the potential for ongoing safety.

Because most people writing about MSBP get involved in the most serious cases it is not surprising that they frequently recommend removal of child victims from the home. Kaufman et al[3] stipulated that in all cases the child should be removed immediately. Likewise, Kinscherff and Famularo[4] have been strong advocates for removing the child, and in extreme cases recommend termination of parental rights. Rosenberg[5] wrote, "Children who are victims of Munchausen syndrome by proxy should be placed outside of the home. Doing otherwise is an act of wishful thinking, and is not based on any data which reassures us about the child's safety." Alexander[6] states, "Out of home placement should be recommended if the diagnosis is strongly suspected." Souid et al[7] wrote that once MSBP has been recognized the victim and all siblings should be removed permanently.

The question whether the child should remain in the family once abuse has been identified has been with us since the very first efforts to treat medical child abuse. In the 2 cases we discussed in the introduction to the treatment section we have examples of 2 answers to the question. Waller[8] related that the child he treated remained in the custody of his father while his mother was hospitalized, thereby effecting a temporary separation from the perpetrator. However, in the case described by Nicol and Eccles,[9] the mother, under threat of losing custody of her child, agreed to treatment and the child and mother stayed in the home. Despite the advice that separation should be considered in many or all cases of suspected medical child abuse, there are also case examples of children treated in the home environment.[10-12]

As we have observed, medical child abuse represents a spectrum of conduct from mild to severe. So, while we would agree with our colleagues that separation is absolutely necessary in some situations, in the day-to-day practice of pediatrics there will be many times when a child is suspected of being abused medically where immediate removal of the child is not required. In our sample, only 29 (34%) of the children were removed therapeutically, and in only 5 (17%) of the cases did the perpetrator permanently lose parental rights. In the 2 cases where the victims died, the medical abuse of the dead children was discovered only *after* another child in the family was determined to be medically abused.

Use the Minimum Intervention Necessary

If we are not about to take every child suspected of being abused medically from his or her home, how can we ensure long-term cessation of the abuse? It stands to reason that preventing reoccurrence of abuse is an extension of stopping the abuse and the same principles apply. It is best to use the minimum amount of intervention necessary to guarantee the safety of the child.

We must remember that the child is the primary patient, not the child's parents, or even the family unit. It is the child who has experienced harm and needs care and protection. We know that children belong in families and that there is a customary assumption that parents speak for their children; that they act in the best interests of their children. Most of the time this is correct and the welfare of the child parallels the beliefs and desires of the parents. But once we have determined that the child has been harmed or is in danger, we need to reconsider this assumption. It is no longer possible to assume that appropriate medical treatment and parents' wishes go hand-in-hand. The ultimate goal is to realign these 2 things and return medical decision-making to the parents, while ensuring ongoing safety for the child. To do so, we have to change the decisions and choices made by family members.

If we cannot guarantee the safety of the child within the context of his or her immediate family, we cannot just walk away saying, "It's your child, do what you want." Society allows wide latitude for parents raising their children. No one would question them wanting to teach manners, deciding to home school, passing on the family's religious beliefs, or defining appropriate dress standards. But in cases of medical abuse, we have already decided that the child's fundamental well-being is in danger and steps must be taken to protect the child from his or her family's actions.

This is where we apply the concept of minimum intervention necessary. At one end of the options available to the medical community in consort with social and legal institutions, the child can be separated from the family and parental rights terminated. However, there are many other potential interventions available before reaching this stage. An analogy, albeit inelegant, would be to consider a child breaking his leg in a bad motor vehicle accident. Before a surgeon decides to amputate the child's leg, there are many treatment options available to him, some of which may not even involve surgery.

In the previous chapter we offered an example of a mother who wanted her child to be in a wheelchair after the child sprained her ankle. Preventing reoccurrence of the abuse is an extension of stopping the abuse. The approach we used with this mother represents the minimum intervention. We used education. We told her that, after consulting with the other doctors involved in her care, we were convinced the girl would heal faster using a soft boot on her ankle than she would riding in a wheelchair. We countered the mother's belief that her daughter was suffering so severely that she needed to be transported painlessly with a medical fact. We told her that encouraging her to lead her life as normally as possible would be more helpful in her recovery than treating her as an invalid.

Education is a staple in medical care. Particularly in pediatrics there is a well-established tradition of giving parental guidance regarding medical conditions and child development. Many times parents ask for and receive information from their doctors and use it effectively. Of course, physicians also know that the advice they offer may not be followed. Education is a powerful tool in the medical armamentarium, but many times not an effective one. How many injunctions from physicians to lose weight, exercise, and stop smoking go unheeded? Such may well be the case when offering new information to parents who are harming their child by advocating for dangerous medical treatment. Education is an early step representing the least forceful means to bring parents around to where they are acting in the best interests of their child. If ongoing education can prevent reoccurrence of the abuse, then there is no need to use a more intrusive intervention.

The steps we offer here in the progression of efforts to stop medical child abuse are representative, not inclusive. We offer examples of interventions knowing that many others are available. For example, once a parent has received an alternative explanation that is based on established medical principles, and this has been ignored or disputed, we can assume that more influence is needed to ensure the child's safety. The next step we refer to as *persuasion*.

The basic form of a persuasive intervention goes like this: "Mrs Jones, I know you do not agree with my advice but I (we) want you to follow it anyway." The "we" in this sentence can be "your doctors," "your husband and I," "your parents, your husband, your doctors, and I," or any other combination that makes sense. Of course, for this intervention to be successful the person being asked to change her behavior must sincerely believe that everyone involved in "we" is in agreement. The most difficult part of using a persuasive intervention is lining up all of the parties doing the persuading beforehand, making sure they are in agreement and willing to stand behind the statement.

Asking someone to change his or her behavior only works if the person to whom the request is made wants to preserve the relationship with the person making the request. If a person does not care about you or anyone in the "we" position, that person will not be motivated to do what you want them to do. People are social beings and they respond to their social network. It is a rare person who can hold a belief or conduct a course of action contrary to the position held by all the significant people in their life.

Usually, we bolster our beliefs by saying either out loud or to ourselves, consciously or unconsciously, that we are right because those close to us believe in a similar way. Take, for example, a mother who believes she is being a "supermom" by allowing her child to go to school in a wheelchair. If the significant people in her life tell her that doing so indicates she is a "less than perfect mom," she may well be persuaded to change her belief and her actions.

Beliefs are powerful things. They are buttressed by logic and illogic alike. They can persist for decades and even from generation to generation. And they can, paradoxically, change overnight. In treating medical child abuse we often find we are dealing with parents who believe they are doing the right thing for their children. It is one thing to stop the abuse. It is another to prevent the abuse from reoccurring in the face of persisting parental beliefs. If we can, through education or persuasion, modify the belief system underlying the behavior of a parent that is hurting her child medically, then we have a good chance of reestablishing a partnership with the family for the benefit of the child. If neither of these strategies is successful, then we need to increase the intrusiveness of the intervention.

A stage beyond persuasion in the process of providing for the ongoing safety of the child can be called "giving a potentially painful choice." With persuasion the consequence for not allowing oneself to be persuaded is the possible loss of relationship with the person or persons asking you to change. No other possible consequence is necessarily stated. But if this is not enough to motivate a person to modify his or her beliefs and behaviors, stating other possible consequences might have more impact.

Scott was an 11-year-old boy whose mother was convinced that his unruly behavior at home was the result of porphyria. She told her pediatrician that Scott had undergone a profound personality change that could only be explained by a significant medical illness. We enrolled him in our treatment program. For the first few days, his mother had difficulty getting him up in the morning so he could arrive at the program at a reasonable time. Once she solved that problem, we found his behavior to be quite acceptable in our environment. He acted like a normal boy, although sometimes truculent, and had no episodes of abnormal behavior. We consulted an endocrinologist and did a preliminary porphyria screen that was, as expected, totally normal. We presented these results to his mother and she told us, based on her search on the Internet, that we had failed to test for several extremely rare subtypes of the disease. She also volunteered to take videotapes of his behavior at home so we could see what she was concerned about. The next day she returned with a videotape that documented Scott being provocative and disrespectful to his mother in a very calculated way. On watching the tape, it was obvious to us that he was pretending to be out of control. He walked around the living room picking up and breaking objects that belonged to his mother while leaving his own possessions totally intact.

We scheduled yet another meeting with his mother to discuss our results. As a professional who worked with children, the mother herself was a mandatory reporter of child abuse. She knew that being investigated for child abuse would not only cause her personal discomfort but also significant professional problems. Less than a minute into our meeting she said, "I bet that you are going to say that Scott's problem is all behavioral." We replied that indeed we felt his behavior was under his control. Next she said, "Don't you dare report me!" We told her that, after having considerable discussion among ourselves and with all of the doctors treating her son, we would be legally compelled to report her for child abuse if she continued taking her child to medical specialists for treatment he did not need. She stormed angrily from the office. Through ongoing contact with her primary care pediatrician, we were able to monitor that she ceased asking for excessive medical care for her son. She responded to a clear statement of possible negative consequences by choosing to keep her son safe.

For this intervention to be successful, Scott's mother had to believe that we were not just threatening her with a consequence. She needed to know, and we needed to be sure among ourselves, that we would do what we said we would do, namely report her for child abuse in the event she continued seeking inappropriate medical care. Stating possible negative consequences is more than making a threat. It constitutes outlining a course of action that will occur as a consequence of certain events. The parent is given a choice about whether to experience the consequences.

As is the case with persuasion, the important work that enhances the effectiveness of this intervention happens before it is presented to the parent. The possible negative consequences need to be agreed on by all concerned, doable, and sufficiently onerous to elicit the desired response. Threatening people offers minimal chance of long-term behavior change. Outlining and communicating a probable future environment that makes it important for the family to make a healthy choice has a much better likelihood of success.

Therapeutic responses described thus far have been aimed at parent behavior at the mild end of the spectrum of potential dangerousness for children. Scott was unlikely to die if his mother took him for another consultation with a specialist. Nor would Mary sustain any permanent harm being in a wheelchair for a few days. As the potential harm to the child was not great, interventions by the medical community could focus on reestablishing a therapeutic relationship with the parents.

The strategies suggested up to this point do not have to be conducted in partnership with the community beyond the medical care system. They do not require collaboration with the hospital child protection team, the state social service system, or other representatives of the community. However, once education, persuasion, or information regarding possible negative consequences seems unlikely to offer protection for the child, at the next level, collaboration with the larger system is almost always required.

The next step is to put into effect the negative consequences already outlined. These consequences will be specific to the situation and may include a formal child abuse report, hospitalization of the child, or any other step that is appropriate given the level of danger the child faces.

In the description of the informing session with Alice's mother, father, and grandmother, it quickly became apparent that Alice's mother would not be able to respond positively to the good news we were trying to convey. Alice's father and grandmother were ready to move ahead with us and give only appropriate medical care. However, Alice's mother responded to the news we were trying to give her by reacting as if her world was falling apart. In fact, she required an immediate psychiatric evaluation for possible suicide.

She was seen by a psychiatrist within an hour of the end of the session and quickly hospitalized. This was not a consequence outlined in advance, but it was appropriate given the unfolding circumstances. And it was consistent with the overall message that Alice was not a sickly child, that she needed to get back to a normal life, and that we were requesting and expecting help from the family to make sure that this happened. This response to the informing session was foreseen as a possibility, and we were prepared for it, having already identified a psychiatrist who was standing by to be a psychological support person for the mother.

This is an example of providing for ongoing safety by removing the perpetrator from the family environment. It can be accomplished as a voluntary step taken by the family or as a mandated process prescribed by an agency of the state. However, having an accused person leave the house is not the same thing as providing for safety. She could still be in a position to make medical decisions for the child, or influence the child's perception of medical symptoms. Within days Alice's mother was requesting that Alice visit her in the hospital, and then requested she visit her at the relative's house where she stayed after leaving the psychiatric hospital.

There are many options available aimed at guaranteeing safety. We have had family court justices mandate that only the father could take his children to the doctor or make medical decisions. In one situation a case manager for an insurance company would not authorize payment for any medical service that was not approved by the primary care physician coordinating the child's care. After running up several thousand dollars worth of uncompensated medical expenses, the family modified its use of medical services.

Using the Medical Record to Promote Ongoing Safety

We saw previously how important it is in establishing whether a child has been medically abused to have good information in the medical record. It is equally important once medical abuse has been identified to make sure that the medical record reflects the need to give ongoing appropriate medical care. Physicians are often cautious about what they document. They know that anything in the medical record can be read by the patient and might be subpoenaed for some future legal purpose. Because of this they often use innocuous language.

Once medical abuse has been identified and brought to a halt, the medical record can be a powerful tool in making sure that it cannot be resumed. We suggest using the same openness and honesty employed in the informing session when writing discharge summaries, chart notes, and letters to referring physicians. We advocate writing repeatedly in the medical record that a patient has received unnecessary medical care in the past as a result of "exaggeration or fabrication of symptoms on the part of his caretaker." We also find it very useful to document explicitly the nature of the ongoing medical contract negotiated with the parents of the child.

Here is an example of a letter we wrote to the mother of a patient. We gave her a copy, sent a copy to all the treatment providers, placed a copy in the medical record, and forwarded it as well to the director of the emergency department of our hospital.

> Dear Mrs Jones,
>
> We are writing today to summarize the treatment of your son in the Hasbro Children's Partial Hospital Program. As you know Andrew has been with us for the past 3 weeks and we have come to know him very well. We observed him closely, did diagnostic tests, and consulted with all of his prior treatment providers. As we explained to you today, we are very happy to tell you that he does not have a seizure disorder and does not require any antiseizure medications at all.
>
> We know that in the past there have been serious concerns about his health and he has been prescribed seizure medications on several occasions. We also know that at times he received overdoses of these medications and had to be admitted to the intensive care unit. Fortunately, he did not die.
>
> Because he does not have a seizure disorder there will be no need for him to have prescriptions of these medicines in the future. Of course, his neurologist, Dr Nathan, will want to see him in 6 months as a normal precaution. In the meantime, if you feel that he is experiencing something similar to what were thought to be seizures in the past and you need to take him to the emergency department, please remember to take this letter

with you. The doctors can get access to your medical record and make sure that Andrew gets exactly the treatment he needs and is exposed to no dangerous treatment that he does not need.

Sincerely,

Our intent with a letter like this is to solidify the consensus regarding treatment going forward among medical care professionals involved with the family. We also want the family to understand that it has a responsibility to work with the medical community to keep their child safe. An emergency department physician seeing this letter and reading the discharge summary from our program in the medical record is very unlikely to give an emergency treatment for a seizure disorder that has been evaluated and found not to exist. Without this documentation Andrew's mother could give a convincing history to a doctor who has not seen him before and start the cycle of prescribing unnecessary medication all over again.

Out of Home Placements to Ensure Ongoing Safety

Hospitalization of the child, either for a few days or for an extended period, represents another means of attempting to provide safety for the child. It can be the next step in the minimum intervention necessary to protect the child. It can also be part of a diagnostic plan if more information is necessary to establish a sufficient level of concern regarding protection.

Annie was 3 months old when she first came to the attention of our *ChildSafe* team. Her mother brought her to the emergency department several times saying that she was vomiting and turning blue. Each time, the child was admitted to the hospital and then sent home after no significant symptoms were observed in the hospital. After the fifth hospitalization, the child protection team was consulted. The team recommended that a staff person be assigned to observe the child and her mother continuously. For several days nothing happened. Eventually, the observer was called away for a few minutes. Almost immediately Annie's mother reported that the child vomited. Another day went by until once again the observer was out of the room for a short time. On this occasion Annie's mother called the nurses to show them how her baby had turned blue. Indeed, the child was showing signs of respiratory distress. There was every reason to believe that in the

3 minutes she was alone with the child, the mother had caused her daughter to have difficulty breathing.

In conjunction with the local child protection agency the baby was kept in the hospital and her mother was told she would have to leave. No family members were available when it came time to determine where the baby would live. It was decided that it would not be safe to have the child return to the mother so the baby was placed in foster care. Annie had no episodes of vomiting or turning blue and thrived in the foster care environment. Her mother actively tried to regain custody. Annie and her mother were evaluated at another hospital and once again it was determined that Annie would not be safe in her mother's care.

Eventually, Annie's mother's attorney arranged for an evaluation by a psychologist who concluded that she "…did not meet the profile for an MSBP mother." The lawyer and Annie's mother took this evaluation to a judge who ordered the child returned to her mother's care because she did not have MSBP. Annie's doctors were extremely apprehensive about not being able to provide for the ongoing safety of this child.

It seems logical that having the child in a semi-public environment such as a hospital should serve to decrease the potential for harm. Nevertheless, we have seen numerous cases where children have continued to be subjected to harmful medical care while hospitalized. As early as 1985, Meadow,[1] in his paper on management of MSBP, gave extensive advice about using the hospital to provide safety for a child being abused. Basically, he said that most hospitals are not equipped to keep children safe from abusive medical care or induction of symptoms by their parents. He advocated putting the child in the hospital, but only with special precautions in place such as not allowing parents to visit, or to do so only under strict supervision. Hence, many years ago he warned against having a false sense of security. Medical personnel tend to consider the hospital an extension of their personal environment. We think of the hospital as "our house," and as a place where we can control what happens. However, without special safeguards in place we have seen how children can be harmed within the medical milieu.

An account of our treatment of Alex illustrates some of the difficulty that can be experienced when using hospitalization to provide for safety. Alex was a 7-year-old with recurring mastoiditis treated with intravenous antibiotics.

After several hospitalizations he was discharged with a central intravenous access port in place and received intravenous antibiotics at home. During the course of his treatment he had several episodes of fever, chills, and positive blood cultures, indicating he was having episodes of polymicrobial sepsis (bloodstream infections with multiple bacteria at the same time). These infections were found to occur both at home and during hospital admissions. During his third hospitalization we convened a conference of his physicians and the child protection team. The goal of the meeting was to reach consensus as to whether it would be appropriate to monitor the child in the hospital to make sure his mother was not contaminating his blood through the intravenous site.

No one had ever seen the mother do anything inappropriate. Several nurses had taken part in training her how to use sterile technique while administering medications. The nursing staff concluded that the mother was competent to provide the necessary treatments. But the fact remained that this child had serious complications directly related to his indwelling line, and a possibility existed that the mother could be purposely causing the infections.

In addition to staff nurses, the social worker directly involved, and several house staff officers, there were 6 attending physicians at the meeting including a representative of the hospital ethics committee. These were senior physicians in the hospital, including several heads of departments. The discussion involved every aspect of Alex's medical history and treatment. We reviewed the child's immune status, the types of organisms with which he had been infected, and the frequency of infections. No one had direct evidence indicating that the mother caused the child to be contaminated. His primary care pediatrician said that the mother was extremely attentive to the child and had, for years, called the physician's office almost daily with medical concerns. The infectious diseases specialist concluded that contamination was the most likely cause of the pattern we were seeing. The conference ran on for almost 2 hours.

In the end, everyone except one physician agreed that there was enough evidence for possible abuse and that Alex needed protection. With this near consensus we decided to admit him to the intensive care unit and allow his mother to visit only in the presence of nurses who would be monitoring her behavior. The orders were written. The mother was informed of our decision.

Because she verbally agreed with the treatment plan we did not seek legal protection for Alex from the local child protection agency. Four hours after the meeting the physician who did not agree with the plan convinced the primary care pediatrician to transfer the child to a hospital in another city. Fortunately, our pediatric infectious diseases doctor was able to communicate with his counterparts at the new institution. The new hospital put into effect our supervisory suggestions and removed the central line within 2 days. Two years later Alex has not had any episodes of polymicrobial sepsis, but has remained a very frequent visitor to his pediatrician's office.

This example demonstrates several important points. The first is how difficult it is to keep the child safe even in the hospital. The second is how difficult it is to create a therapeutic web of safety around the child. We identified possible abuse, hospitalized the child to stop it, and then attempted to put in place a plan to guarantee ongoing safety. We decided that the minimum level of protection necessary was to supervise the mother at all times while she was with her child. We knew that to make this happen within the hospital we needed the cooperation of many people including those who wrote orders and those who worked directly with the child. The nurses were in complete support of the plan. Yet the disagreement of one physician (who was not directly involved in the child's day-to-day treatment) out of the 6 physicians was enough to allow the protective web to fall apart.

The physician in question is well known for his empathy and loyalty to patients and their parents. The parents of his patients are, likewise, extremely loyal to him. In this case, despite an infectious diseases attending giving his opinion that there could be no other cause for this infection, the medical evidence was insufficient to convince this doctor that the patient's mother should be suspected of tampering with the child's intravenous line. By engineering the transfer, he took the side of the child's mother against the group of hospital doctors and nurses, even if it meant possibly putting the child at risk.

Fundamentally, hospitalization or separation from the family cannot be considered more than a stopgap measure in protecting children from medical child abuse. We must still be prepared to do whatever it takes to guarantee the child's ongoing safety, and hospitalization may not be enough.

Medical Foster Care

Medical foster care has been suggested as an alternative to long-term hospitalization.[6] We have had positive experiences using medical foster families as a transition in the process of reunifying children with their families of origin. We cannot say enough about what foster families can accomplish in providing a normalizing environment for children who have been highly medicalized over months or years. One family we used repeatedly provided the perfect environment to complement our therapeutic efforts on behalf of several very compromised children. The mother in the foster family was a registered nurse and was able to discern between worrisome medical symptoms requiring treatment and learned behaviors that were best left unattended.

We met Dan when he was 14 years old and hospitalized with paroxysms of uncontrollable vomiting. He would vomit every half-hour for several hours and make himself severely dehydrated. Before long it became apparent that he lived in an emotionally charged home where his parents were constantly at each other's throats. Sitting in a room with the 2 parents was painful even for non-family members. The atmosphere was corrosive. In the hospital Dan would pull himself together, begin eating again, and then receive a visit from his parents, starting the vomiting cycle once more. Eventually he was being fed through a nasogastric tube and when this didn't work, he was given a weighted nasal jejunal tube. One time while his mother was visiting he began throwing up. She panicked, and tried to jerk the tube from his nose. He was discharged from the hospital to our day treatment program but his mother disagreed with everything we tried to do to help him. We concluded after only a few days that we could not guarantee his safety when he went home with his mother each day after the program.

We advocated for his hospitalization on an adolescent psychiatric unit, where he stayed for more than a year. Every time he became eligible for discharge and began having visits home, his vomiting would start anew.

During his psychiatric hospitalization, a court proceeding resulted in his being declared a victim of MSBP in a court proceeding. When it came time for him to leave the hospital and return to our partial hospital program, we called on our favorite medical foster care home. Dan attended the day treatment program during the day, lived in foster care at night, and we continued family therapy. By this time his parents were separated and we met with Dan alternately with his father or his mother. His foster family, particularly his foster mother, became an island of sanity. We were only able to guarantee his ongoing safety by knowing he could return each afternoon to an environment that was emotionally and medically stable. Eventually Dan declared his own divorce from his mother, began his long-delayed growth spurt, finished high school, and went off to college. Midway in this process he went to live with his father, saying he would resume his relationship with his mother at some future date when he felt his health would not be compromised.

Termination of Parental Rights

At times during the course of his long treatment there was a restraining order preventing his mother from contacting Dan. There was never an attempt made to terminate parental rights. When is it appropriate to have the courts declare the legal parental relationship null and void? How bad do things have to be before we entertain this final step?

Dan was already a teenager when he developed psychogenic vomiting. He was an intelligent young man, sensitive to his relationship network and, although ambivalent, able to participate in the often painful emotional process of defining his relationship with his parents. With significant help from those of us who rallied to his cause, he was eventually able to more or less protect himself. What about children without so many assets? Would we be more likely to advocate for termination of parental rights for a young child with multiple handicaps, and few or no verbal skills? Or is this precisely the child who needs to maintain a relationship with birth parents?

Early in his career Jones[13] wrote the paper, "The Untreatable Family." He defined an untreatable family as "…one in which it is unsafe to permit an abused child to live." He reviewed the available data regarding children being re-abused in families while under treatment and outlined the factors that lead to poor outcome. Perhaps the most important contribution made by this paper is this: It gives helping professionals permission to state that not every family situation is treatable. Following are the categories of families he described who do not respond well to treatment:

1. There are some families who simply will not change. They do not intend or want to change.

2. Some parents persistently deny abusive behavior in the face of clear evidence to the contrary.

3. Some families cannot change in spite of a will to do so. There may be a subgroup here of families that is willing to change but sufficient resources to help this subgroup are not available.

4. Some parents can change, but not "in time" for the child's developmental needs. For example, a 6-month-old baby's abusive parent may become less impulsive and dangerous after 2 years of treatment, but in the meantime the baby has developed a strong attachment to a surrogate parent.

5. Similarly, other parents may change in time for the next child to remain with them, but not for the index child.

6. Finally, there is the category of untreatable parents who fail to respond to one treatment approach but who may be amenable to another agency or approach.

Jones makes the point that declaring a family untreatable is not the same thing as saying the parents did not deserve treatment. While parents may deserve treatment it should not be at the expense of the child whose welfare is sacrificed on their behalf.

Defining Ongoing Safety

How do we know the child will be safe? This is a very difficult issue. Nicol and Eccles[9] addressed this question more than 25 years ago. They concluded that they needed to get objective confirmation for any claims of success of treatment, that statements by the family were a starting point but that the safety of the child required having objectives in place that could be measured. In making these comments these authors specifically noted the parallel between treatment of medical abuse and treatment of other types of child abuse.

To these comments we add that guaranteeing the safety of the child is an ongoing process. The fact that a child is safe today may say little about tomorrow. A continuous effort is needed to reevaluate the child's safety on a continuing basis. Once medical abuse is stopped, the best way for a child's ongoing safety to be monitored is have a single "medical home", where an informed primary care physician who understands the child's past problems is in charge of managing ongoing care. The medical home provides for continuity, safety, and moderation. The American Academy of Pediatrics recommends that every child with special medical needs have a medical home where he or she will get uninterrupted care for illnesses as well as preventive care.[14] This is equally important for a child who has been medically abused in the past and returned home after the doctor-patient relationship has been healthily redefined.

Many families with whom we have worked have stopped exposing their child to medical danger. Earlier we stated that successful treatment should be defined from the perspective of the child having the ability to grow in a loving and supportive environment to productive adulthood. Although not always successful, we can point to many children, like Dan, who are well on their way to achieving this goal.

References

1. Meadow R. Management of Munchausen syndrome by proxy. *Arch Dis Child.* 1985;60(4):385-393
2. Ayoub CC, Deutsch RM, Kinscherff R. Munchausen by proxy: definitions, identification, and evaluation. In: Reece RM, ed. *Treatment of Child Abuse: Common Ground for Mental Health, Medical, Legal Practitioners.* Baltimore, MD: The Johns Hopkins University Press; 2000:213-225
3. Kaufman KL, Coury D, Pickrel E, McCleery J. Munchausen syndrome by proxy: a survey of professionals' knowledge. *Child Abuse Negl.* 1989;13(1):141-147
4. Kinscherff R, Famularo R. Extreme Munchausen syndrome by proxy: the case for termination of parental rights. *Juv Fam Court J.* 1991;5:41-53
5. Rosenberg DA. Munchausen syndrome by proxy: currency in counterfeit illness. In: Helfer R, Kempe R, Krugman R, eds. *The Battered Child.* 5th ed. Chicago, IL: University of Chicago Press; 1997
6. Alexander R. Medical treatment of Munchausen syndrome by proxy. In: Reece RM, ed. *Treatment of Child Abuse: Common Ground for Mental Health, Medical, Legal Practitioners.* Baltimore, MD: The Johns Hopkins University Press; 2000:236-241
7. Souid AK, Keith DV, Cunningham AS. Munchausen syndrome by proxy. *Clin Pediatr (Phila).* 1998;37(8):497-503
8. Waller DA. Obstacles to the treatment of Munchausen by proxy syndrome. *J Am Acad Child Psychiatry.* 1983;22(1):80-85
9. Nicol AR, Eccles M. Psychotherapy for Munchausen syndrome by proxy. *Arch Dis Child.* 1985;60(4):344-348

10. Haddad E, Lapeyraque AL, de Pontual L, Landthaler G, Bocquet N, Baudouin V. Clinical quiz. Loin pain haematuria syndrome. *Pediatr Nephrol.* 2002;17(3):217-219
11. Griffith JL, Slovik LS. Munchausen syndrome by proxy and sleep disorders medicine. *Sleep.* 1989;12(2):178-183
12. Lyall EG, Stirling HF, Crofton PM, Kelnar CJ. Albuminuric growth failure. A case of Munchausen syndrome by proxy. *Acta Paediatr.* 1992;81(4):373-376
13. Jones DP. The untreatable family. *Child Abuse Negl.* 1987;11(3):409-420
14. The medical home. *Pediatrics.* 2002;110(1 Pt 1):184-186

Chapter 12
Treating the Physical Consequences

Children are inextricably involved with their families and learn not only the expression but also the experience of emotional and somatic symptoms from their family members' modes of experience and communication. If the family's mode of expressing tension or distress is through physical symptoms, including full-blown somatization disorder, the child is significantly at risk for developing more unexplained physical symptoms and more psychiatric disorders than is a child in a family that does not have this pattern. —Krener, 1994[1]

Introduction

After identifying abuse, stopping it, and working to ensure that it will not happen again, we are left with the task of treating the child's physical and psychological sequelae. This is what people often mean when they refer to "treatment of child abuse." For medical child abuse it means stopping the harmful medical treatment, ameliorating any damage done, and addressing the emotional consequences.

In this chapter and the next we face the central paradox in child abuse treatment. Must we sacrifice the child for the sake of the family or sacrifice the family for the sake of the child? In truth, we want to do neither. We want to restore the child to both physical and emotional health while maintaining a viable family in which the child can remain safe and develop normally.

Families are living collections of people bound to one another by birth, marriage, circumstance, and intense emotional bonds. Families are born, grow, change, and fall apart. People in a family face the world together, meeting challenges big and small, sometimes successfully and sometimes not. Being part of a family carries with it an obligation to other family members, and the right to draw strength from others for one's own benefit. Family members have particular roles, responsibilities, and obligations to one another.

A family is a protective cocoon within which children are nurtured and grow to adulthood. Within this environment a child comes to learn about the world, its dangers and its challenges. More than anything else the child learns to trust, to expect help from the family in negotiating his or her surroundings.

Child maltreatment occurs when parents fail in their obligation to keep children safe. The safety of children is not relegated exclusively to parents, but primarily so. Despite the best efforts of caretakers, children still can come to harm. But parents and families are the first line of defense. Parents cannot keep their children safe from every threat all the time. Children need to learn how to pick themselves up when they fall. They need to make mistakes and learn from them. But it is the family's obligation, and particularly the parents, to know when and how to protect their children from harm.

As noted earlier, abusive parenting is defined by the larger society. Most of us live in families and watch as other families around us deal with the world, each in its own way. Surely families are subunits of the larger family that is humanity. When the subunit does not function properly it affects the larger family—the society we live in. When a family fails in its duty to protect its children some of us step forward to provide assistance and, if necessary, take over the responsibility of keeping those children safe.

But before we get to this point, before we offer help or take over, the damage may already be done. A child hurt in his family not only experiences the broken bones, or emotional pain, but also feels betrayed. This betrayal is often the most important aspect—a child losing faith in the family, the primary social institution charged with helping him or her to grow and prosper. Child abuse represents a failure of a family to fulfill its most basic contract, its obligation to its children.

So how do we go about treating the physical and psychological effects of abuse? Certainly we need to fix the broken arm, reverse the consequences of the actions of parents. But we also need to reconstruct the family to its most functional state possible, reinstitute safety provisions, and somehow help the child learn to trust again.

The Hasbro Children's Partial Hospital Program

We treat medical child abuse in a specialized therapeutic environment.[2] The Hasbro Children's Partial Hospital Program (HCPHP) is a family-centered, multidisciplinary treatment setting for children with both medical and emotional needs. It functions 8 hours a day, 5 days a week. Parents bring their children each morning, as if taking them to school, and pick them up each afternoon.

Children suspected of being abused medically make up only a small portion of the patients in HCPHP. Typical patients in the program are children with diabetes, abdominal pain, eating disorders, neurologic problems, or just about any other childhood illness that can be complicated by significant emotional issues. The children we treat have often been ill for a long time. They frequently have been in and out of the hospital, or have been seen many times in an outpatient setting. Usually the child's illness has taken on a life of its own, and the entire family is organized around it. Our task is to take control of the illness and give that control back to the family.

The staff, including pediatricians, child psychiatrists, psychologists, social workers, psychiatric and pediatric nurses, nutritionists, teachers, and milieu therapists, works together to create a therapeutic environment. The staff functions as a team of people, collaborating with one another, each making his or her own contribution, and creating an atmosphere where children and their parents can make healthy choices.

We have a basic treatment model that we apply broadly but modify for each individual child. Rarely do we need to make a new diagnosis. Usually children come with clearly identified medical problems and obvious medical solutions. Unfortunately, the child and his or her family have not been able, for a host of reasons, to put treatment into effect that allows the child to lead as normal a life as possible given the medical condition. A teenager with diabetes may know how many grams of carbohydrates to eat for each meal. Her parents may know how important this is for the long-term survival of their child. Nevertheless, the diet is not followed and the child's metabolism spirals out of control. We invite the teenager and her family to join with us in taking back control. We empower the parents to help their child. We empower the teenager to take control of her illness.

When a child with suspected medical child abuse comes into the program, we approach the situation in the same way. We take medical symptoms seriously. We assess the emotional effects of the illness on the child and family. We determine what factors are keeping the family from having a normal life. We invite families to join with us in the search for a new balance between the medical symptoms and the emotional health of the family.

The program's philosophy is based on family systems theory. We believe that each family is a living entity, that events in the life of the family affect family relationships, and that family relationships affect events in the life of the family. Symptoms and behaviors coexist in a context of relationships. How family members relate to one another affects the choices they make. Each family comes to us with a set of shared beliefs, and a "narrative," a story about how they have come to be organized in general and, in particular, around the child's medical illness. We listen to and try to understand this narrative. We need to begin treatment with the family reading from the same page of the life story they relate to us.

Once we have determined to the best of our ability where the family is functioning with the illness, we offer to have the family join us in finding ways around the places where they have become stuck in the past. This process is the same with the child experiencing medical child abuse as it would be with another having pseudo-seizures, uncontrolled asthma, or functional abdominal pain. The family presents its view of reality to us. We do our best to understand it, and then we offer to incorporate their real world into our larger health-promoting context.

We tell families at the beginning of treatment that we expect the family to come away from the program organized differently, having new responses to the child's symptoms and illness and new ideas about what they can do to help. We say that we will be successful only when the family comes to believe that things will not go back to the way they were before, and that they can contend effectively at home with the challenges presented by the illness.

Because we are a medical treatment center, families struggling with medical conditions, as well as families suspected of medical child abuse, feel welcome. We speak the language of medical symptoms. We offer diagnostic tests. We read medical records. We define success in medical terms.

We tell families that we operate as a team. We say that success depends on how well the team works together. We ask the family to join the team, and we give parents responsibility as leaders of the team. We say that no decisions will be made without consensus. We stipulate that consensus is often difficult to achieve and that discussion, even including conflict, is normal between team members. We maintain that if we are not being successful at getting control of the illness, we must reevaluate how we are working together as a team and, in some cases, it is necessary to make the team larger. This means the team can eventually consist of our staff, immediate family members, extended family members, school personnel, church leaders, neighbors, friends, and specialty physicians, depending on the needs presented. In certain situations the team can even include state child protection workers.

The bigger the problem, the bigger the team will be. But the larger the team becomes the more possibility exists that there will be disagreement between team members. Success comes from consensus. Consensus results from people communicating with one another openly and honestly. Honesty is a precondition for arriving at consensus but does not guarantee that all parties will come to agree with one another. We need straightforward communication. Without it, any agreement reached is not truly binding. As staff we pay close attention to our own open and honest communication with each other, with family members, specialty care providers, and anyone else we bring into the team helping the child. We ask for clear, honest communication in return.

Because a defining characteristic of medical child abuse is the introduction of false information into the doctor-patient relationship, we can expect that establishing this collaborative relationship will be most difficult with this group of patients and their families. And it is. But it is also an ongoing issue with many of the other families we treat as well.

For example, Molly was referred to us as a teenager who had an eating disorder, namely bulimia nervosa. But because of the interactions between her mother and physicians attempting to care for her, she also was identified as a possible victim of Munchausen syndrome by proxy (MSBP). Molly swore to her mother and to her pediatrician that she was not vomiting. Her mother believed her and had frequent arguments with medical care providers asking them to find another reason to explain her child's chronically low serum potassium level. The fact that her parents occasionally found plastic bags filled with vomit hidden in their daughter's room would temporarily affect their judgment about her truthfulness. Her mother, following such an episode, would admit to us that she could understand why people were concerned that Molly might have bulimia. Then, in the car on the way home, Molly would begin to work on her mother, pleading with her to believe her and not the doctors. The next morning, her mother would arrive asking for another consultation because, "I have to believe what my daughter tells me."

Although Molly was referred to us as a possible case of MSBP, we did not sense that she had received any unnecessary medical care. Her doctors felt that her family was difficult to work with but they had not given in to requests for inappropriate treatment. We did not feel she met criteria for medical child abuse. But we still had to make a significant effort to incorporate her and her family into our health-promoting network. Several times Molly talked her mother into not bringing her to the program. A day or two would go by before the mother realized once again that she needed our help.

Eventually, after receiving a consistent message from us for several weeks and having evidence, such as plastic bags full of vomit that supported our position, Molly's mother came to trust us and came to believe that we were telling her the truth regarding her daughter's illness. We were able to convey to her that we understood why Molly was vomiting and then lying about it, that it was part of the illness, and that it was her mother's responsibility to join with us in helping Molly get back in control of her life. Slowly, she joined with us against the illness. Only then were we able to enlist Molly in the fight against her bulimia.

This example is characteristic of the model we apply for most children treated in the HCPHP. Families enter the program saying that they do not know what to do. Even though they may have been told what to do by medical treatment providers, they feel stuck. They tell us they have tried to do what the doctors prescribed but that it didn't work. Inherent in almost every situation is an unresolved conflict and a lack of consensus about what to do next. The conflict might be between the child and his or her parents, between the parents, between the parents and their doctor, or even between physicians attempting to treat the same child. Because of the unresolved conflict the family feels "damned if they do and damned if they don't." The result is a static situation where the illness continues unabated.

Our job is to understand the conflict and create a therapeutic patch around it. The conflict may be expressed on a rational level. Usually, however, there is discrepancy between the rational and the emotional meaning of the communication between parties. A father might say to his wife that he understands why she is treating her son in a certain way but be furious with her at the same time about what she is doing. She can respond either to his expression of understanding or to his anger, but the same response seldom is appropriate to both messages. She can react to her child's illness by giving treatment that her husband "understands" while knowing at the same time that he will become angrier with her as she moves forward. At a certain point the balance might shift in her mind making it more important for her to have her husband be less angry than to carry on with her medical treatment. The result is a situation where no one knows what to do next.

This is only one example of a potential unresolved conflict. There are as many varieties as there are families. We expect there will be differences of opinion and that arriving at consensus will most likely be difficult. We also expect that once the family reaches a crucial turning point and begins to see the world in a new way, it can rapidly move ahead to take control of the child's illness.

In the anecdote describing Molly and her family, we see several ongoing conflicted views of the world. Molly's mother felt that a mother and daughter should have no secrets from one another. If this were true then her daughter could not lie to her. Consequently, as a good mother she should believe everything that her daughter told her. Molly felt that her mother was trying to control her life. She loved her mother and felt close to her, but to keep her mother from running her life she had to lie to her. For their part, her medical care providers wondered aloud how a mother who was so obviously attached to her daughter, and cared so much about her, could make decisions that could potentially lead to her daughter's death. If they expressed these concerns with the mother, she felt attacked and justified in doubting their judgment. These differences, these inherent paradoxes in interpreting reality, allowed a static, unresolved, painful situation to persist. Each attempt to move forward elicited actions that blocked movement.

We use the same basic treatment model with medical child abuse as we do with other illnesses treated in the HCPHP. Another example is how we treat anorexia nervosa. As do others having significant success treating adolescent eating disorders,[3,4] we use parent empowerment as a significant aspect of our treatment. We tell teenagers and their parents that we honestly believe that without food children die. We say that, for a certain group of teenagers who have significantly restricted their food intake, food is medicine. We maintain that it is not open to discussion whether a child should take medicine that can cure a potentially fatal illness.

We have known for decades that children with anorexia nervosa usually eat while in the hospital but stop eating when they go home. In the hospital they get an unambiguous message that eating is expected, required, and will happen whether they like it or not. This is not the case once they return home. In the HCPHP there are no secrets. We partner with parents in full view of their adolescent children to reach consensus regarding what is healthy eating and what is not. Their teenager will often suggest that limiting food is healthy and that restricting food intake and being thinner is necessary for their self-esteem, promotes acceptance into a social network, or gives them a sense of control over their lives. For the anorectic teenager, these beliefs take on a life of their own. The adolescent often loses any semblance of connection with the real world. We collaborate with their parents to carry the message that, in addition to or in spite of all the reasons offered by the teenager, healthy eating involves taking in an appropriate quantity and variety of foods and that this is not negotiable. Our success with treating adolescent anorexia is in direct proportion to our ability to partner with the parents to put into effect this consensus about healthy eating.

We tell the parents we are on their side and expect them to be on our side as we struggle to make their child healthy. The partnership we create is based on being honest with one another, recognizing when we need to work harder to arrive at consensus, and keeping the health of the child as the primary concern. We do the same thing with children who are victims of medical child abuse. Treatment of medical child abuse differs in degree, but not in kind, from treatment of other children with illnesses who come to our program. All the families come to us feeling out of control. All of them feel their child is ill and that treatment is not working. Many come to the program in conflict with their medical care providers. Most insist they have tried everything, and that nothing works. Many have strange beliefs or offer inaccurate or false information.

The difference between the greater part of our children and families and those in which children have received harmful medical care at the insistence of their parents is sometimes not very great. Apart from the extreme situations where a parent is inducing illness (assaulting the child) or fabricating test results, the difference can be a matter of degree. In the cases where parents are directly causing harm we move quickly to protect the child. For the others who significantly exaggerate symptoms or refuse to adhere to standard medical treatment, we act to enlist the support of the family to change and establish healthy habits and attitudes. Medically abused children have received harmful medical care caused by parents who refuse or are unable to moderate their behaviors. Most families that accept our treatment come away feeling more in control of the illness that precipitated the admission. Sometimes we are not successful. In some cases we decide the child may need to be protected from caretakers. With these we move to involve the child protection community.

We begin treatment with all families pretty much the same way. We invite them to share their lives with us. At the beginning we assume that parents want the best for their children. We assume that they want their children to be healthy, but that differences may exist about their idea of what constitutes good health.

For most children victimized by medical abuse we can form a partnership with the family based on these principles. There is a minority of families where we try to incorporate everyone, including the offending caretaker, and fail. In one such case we were able to save the child but not the parent. A girl with a chronic liver disease that affected her entire life was hospitalized after it was found that her mother was inappropriately dispensing medication and then lying about it. We worked for several months to bring the parent into a functioning partnership with the doctors. At a certain point we determined we were not making any progress and decided to recommend medical foster care. We testified in family court to the necessity of having the girl receive medical care in a consistent way. She thrived in medical foster care and began functioning at a much higher level than she had been able to accomplish in the past. She continued to have supervised visitation with her mother. Her father, who had long been kept at a distance, once again entered her life. Several months after she was removed from her mother's care, her mother committed suicide.

The treatment of Laura and her family offers an extended example of our treatment approach, and many of the difficulties this treatment entails. We have made several references previously to Laura and her family. She was a participant in our program periodically for more than 6 months. We learned a great deal from her and her family.

Laura

As noted earlier, Laura was 10 years old when she first came to us. A psychologist who was attempting biofeedback treatment for chronic abdominal pain referred her. It quickly became apparent that abdominal pain was only one of many issues plaguing Laura and her family. During our first meeting her mother said that her goal was to have Laura "…not take so many medicines." She brought with her a large paper bag filled with medication containers and a list of medications and daily treatments written by a nurse who, incidentally, provided 40 hours of in-home nursing care per week.

The paper bag contained medicines prescribed to treat a wide variety of illnesses. In total there were more than 30 different prescriptions. Laura took medicine for asthma, hypothyroidism, headaches, a seizure disorder, gastroesophageal reflux disease (GERD), depression, attention-deficit/hyperactivity disorder (ADHD), constipation, diarrhea, seasonal allergies, easy fatigability, immunodeficiency, and frequent infections thought to be secondary to immunodeficiency.

She had a central line in place through which she received antibiotics and intravenous immunoglobulin (IVIG). She also had a gastric tube through which she received hypoallergenic formula and milk of magnesia purportedly to keep her well hydrated and to avoid constipation. The consequence of receiving fluids overnight and a daily laxative via her gastric tube was that she wore diapers to bed and awoke each morning both wet and soiled.

She attended school infrequently due to her many medical illnesses and doctor appointments. Although she performed in school at grade level, she carried a diagnosis of developmental delay. She was overweight, rather clumsy, and socially inept. She and her mother had frequent arguments, and her mother maintained that Laura was spoiled because she had been ill so much. One of the reasons her mother gave for wanting Laura to be on fewer medications was that getting her to follow so many different medical regimens was becoming more and more difficult. The function of the in-home nurse was to administer medicine, do various medical treatments, and provide an emotional buffer between Laura and her mother.

As part of the admission to the HCPHP we completed a thorough history and physical examination. Laura's mother told us the story of her long, complicated relationship with medical care providers. Her child had been treated for illnesses involving almost every organ system of her body. For example, she told us about Laura's numerous fractures, including broken arms and legs and a broken back. Laura was actively seeing 7 different pediatric subspecialists and had a coordinating primary care pediatrician whose role it was to make sure that all of her doctors communicated well with one another.

Laura's mother readily gave us permission to review medical records. We began collecting documents from a number of hospitals and physicians. The records gradually accumulated. We began the record review starting with her birth. The table documenting her medical events grew longer and longer. We looked for patterns of utilization. For example, her doctors had performed surgery on her 15 times, not counting biopsies and other minor outpatient procedures. She had received dozens of x-rays of her abdomen looking for signs of constipation with no studies read as confirming obstruction or impaction. There were numerous hospitalizations, some lasting as long as a month. Her central venous line had been in place for 6 years and the gastric tube had been inserted when she was 4 years old. We found that Laura had been evaluated for trauma to her back, legs, and arms. X-rays had been obtained, and none of the radiographic images showed evidence for fracture. There were notes describing Laura being temporarily immobilized because of her complaints of pain, but her mother's story that "Laura was always breaking bones" did not stand up to scrutiny.

From the treatment records, we were able to estimate that the total cost of her medical care had exceeded $3 million.

We called the other doctors involved in her treatment. Several acknowledged that a few years previously there had been discussion of MSBP. An equivocal test suggesting possible mitochondrial disease allowed the multiple specialists to put on hold the consideration of MSBP. Her doctors depended on the mother's history of easy fatigability, recurrent pancreatitis, developmental delay, muscle weakness, seizures, and chronic constipation to support the diagnosis of mitochondrial disease. She turned out to have none of these symptoms on direct observation. The picture that emerged from talking to the medical care providers and reviewing the records was that Laura's mother frequently took her daughter for emergency care that resulted in more and more specialty evaluations. A headache could not be ignored or treated with a tablet of acetaminophen. Her mother responded to any symptom Laura mentioned as if it were a catastrophe. The physicians all commented on how dedicated this mother was to her daughter, how she always tried her best to follow prescribed medical treatments. In their offices she was not a hysterical mother, just persistent. And she carried information from one office to the next in a way that always made things sound worse.

We related earlier that we discovered in an old hospital chart how Laura acquired the diagnosis of recurrent pancreatitis. Laboratory values that would indicate an inflamed pancreas were never abnormal. Her attending physician had no concern about pancreatitis and did not mention it in the discharge summary. One month after discharge, Laura was seen by several specialist physicians who all included pancreatitis in the history section of their evaluations. From that time forward the medical record includes references to recurrent pancreatitis. We assume the medical student who interviewed the mother during the hospitalization heard "pansinusitis" as pancreatitis and repeated it back to Laura's mother. She then included it in the history she offered to subsequent physicians just as she told us about Laura's many broken bones.

By the time we began treating Laura, she had learned to be sick in many different ways. She used her symptoms to control the world around her, knowing that her mother could not resist responding to a medical symptom with maximum attention. She would go to the school nurse an hour after school began and complain of a headache. Her mother would come to school and take her home. She would complain of being tired and her mother would be unable to get her up to bring her to the treatment program. We spent many months with Laura and her mother and her symptoms were always many times more dramatic in her mother's presence. Once her mother left for the day Laura became a normal 10-year-old, taking part in all activities. If she complained of a headache or abdominal pain, we made a brief assessment and encouraged her to rejoin the group, which she did with no difficulty. Of the many times she complained of pain, not once did the pain keep her from taking part in a desired activity.

Apart from her hypersensitivity to her daughter's physical complaints, we found the mother to be reasonable, responsive, and thoroughly invested in the welfare of her child. She made very few demands on us, and there was no sense that she was receiving nurturing from her interactions with the medical care system. There was no doubt that her daughter had received unnecessary and harmful medical care and that she had participated in making it happen. Her defense was always that she was "just following doctors' orders." In the thousands of pages of medical records and the many months of direct observation we saw no evidence that she had induced illness in her child. And there were no examples of falsifying medical records or laboratory tests. There was a long-standing pattern of exaggeration of symptoms and persistent requests that doctors do more to help her daughter.

We decided to treat Laura as we would any other participant in the partial hospital program. We accepted the stated goal of the parent to decrease the number of medications and treatments. To do this we observed Laura medically for several days and checked out every symptom described by either child or parent.

We acknowledged that we would first try to undo the physical consequences of the abuse within the existing family network. It was clearly apparent in our discussions with the specialty physicians that they were not ready to support us in making a report of child abuse and separating the child from her family. We were far from having a consensus that much of her care had been unnecessary and harmful. From our analysis of the medical record, we did not have confirmation of illness induction that would be admissible as evidence for physical child abuse. Instead, we had a mother who "always did what the doctor said" and physicians who confirmed this behavior.

We did not know in the beginning if Laura's mother would accept a revised treatment relationship with her doctors that substantially changed how she sought medical care. Also, we did not know if Laura would be willing to find other ways of getting what she needed or wanted besides exhibiting physical symptoms. But, on both counts, this is what we set out to do.

The stated goal of the family was to decrease the number of medications. We could only accomplish this goal if we had the full support of the existing medical care personnel treating Laura. In addition to our telephone calls we sent an introductory letter to all of the physicians involved in her care stating that she was attending our program 5 days a week, 8 hours a day, and we wished to see if we could simplify, with their approval, her medical regimen. In doing this we set the stage to systematically remove her multiple diagnoses and treatments, one illness at a time.

We judged the central line to be the most dangerous form of medical treatment that Laura continued to receive. Through her central intravenous access she was receiving IVIG and antibiotics for an immune disorder. She had been receiving IVIG for many years. We repeated her immunoglobulin profile and noted that it was essentially normal, as it had been on several previous occasions throughout her life. We spoke with the infectious diseases specialist, who had no objections to discontinuing the treatment saying that he was unsure whether it was necessary and one way to find out would be to stop it. Next we wrote a letter to all of the specialists bringing them up to date regarding our observations of Laura, and our discussion with the infectious diseases specialist. We communicated our intention to stop the IVIG treatment with the goal of taking out the indwelling catheter. Laura had experienced several episodes of polymicrobial sepsis (bloodstream infections with multiple types of bacteria at one time) shortly after the central line was placed. The fact that several years had gone by with no major complications did not change our opinion that getting rid of this treatment would be the best thing we could do for her. We stopped the IVIG and antibiotic, and on the recommendation of the infectious diseases specialist repeated an immunoglobulin panel at a later time. This once again came back normal, and so her central venous line was removed.

There were many more steps to come. Laura was taking 3 medications for her asthma. On our physical examination we found no signs of reactive airway disease. We monitored pulmonary peak flow values for a week, both with and without exercise and before and after medications, and saw no differences. Our medical record review turned up many references to asthma but no physical examination findings that indicated that anyone had ever heard Laura wheeze. Once again we wrote to our colleagues involved in her treatment requesting evidence that someone had seen active asthma symptoms. No one could verify ever having seen Laura with difficulty breathing. Our next step was to schedule a methacholine challenge. Methacholine is a chemical that when administered as an aerosol irritates the lungs and induces wheezing. Given enough methacholine, anyone will eventually respond with difficulty breathing and abnormal pulmonary function tests. People with asthma respond quickly and dramatically. Laura was particularly unresponsive, evidence that she did not have reactive airway disease. We told Laura and her mother the good news and wrote a letter to all of the consulting physicians telling them we were stopping 3 more medications and declaring that Laura did not have asthma.

One by one we peeled away the diagnoses and their treatments. As we had clear evidence that Laura was neither dehydrated nor constipated, we advocated terminating overnight gastric tube feedings of milk of magnesia and formula. With the permission of her gastroenterologist we began a trial of no nighttime feeding. She stopped having diarrhea in her diaper. We asked if she and her mother would like her to stop using diapers at night. They both acknowledged that this would be wonderful but expressed doubts about whether it could be accomplished. We instituted a bowel and bladder training program and within a week she was completely continent. Her mother donated several cartons of adult-sized diapers to a homeless shelter.

The child psychiatrist who had been treating her for ADHD and depression told us that she might be able to function well in our program without medications but would most likely need to return to using them when she was back in her school environment. A telephone call to her school put us in touch with her counselor and school nurse. They sent us copies of letters they had written to her physicians saying that they saw no evidence for attention difficulties or depression while in school. In fact, they could not believe that Laura was receiving as much medical care as she was getting because they hardly ever saw her truly sick. In addition, they said that their psychological testing showed normal intelligence (ie, no evidence for developmental delay), contrary to a report they had seen from one of Laura's doctors. We stopped the stimulant and antidepressant medications and saw no change in Laura.

We sent weekly letters to the entire list of physicians actively involved in Laura's treatment, updating them on the good news. Occasionally, when we felt it necessary to have more extensive communication with a doctor regarding treatment, we scheduled a personal meeting in his or her office. We expected, eventually, to meet with resistance from Laura and her mother as we took away illnesses. It was a little surprising to find *more* resistance from several of the physicians. In each case we asked what would be the appropriate medical approach to determining whether the treatment was still necessary. The neurologist who had been treating her for seizures requested a videotaped 24-hour electroencephalogram (EEG) before considering a taper of her antiseizure medications. He also wanted another EEG done once she had been off medications for a month, even though previous EEGs had been normal. We scheduled the tests and discontinued the anticonvulsant medication.

Over the course of 4 months we were able to eliminate most of the illnesses and medical treatments. The central line was surgically removed. We wanted to close the gastric tube opening as well, but Laura's mother insisted that we wait a number of months after it was no longer being used before closing it.

Her refusal to acknowledge that Laura did not need the gastric tube was an early sign that we were getting to the point where she may not be able to go along with us. We had regular meetings with her and we systematically reiterated that Laura was much healthier than she had ever imagined. She wanted to believe us but at the same time had spent a decade defining her life and the life of her daughter around medical treatments. Eventually Laura was left with a positive diagnosis, confirmed by pH probe testing, of GERD and allergic rhinitis activated by spring pollens. Her medication list consisted primarily of vitamins and treatment for her GERD. We discharged her and sent her back to school anticipating that old behaviors might return.

We received word a month later that Laura was in the emergency department of the local hospital with complaints of severe headache. Finally we experienced the crisis that we felt was coming. Laura's mother wanted to follow the advice of the emergency department physician who, after seeing her daughter one time, began treatment for severe migraine, even though this was contrary to what her established medical team was saying. Once again, at a time of stress, Laura complained of pain and her mother responded by going to an emergency department, and relaying a less than accurate medical history. The physician, who had never seen the child before, prescribed medication that was not necessary. When her doctors, including us, asked her to discontinue the new medication, the mother threatened to fire all of us and find someone who could "…really help my daughter." It was at this point that we informed her that if she continued to take her daughter to doctors, someday Laura would die from medical treatment that was not necessary and that it would be her fault.

If she had gone through with her threat to terminate her relationship with her medical treatment team, we were prepared to file a report of child abuse. By this time, a number, if not all, of the treating physicians were supporting us. Fortunately we were able to resolve the conflict. Laura's mother acknowledged that her daughter was healthier than she had ever been in her life. She agreed to stay with the existing treatment team.

When we began treatment with Laura and her family we thought it highly unlikely that the medical and legal community would agree with us that she needed to be protected from her mother. There were several prominent doctors prepared to stand up in court on behalf of the family. We did not think we could make a case with child protection to remove Laura from her family for her own safety. It is possible that, had we been able to effect the removal, we might have eliminated medical treatments much quicker and eliminated the gastric tube months earlier.

When Laura left our program, we discharged her into the care of a very competent primary care pediatrician who understood the true nature of Laura's past illnesses and her relationship with her mother. Several months later she moved to another state and we communicated with the physician the mother identified who would be assuming Laura's care. We had word 2 years later that Laura was doing well.

We have said that the goals of treatment of medical child abuse involve identifying it, stopping it, having some assurance that it will not resume, and reversing the consequences of the abuse, all while attempting to maintain the integrity of the family. While there are no assurances that Laura and her family might not return to old patterns, we feel we have come a long way toward accomplishing these goals.

Starting Treatment at Different Places

We began treatment of Laura and her family with the mother's goal to decrease the number of medications. Each family comes to us in a different place. The treatment of the physical consequences of abuse consequently begins in many different ways. As a medical professional it is necessary to give only beneficial treatment. Medical judgment is involved in how quickly to stop treatment and when to try to reverse the negative consequences of prior treatment. Obviously, life-threatening treatment should be ended first. It becomes a balancing act whether this can be accomplished without removing the child from the family.

Children receiving unnecessary medical care can have both direct and indirect physical consequences of that care. They can experience side effects of medications, complications of procedures, and physical consequences from unnecessary surgery. If the child has been removed from the family and remains in the hospital, unnecessary medical care can often simply be stopped. We can withdraw medications, remove central lines, and encourage children to get out of their wheelchairs and walk.

Alice, the youngster described previously whose mother felt she had ulcerative colitis and immunodeficiency, represents a good example of how quickly a child can improve if unnecessary treatment is stopped. Within days of her mother no longer having a direct influence on her perception of medical symptoms, she not only defined herself as healthy and made significant social progress, but she stopped complaining of any significant symptoms. All treatment was simply halted.

Brian, however, was not as fortunate. He was removed from his parents' care after a judicial proceeding declared him to be the victim of MSBP. At the time of his hospitalization at age 4, he was severely malnourished, unable to walk independently (his mother carried him everywhere), had minimal speech, and vomited whenever presented with food. His medical care providers determined that he had learned to vomit through the persistent expectations of his mother that he would do so. A gastric tube had been surgically placed when he was 6 months old. In retrospect, there is little medical evidence that he had any underlying medical condition that would have required this measure. His symptoms were the result of the home environment.

We met him when he was 7 years old. At that time he had been separated from his family for almost 3 years. Before coming to us he spent more than a year living in the hospital and being fed through his gastric tube. The same formula he was previously receiving at home, when given in the hospital, allowed him to grow slowly but steadily. Although small in stature, he was a bright child, full of energy and physically competent. Even though he was capable of taking food by mouth, he chose not to and entered into treatment with us to learn how to eat again. While in our program, he lived in medical foster care, first with one family and then with another.

Eventually, although it took nearly 9 months, Brian reestablished normal eating patterns and was reunited with his father. In this case, removal from the noxious environment of the home was only the beginning of a long rehabilitative process. Brian, after years of suboptimal nutrition, will more than likely always be significantly smaller than his brothers. In this case the abuse he experienced in his early years will have a permanent effect.

Treating the Physical Effects of Medical Abuse Without a Partial Hospital Program

In this chapter we have described in some detail our program for treatment of medically and psychiatrically ill children. We are aware that around the country, availability of such programs is limited. We have what we consider to be a nearly ideal environment in which to address the multifaceted issues involved in the treatment of medical child abuse. We can deal with most *medical* symptoms within a *psychiatric* treatment milieu. How does this translate to situations where such resources are not available?

The philosophical basis of what we try to accomplish is available in many less structured settings. We advocate creating an accepting environment that incorporates the family at its level of functioning. We discuss the importance of promoting honest, open communication among staff and between staff and families. We assess the family belief system in a nonjudgmental way and communicate to the family respect for how they may have arrived at their present situation. We accept presentation of medical symptoms at face value but investigate them in an evidence-based manner. We also are continually prepared to discuss with the family the need to renegotiate the doctor-patient relationship. These are all general principles that most pediatric practice environments can do or strive to accomplish.

While the general treatment principles are not dissimilar to those found in other treatment settings, we do have the opportunity to spend much more time with each individual child and his or her family during the course of a treatment period that can last from days to weeks. And during this time we can foster trusting relationships that allow us to open doors for families to new possibilities. The typical pediatric outpatient setting may be appropriate for identification of medical abuse, and in some cases making the first efforts toward redefining the doctor-patient treatment relationship. In other cases the local pediatric hospital environment may be a more appropriate setting.

Hospitalizing a child increases the intensity of the intervention and provides a message to the family that something significantly different needs to occur.

Pediatric hospital units vary greatly across the country in their ability to deal with psychosocial issues. The availability of child psychiatric consultation and the sophistication of the staff affect their ability to address issues of medical child abuse in a empathic but objective fashion. Experience with each case will make it easier for the unit to respond to the next. We recommend creating a working group including pediatricians, house staff, nurses, and child psychologists or psychiatrists to prepare the unit for the emotional confusion resulting from the treatment of children being harmed by their medical care. The first several times a unit faces these challenges, the potential exists for a profound lack of consensus about how to proceed.

Before we return to discuss strategies about how to generate consensus in groups of physicians collaborating to treat medical child abuse, we need to continue by discussing treatment of the emotional consequences.

References

1. Krener P. Factitious disorders and the psychosomatic continuum in children. *Curr Opin Pediatr.* 1994;6(4):418-422
2. Roesler TA, Rickerby ML, Nassau JH, High PC. Treating a high risk population: a collaboration of child psychiatry and pediatrics. *Med Health R I.* 2002; 85(9):265-268
3. Lock J. Treating adolescents with eating disorders in the family context. Empirical and theoretical considerations. *Child Adolesc Psychiatr Clin N Am.* 2002;11(2):331-342
4. Lock J, Le Grange D. Can family-based treatment of anorexia nervosa be manualized? *J Psychother Pract Res.* 2001;10(4):253-261

Chapter 13

Treating the Psychological Consequences

Each time I review my medical records, I go through a period of mourning for a childhood lost. In the name of sickness and at the hands of medicine, I am disfigured with permanent physical scars. Because of distorted motherly love, I continue to battle deep emotional wounds. —Bryk, 1997[1]

Introduction

Mary Bryk,[1] in her article published in *Pediatrics,* described how from the ages of 2 to 10 her mother systematically hit the bones in her arms and legs with a hammer, sometimes as often as 3 times per week, leaving bruising, inflammation, and abrasions that fit no pattern of ordinary childhood disease. She had cellulitis that did not heal for years because her mother contaminated the wounds with dirt and other foreign substances. Her mother took her to the doctor and lied about what had happened. When Bryk was 10 years old she told her mother if the abuse did not stop she would tell the truth to her teachers and doctors. Her mother stopped abusing her, but then began giving "hammer treatments" to a younger brother.

Bryk grew up, became a nurse like her mother, and as an adult began to look back to see if she could make sense of what had happened to her. She called what she experienced *medical abuse.* To this day she has the scars of the injuries induced by her mother, both physical and emotional. The physical consequences consist of significant muscle wasting and large scars on her extremities. (Her article includes photographs of her injuries.) The emotional consequences were even more serious. As a child she was *physically* abused, and then taken to the doctor for extensive medical treatments, her *medical* abuse.

Looking back on her childhood she remembers being confused and angry about what her mother was doing to her. Her mother was causing her pain for no reason a little girl could understand. Her mother described the beatings as "treatments." As an adult she tells about trying to discuss her childhood with her mother and other family members. Her parents discounted her story despite there being both physical evidence and medical documentation establishing the authenticity of the attacks. The early betrayal became permanent.

Although every child wishes his or her family to be faultless, there is always evidence of imperfection in daily life. Prior to adolescence children often idealize their parents, looking past their faults and seeing only what they want to see. During early adolescence, in the normal course of psychological development, a child's view of his or her parents changes from, "I've got the best daddy in the whole world!" to "My parents are so mean!" This change is normal. But what about children whose parents don't even meet the minimum standards for keeping them safe? What is the "normal" reaction, the understandable adaptation, to having a mother who hits you with a hammer? What should a little girl think or do or feel when her mother purposely injures her and then takes her to the doctor pretending that she doesn't know how it happened?

Here we discuss the emotional consequences of medical child abuse. We agree with others that the emotional consequences of medical abuse parallel those of other forms of child maltreatment.[2,3] Numerous studies confirm that victims of child abuse suffer from attachment problems, post-traumatic stress disorder (PTSD), depression and anxiety disorders, and are prone to having difficulties in adulthood with drugs and alcohol.[4] While it is beyond the scope of this work to detail treatment for the effects of all types of maltreatment experienced in childhood, most of the principles of treatment of other forms of abuse apply to medical abuse as well.

A child who grows up in an unsafe environment comes to expect not to be protected. One learns trust by being in a relationship with someone who is trustworthy. Most people grow up in a network of relationships where predictable things happen. They know that the adults in their lives love them and will keep them from harm, at least most of the time. We learn to be social creatures within this early environment where members of our family pass us back and forth, each assuming responsibility for our safety. We come to learn that no one will drop us. A child who misses this early experience learns not to trust and has difficulty forming relationships in future life. One of the few attempts to interview adult victims of medical abuse makes this point.[2] Inability to make relationships is a significant handicap and in its extreme form is referred to as *attachment disorder*.

Everyone experiences bad things in life. We all need to learn how to cope with adversity. As small children our repertoire of coping skills is meager so we rely on the adults around us to run interference, to cope for us. As we grow up we learn more and more ways to deal with traumatic events. There is always the possibility that traumatic events will overwhelm our ability to cope. When this happens we fall back on more primitive coping skills. We go back to what used to work in the past, to the strategies that we learned when first dealing with the complexity of life. This constellation of primitive responses to overwhelming trauma has come to be known as *PTSD*. It is the most frequent emotional consequence of child abuse. In addition, many children and adults who have been experiencing PTSD symptoms for a significant length of time come to feel depressed or anxious. It is not uncommon to find people in treatment for depression or anxiety who also have significant histories of child abuse. In fact, children abused in multiple ways in the first years of life have a greater chance of being diagnosed with a major depression in early adulthood.[5]

In addition to attachment difficulties and the responses children make when they find themselves unable to cope with trauma, a third category of psychological response to abuse is to develop thinking patterns and to learn behaviors that are consistent with one's life situation. These thoughts and behaviors make life somehow seem normal. For example, a child sexually abused by her stepfather can come to believe that she somehow caused him to molest her. Taking personal responsibility for the abuse can substitute for her having to consider that she may be the victim of atrocious violation at the hands of her caretaker. We call these thoughts *cognitive distortions*. From the viewpoint of a clinician who has not experienced what the child has gone through, thinking that the child caused her father to sexually molest her might seem to be a distortion. But from the child's perspective it seems totally consistent. Something happened to her and this idea allows her to make some sense from her childlike point of view. Likewise, a child who has been sexually abused is more likely to act out sexually with peers.

These thoughts and behaviors, while somewhat protective, can also lead to significant difficulties.

These 3 broad categories of psychological responses to abuse occur both with medical child abuse and with all other forms of child maltreatment. Attachment/relationship difficulties, PTSD symptoms, and cognitive and behavioral distortions are all common responses to abusive behavior.

Our approach to the treatment of medical child abuse begins with the child, involves family members who love and support the child, and then extends to the perpetrator of the abuse if that person desires to have an ongoing relationship with her child. Others writing about treatment of Munchausen syndrome by proxy (MSBP) have indicated that treatment refers to the psychotherapy of the adult perpetrator.[6] Parnell and Day[7] describe in detail the process of forming an individual psychotherapeutic relationship with adults who harm their children by getting them unnecessary health care.

Attachment Difficulties

Attachment difficulties range from mild to severe. At the mild end we find difficulty making friends or having low self-esteem. At the severe end of the spectrum, children diagnosed with reactive attachment disorder[8] are often those with the worst early childhood experiences. Reactive attachment disorder is found in children who grow up in orphanages, children taken from their parents at a very early age who have cycled through many foster homes, and children who have experienced severe abuse at the hands of their caretakers. Children with reactive attachment disorder will either not have anything to do with an adult, or will climb into the lap of anyone available. The *Diagnostic and Statistical Manual of Mental Disorders, Fourth Edition (DSM-IV)*[8] describes this later characteristic with this language: "…diffuse attachments as manifest by indiscriminate sociability with marked inability to exhibit appropriate selective attachments (e.g., excessive familiarity with relative strangers or lack of selectivity in choice of attachment figures)."

Brian, the child taken from his parents when he was 4 years old, exhibited some features of reactive attachment disorder. This is the boy we taught how to eat when he was 7 years old. He had lived most of his life not with his family, but in the hospital and a series of foster homes. He got on well with adults. While he was not particularly compliant, he was charming and verbal. Brian had superficial attachment with a large number of caregivers, including staff from the Hasbro Children's Partial Hospital Program (HCPHP). It did not seem to matter who the adults were as long as they appeared reasonably well meaning. He saw his parents during supervised visitation sessions and observers described his attachment to his parents as superficial as well.

His lack of attachment presented a problem in his treatment. He was dependent on a gastric tube. He could eat normally but in practice he would take a small amount of food in his mouth, taste it for a minute, and then spit it out. He first began getting fed through a nasogastric tube when he was a few months old. A feeding tube was placed through his stomach wall at age 6 months. He missed the developmental window when children learn how to eat. Training older children to eat who have missed this stage in maturation can be a challenge. With Brian his attachment issues made it more complicated.

Wanting to please important people in their lives usually motivates children. For Brian, one person was not particularly more important than anyone else. Ordinarily, we would work with him and his family to encourage him to eat to please his parents. In the absence of his parents, hospital staff provided only a pale approximation of the degree of relatedness that would usually motivate a 7-year-old boy. While we were eventually successful in helping him learn to eat normally, it took much longer than we expected.

In its more severe forms, reactive attachment disorder is very difficult to treat. It takes many months and years of consistent loving experiences with close people in one's life to make up for what was missing in the early months of childhood.

We have seen that a child who experiences maltreatment in one area of his life is often maltreated in other areas as well. A child who is physically abused might also be sexually molested. Bools and colleagues[9] found that children who fell into 1 of 4 categories of MSBP symptoms (poisoned, smothered, seizures, or other) often had other child abuse experiences. But having said this, most children who experience medical abuse are attached to their parents. In many aspects of their lives (eg, being fed regular meals, getting a bedtime story, receiving hugs and kisses, and learning not to run out into the road), these children lead normal lives. It is more likely in the arena of illness expression that the relationship between parent and child gets distorted.

Post-Traumatic Stress Disorder

It is useful to think of PTSD not as an illness but as an adaptation to a difficult life situation that has overwhelmed one's coping mechanisms. By *DSM-IV*[8] definition, PTSD includes factors in 3 different symptom categories. Some of the factors are associated with reexperiencing the painful event over and over again—the so-called flashback phenomena. The second group of symptoms has to do with trying to avoid memories of painful experiences. The third group is arousal symptoms, the heightened sensitivity to stimuli associated with a traumatic event.

How might this function in the life of a real child? A little girl stopped breathing and received an emergency intubation, a tube passed through her throat and beyond the vocal cords that allowed a respirator to breathe for her.[10] Both the experience of stopping breathing, and also the tube being pushed down her throat, took place while she was conscious. She was extremely frightened. Afterward, she repeatedly drew pictures of a tiny figure with something protruding from its mouth. She refused to talk about the drawings or about the time she was in the hospital. Every time she saw a nurse or a doctor in a white coat she began to scream. She was completely inconsolable any time a doctor tried to examine her, especially if she was asked to open her mouth.

The repeated depiction of a scene similar to her trauma in her drawings and play are a small child's way of reexperiencing the event. Even though she was able to draw the event over and over again, her refusal to talk about the image or anything else having to do with the intubation falls under the category of avoidance. And her hypersensitivity to medical examinations counts as an arousal symptom.

These 3 types of symptoms—reexperiencing, avoidance, and hypersensitivity—are the hallmarks of PTSD. They are the coping mechanisms humans fall back on when nothing else seems to work. The avoidance symptoms, for instance, are a form of denial, an attempt to block all thought from consciousness that would bring back painful memories. The reexperiencing symptoms are commonly felt to be the human organism's primitive attempt at problem-solving. It is as if the little girl thinks at an unconscious level that if she draws the picture just one more time she will come to understand why there is a tube in the little figure's throat. The arousal and hypersensitivity symptoms are directly tied to the fight or flight response, the autonomic nervous system's way of preparing us for action to deal with a potentially dangerous situation.

By definition PTSD can be diagnosed only when symptoms have continued longer than 1 month after the onset of the traumatic event. In fact, PTSD symptoms can continue for many years. There may also be a significant lag time before PTSD symptoms appear. While PTSD is commonly felt to result from a specific life-threatening, or perceived to be life-threatening, event the same constellation of symptoms are seen in children and adults exposed to a prolonged series of events which, although unpleasant, might not be life-threatening. For example, children who have been sexually abused often have PTSD symptoms even though a knife was not held to their throats.

Rather than dictating that the traumatic events need be life-threatening, it would be more accurate to describe them as "completely overwhelming." Bryk was pounded with a hammer several times a week for many years. It is unlikely that any single episode was, in fact, life-threatening. But the experiences taken as a whole overwhelmed her ability to understand, cope, or survive using her own skills. From her description it is clear that she experienced symptoms of PTSD.

One of the few studies that looked at long-term consequences of medical abuse confirms that victims have similar responses to that of other forms of child abuse. Libow[2] interviewed 10 adults who contacted her after identifying themselves as victims of medical abuse. She documented high levels of PTSD symptoms, difficulties with self-esteem, symptoms of depression and anxiety, and difficulties in relationships. Many of the adults related ongoing issues regarding whether to trust themselves to seek medical care appropriately. None of these subjects received treatment for abuse during childhood.

The treatment for PTSD is aimed at helping the individual to go back to the precipitating event and learn to cope successfully. It is not necessary to experience the event again in real life. Rather, the individual needs to think through the event psychologically and emotionally and have an understanding of how and why the traumatic event took place. The child or adult needs to "make sense" of what happened and, in doing so, to become desensitized to the memory.

Many times adults viewing traumatic events that happened in childhood must come to recognize that when they were young they only used those coping skills available to young children. It is no wonder they were unable to deal with experiences that were beyond the psychological resources they possessed at the time. It was the responsibility of their *family* members to fill in the gaps in their management strategies while providing for their safety.

Post-traumatic stress disorder symptoms represent a fallback adaptation when other resources are not sufficient. Unfortunately, denying that events took place, reliving them over and over in one's mind, and being overly sensitized to one's environment are not very effective ways of dealing with painful episodes in one's past. Instead, PTSD sufferers find themselves in a kind of time warp, perceiving the world as they did when the traumatic events were taking place. If the trauma took place in childhood they experience the reality of the events through the eyes of a child. They carry this reality forward. It is this view of the world that needs to grow and change for them to find peace.

Adults in individual and group therapy specifically aimed at dealing with the effects of childhood abuse undergo a process of looking at what happened to them, remembering what they did in response, and using their current, adult understanding to see why they were unable to cope at the time. Group therapy is especially helpful because group members, even though they share similar life events, are able to look at each other objectively. They can see things for other group members that they cannot see for themselves.

When adults are able to look back at a childhood abuse experience and say that (1) a bad thing happened, (2) they did the best they could under the circumstances, and (3) people charged to keep them safe should have done a better job, then they are on their way to emotional equilibrium. In the process the reality of the present takes over from the reality of the past. Reality as seen through a child's eyes is replaced by reality as seen by adults functioning in the here and now.

We mentioned previously that people who experience PTSD symptoms for a considerable length of time often find themselves depressed or showing symptoms of an anxiety disorder. When this happens depression and anxiety disorders are considered comorbid with the constellation of symptoms that make up PTSD. Medications commonly used for depression and anxiety often can be helpful. Medications do not cure traumatic memories but they do allow patients to decrease their levels of depression and anxiety while proceeding with difficult therapy.

Here is how Bryk[1] describes her therapy:

> Therapy was not easy. Although I always had memories of what my mother did to me, I had never talked to anyone about it. To speak out loud and relive these memories brought to the surface feelings I had spent thirty years trying to stifle. Along with individual therapy I also attended group therapy with other female survivors of childhood abuse. There, I learned I was not alone in my pain. Therapy was a safe place to vent feelings and learn how to set boundaries. *The final piece of the puzzle was learning that the abuse I suffered had a name.* I had always felt that my experiences were different from others in the group and I finally understood why; the medical abuse I experienced was a deliberate, premeditated act; the physical abuse that other group members experienced was more impulsive and reactive. My recovery progressed rapidly from then on.

Adults who are trying to recover from the effects of childhood sexual abuse share Bryk's feeling that their abuse is different from those who were beaten by their parents. As is the case with medical abuse, sexual abuse is often premeditated and deliberate and can go on for many years.

Children experiencing symptoms of PTSD in the present cannot look back on their trauma from the perspective of an adult. They still have partial coping skills and incomplete abilities to deal with the world based on their age, cognitive talents, and other resources. Treatment of PTSD symptoms in children, therefore, requires us to understand the talents available for each specific child and then create a therapeutic environment around them to allow them to use those coping skills, but also compensate for the coping skills they have not yet developed. The most appropriate people to offer these resources are the child's parents and other close family members.[11] Therapy is most effective when the family is mobilized to do the job that should have been done in the first place.

Children come to understand the world through their own eyes and the eyes of those who are close to them. Reality for the child is the world he shares on a verbal and emotional level with his mother, father, and other family members. He learns to manage life events from this source. Medical illnesses and symptoms are a part of that reality. If the child has become "completely overwhelmed" there is a good chance that his family unit shares that sense of inability to cope. The family systems based treatment as outlined in the description of the HCPHP is designed to encompass the child, the medical symptoms, and the family to allow them to develop new management strategies.

Any treatment that allows a child to feel competent and to recapture a sense of control over his or her surroundings will be helpful in undoing the psychological consequences of abuse. In some cases merely stopping the abuse will be all that is necessary. In other situations, individual or group psychotherapy can be helpful. But in the long run, the child will most likely live in a family environment, sharing the reality of that family. It is at this level that he eventually must feel comfortable. For this reason we recommend family-based treatment.

Treating Cognitive Distortions and Behavioral Symptoms in Children

We began this discussion by asking what a child's normal response would be to an abnormal situation. Here is a description offered by Ayoub and colleagues[12] of children victimized by MSBP: "Across the developmental spectrum, children victimized by MBP exhibit considerable need for extensive control over their environments, which can supersede their desire to form attachments. They often continue to be hypervigilant long after they are in a safe alternative placement. …Notable is the 'chameleon' quality of many MBP children's responses to those around them. They often react differently in different contexts and seem to be attempting to anticipate and conform to the expectations of the adult or child with whom they are speaking." While this depiction is based on anecdotal information, it seems consistent with how a normal child would respond to an abusive environment.

In everyday life we expect to be healthy most of the time. Becoming ill is unusual. Every family has its own way of responding to illness in one of its members, but in most cases, the response includes special treatment. Once someone has been declared ill, the family reorganizes around that person and a whole series of activities and expectations are set in motion. As a result, a normal response to being told that one is sick is to feel sick. A small child told he is sick on a regular basis begins to think and act like a sick person. In the description of Laura in the last chapter we saw how she came to live the sick role and use it to control her environment.

Parents who maltreat their children seldom announce to the world that they are doing so. Nor do they tell their children that their behavior as parents is inappropriate. Rather, they often find logical justification for their actions. Fathers who beat their children often characterize their actions as beneficial for the child, or at least as a deserved consequence for the child's actions. Adults who sexually molest children sometimes have similar explanations such as, "I was just teaching her about sex." Likewise, parents who expose their children to harmful medical care almost always explain that they are doing so to benefit the child.

If the abuse is experienced within this context, it is not surprising that children come to think of the medical care as necessary or helpful. Going to a doctor and receiving unnecessary and painful medical treatments becomes incorporated in the child's mind as, "It's what we do in our family."

Gregory[13] recounts what it is like to grow up in such a family. As the story unfolds we can share with her the experience of realizing what was happening to her was not typical. Her perspective seems to shift back and forth between looking through a child's eyes, almost thinking she comes from a normal family, and then coming up against an antithetical vision as she employs an adult viewpoint. As did Bryk, Gregory documents her story using excerpts from her own medical record.

We once lectured about medical abuse to a large audience in the Midwest. At the end of the talk a social worker approached us saying that he had been ill constantly during his youth. He had juvenile onset diabetes that his mother, a nurse, managed for him up to and including the night before his wedding. He told us he had been in and out of the hospital multiple times because his diabetes was in such poor control. The day before his wedding he had a life-threatening hypoglycemic episode after his mother gave him his insulin shot. He ended up in the hospital. Despite being in the hospital he wanted to get married. His bride and the minister came to his hospital room to perform the wedding ceremony. When he left the hospital, instead of returning to his parents' home, he moved to an apartment with his wife. From that day on, he managed his illness himself. Within weeks he realized that his diabetes was actually quite easy to treat. He told us he had been in good control ever since his wedding day. He said he now looked back on his childhood as if through a new pair of glasses, certain that his mother had been abusing him consciously through her management of his illness.

This revelation phenomenon is commonly seen in other types of child maltreatment as well. Adults sexually molested as children often are surprised to learn that what happened to them is against the law and could result in a long prison sentence for the perpetrator. After all, activities that took place within the context of their family were interpreted as "normal." Because of this, undoing the effects of child abuse begins with determining how the adult looks back at the world of his or her childhood, and then beginning to contrast this view with one shared by the general population.

What we call *cognitive distortions* often seem completely logical within the shared belief system of the family. For example, a parent who believes she can read her child better than any doctor feels perfectly justified in finding a new physician if her doctor does not agree with her. We call this *doctor shopping,* with the implication that it is a way to defeat the medical care system. For a mother with this belief system, it is merely doing what she has to do for the sake of her child. And her child feels equally justified in going along with his mother. Similarly, as a child gets older it is common to see him or her participating in the illness behavior.

This participation might range from exaggerating symptoms to actual fabrication of symptoms or illness. It is reasonable to assume that people who grow up to see the world in terms of somatic symptoms begin that process in childhood. Sanders[14] described what she called "symptom coaching." She outlined the child's participation in the illness behavior as a gradual process of increasing collusion from naïve child, to passive acceptance, to active participation and, eventually, active self-harm.

Libow[15] has written about how adults and older teenagers come to engage in illness fabrication behavior. She states that a case can be made that adults who fabricate illnesses often were victimized medically in childhood. She discusses what she calls "blended cases" where illness is not only fabricated by an adult but also produced by the child.

We have already discussed several examples of children colluding with their parents in producing symptoms. Scott, the boy whose mother felt he had porphyria, acted out a particularly strange, silent tantrum that his mother caught on videotape. This "evidence" seemed oddly convincing to his mother that her son was suffering from a rare disease. Richard, the boy whose daily temporary paralysis kept him from going to school but yielded to a desire and an ability to ride in bicycle races in the afternoon is another example.

Alice, the girl whose symptoms disappeared when her mother was removed from the home demonstrates another facet of this interactive phenomenon. Several months after she was placed in the custody of her father, she was again allowed regular visits with her mother. She would return from visits with her mother complaining of symptoms of abdominal pain, reminiscent of the time when we first met her. In a day or two her symptoms would subside only to reappear after the next visit. A significant aspect of the mother-daughter relationship consisted of Alice having symptoms and the mother responding with attention and sympathy, which, of course, led to her having more symptoms, at least in the presence of her mother.

Treatment of the thoughts and behaviors resulting from the medical victimization of the child is directed at helping the family reorder their belief system. A child who has received multiple messages for many years that feelings are communicated through physical symptoms needs to get an alternative message not just from his medical treatment team but also from his family. Families who find themselves on the medical abuse spectrum have become isolated from the mainstream. They interpret bodily sensations, feelings, and responses to normal physical events in a way that sets them apart from most other families treated within the medical environment. Treatment consists of bringing them back into the mainstream.

Treating the Non-Perpetrator Parent

Caretakers, usually fathers not actively involved in committing medical abuse, have been characterized as domineering, absent, or detached, as well as well-meaning but ineffective.[16] Fathers in medically abusive homes have been said to have histories of domestic violence and drug and alcohol abuse.[12] They have also been accused of sometimes enabling the abusive behavior[17] in their spouses. The variation in descriptions is quite extensive.

While fathers in families where medical abuse is taking place may have some or all of these characteristics, it is equally accurate to describe them as being stuck in a bad situation along with everyone else.

Do fathers know about medical abuse taking place in their family? This question can be asked of families in which any type of abuse is occurring. Why did the wife not stop her husband from shaking the baby? Did the parents know that the grandfather was sexually abusing their child? Did they stand by and let it happen, or did they truly not know? From a therapeutic standpoint these questions are important but not as important as whether people are ready, once abuse has been identified, to accept help from outside the family.

Bryk describes telling her father when she was still a child that her mother was abusing her. Her father immediately confronted his wife who vehemently denied the allegation. He then gave his daughter a stern lecture about lying. Bryk states that as an adult she told her father that her mother was inducing illness in herself and even showed him where the hammer was hidden in the parents' bedroom. He refused to believe her. Did he know what was happening? If he was told his wife was hitting his daughter with a hammer and accused his daughter of lying, would he then be complicit in her abuse, or should he be considered loyal to his spouse?

Most families arrive at some sort of equilibrium involving the division of labor between roles of parents. One parent may be more actively involved in handling the finances of the family. Another might be more responsible for providing for the daily needs of the children. Families usually assign responsibility for obtaining medical care to one parent rather than another, and mothers often take on this role. Deciding when the children are sick, making doctor appointments, and dispensing medications all represent a significant responsibility. By honoring a spouse's commitment to the health of the family, a husband is showing respect for his wife.

Alice's father told us that he had been concerned about his children receiving inappropriate medical care for many years. He said he had felt powerless to do anything about it, as this was clearly defined as his wife's responsibility in the family. Yet he was immediately willing to step forward and become the child's primary caretaker when given the opportunity. The court awarded him temporary custody of all of his children. Within a few weeks, he reorganized his work schedule and filed for divorce.

Treatment for the non-abusing parent, like treatment of the child, is best done within the family system. It begins with offering the parent an opportunity to help bring the family back into the mainstream. If the non-offending caretaker is not ready or able to participate in this process, resources can be brought to bear to assist him. Extended family members, in-home psychological resources, and family therapy all have a place in helping the family, including the father, set right its relationship with the health care system.

Treating the Perpetrator

Treating the perpetrator of medical child abuse is really no different from treating a parent involved in maltreating her child in any other way. Once the abuse has been identified and the child has been protected from further abuse, we need to evaluate if the abuser can be trusted with the child. We need to know what her motives were, how she interprets her past behavior that left the child at risk, and whether she is willing to take responsibility for her actions that made her child vulnerable. It is hard to imagine trusting a child with a parent who does not believe, as we do, that the child's life was in danger. We could say the same thing about a father who sexually molests his daughter. If he cannot share our understanding that what he did was extremely harmful to his daughter, it is hard to believe he would have the motivation not to repeat his actions. It is for these reasons that we maintain that the motivation of the perpetrator of medical abuse is just as significant as the perpetrator's motivation in any other kind of child maltreatment.

What is different is the nature of the excuses used by the perpetrator of the maltreatment. Instead of those we commonly hear from physical, emotional, or sexual abusers, the perpetrator of medical child abuse is likely to fall back on explanations that her behavior was motivated to promote the health of her child. One of the important early steps in the treatment involves communicating that such excuses do not fit with reality. It is important for the mother to come to understand that what she may have thought was helpful to her child was, in fact, just the opposite. Coming to this point is part of a process. The process can take longer if the child is not in imminent danger. If unnecessary surgery is scheduled for the next week then, in order to protect the child, we must move much more quickly. But in most cases the process can unfold over time.

As stated earlier, in our day treatment program we begin treatment by determining where the family is in understanding the problems they face. We assume that parents want their children to be healthy, and that this includes not getting unnecessary or harmful medical care. We are often justified in this assumption but always stand prepared to offer protection for the child if it does not prove to be the case.

Pam, the child who had surgery at 2 months of age to repair a significant cardiac anomaly, had a mother who was extremely protective of her. She kept a wheelchair available even though Pam had no restrictions on her physical activity. She recalls having been told by the cardiologist that Pam should only do what she felt able to do comfortably. She interpreted this to mean that Pam should not participate in any sports, take part in gym class, or even ride a bicycle. In addition to being a "cardiac cripple," Pam also seemed to show symptoms of a major illness every few months. She had been evaluated for kidney failure, pneumonia, and various allergies without significant findings to confirm the diagnosis.

We first met Pam when she was hospitalized in a child psychiatric facility for evaluation of bipolar illness. She had no significant signs or symptoms of psychiatric illness apart from having been infantilized for the first 10 years of her life. She was anxious to be discharged from the hospital because the family was planning a trip to Disney World. The trip was a gift from a charitable foundation.

We reassured the family that Pam did not have bipolar illness and that it was perfectly OK to make the trip to Florida. They agreed to come for outpatient family therapy when they returned from their vacation. The family wanted help for Pam's behavior. They referred to her as "spoiled" and wanted us to help her be less manipulative.

Everyone perceived Pam as extremely fragile. Even her older sister did not fight back when Pam beat her up because she feared aggravating the presumed heart condition. The father was a person of few words who watched what was happening in his house with a certain detachment. He completely agreed with his wife that above all else they needed to protect Pam from exerting herself.

Over the next few weeks we addressed the question of Pam being spoiled by considering whether it had anything to do with her family protecting her too much. With the older sister leading the way, the parents agreed that it was reasonable for Pam to follow the rules of the family like everyone else. She should pick up after herself, carry her dishes to the sink, even if it meant putting a little strain on her heart.

One day while meeting with the mother alone, she admitted that she felt her overprotectiveness might have made things worse. She described how during the trip to Florida she had visited with her mother and sister who still lived together. Her sister had been in a wheelchair since childhood and her mother took care of her. Pam's mother admitted to always resenting the time her mother spent taking care of her sister and volunteered that the only time she was given equal attention was when she was sick. She later shared this with her husband and began a process of allowing her daughter to live life like a normal girl. She began setting limits on her behavior, not responding every time she called from school wanting to come home, and even taught her how to ride a bicycle.

We recently heard news that Pam was married and expecting her first child. No one was concerned that pregnancy would put any undue stress on her heart.

Maintaining the Integrity of the Family

Family preservation is the term used to justify reuniting children with families where they have experienced abuse or neglect. This process is justified in a number of ways. To begin with, society does not have the resources to take care of all of the children who have inadequate parenting. Orphanages have long since gone the way of almshouses. Children are no longer sent away to be apprenticed to a blacksmith or to work on a farm as cheap labor. Foster homes are a precious commodity. Families are smaller and do not want take in extra children as they once did. When both parents work, an extra child can be a real burden. What is more, there is a philosophical bias, shared by society at large, that a child is usually better off living in his own family, however flawed, than being institutionalized or separated from his parents.

Most would agree that the goal of treatment is to have children remain safe within a competent family. So what does it mean to maintain family integrity? Basically, the therapeutic community must make every reasonable attempt to enlist existing family members to join in the effort to create and maintain an adequately functioning family unit. When one person (or several people) is unable or unwilling to take part in this process, we need to take whatever remaining parts are available and reconstitute the family. Families change all the time. Parents get divorced. People move away or become seriously ill. Children grow up. There is no rule that states that every family has to have a certain number of people.

We evaluated a child for possible medical abuse whose parents were in the middle of an awful divorce. The mother had taken her 4-year-old daughter to hospitals 6 times to get sexual abuse evaluations, accusing her ex-husband of touching the girl inappropriately. She provided as evidence videotape she made of her daughter purportedly disclosing the abuse. Sadly, what the videotape actually revealed was a mother actively coaching her daughter to say incriminating things about her father. The girl looked truly pained when forced to repeat after her mother the accusations. We recommended that the girl not have visitation with her mother until the mother underwent therapy with the goal of understanding how she was harming her child. She had already fired one experienced child therapist who, after seeing the little girl for several months, had concluded there was no sexual abuse. The mother began psychotherapy but steadfastly refused to consider that her child had not been sexually abused. We recommended that until she was able to change this belief, the little girl should live entirely with her father. Family court agreed that the best family unit available for this child at that point in time did not include her mother.

In cases where children have been seriously harmed by medical abuse and removed from their families, is it safe to have them return to the care of the perpetrator? The best evidence available comes from the report by Berg and Jones[18] describing efforts to return children to their families after their participation in a child abuse treatment program in Great Britain. They did follow-up outcome interviews several years after discharge. The children received treatment in the Park Hospital for Children's Family Unit. Berg and Jones followed 17 children from 16 families. Four had been admitted for evaluation only and 13 had been admitted for treatment with the goal of reunification.

The 13 children admitted for treatment experienced non-accidental poisoning, induced failure to thrive, and factitious epilepsy. "Treatment comprised psychological interventions targeted at the parent-child relationship, the quality of the child's attachment to each parent, the abuser's own childhood experiences, and the current social network and family dynamics, together with work with the parental couple." Children were in treatment in the family unit for an average of 7½ weeks.

The 13 children who took part in the treatment were all returned to their parents with whom they were living prior to hospitalization. All but one of the children at follow-up remained with their family. In the one case where the child was removed, the mother subsequently caused bleeding in the ear of her child that resulted in a recommendation that she not be allowed to stay in a parental role. The child continued to live with her father after the parents separated.

The authors commented that they had concerns about the functioning of several families at follow-up, but that generally the children had "reasonably good outcomes." They added a caveat that families accepted for treatment aimed at reunification were screened vigorously for appropriateness at the time of enrollment. In all but one situation the abusing caretaker later demonstrated insight into her role in harming her child. One mother at follow-up refused to acknowledge her part in the abuse, but her child was healthy and developing normally.

Except for the one child, none of the treated children had experienced factitious illness in the intervening time between treatment and follow-up. In addition, none of the siblings of the index children had experienced abuse. The authors concluded that the treatment had been effective. They specifically cited the importance of fathers and stepfathers in the success of the treatment.

References

1. Bryk M, Siegel PT. My mother caused my illness: the story of a survivor of Munchausen by proxy syndrome. *Pediatrics.* 1997;100(1):1-7
2. Libow JA. Munchausen by proxy victims in adulthood: a first look. *Child Abuse Negl.* 1995;19(9):1131-1142
3. Bools CN, Neale BA, Meadow SR. Follow up of victims of fabricated illness (Munchausen syndrome by proxy). *Arch Dis Child.* 1993;69(6):625-630
4. Beitchman JH, Zucker KJ, Hood JE, daCosta GA, Akman D, Cassavia E. A review of the long-term effects of child sexual abuse. *Child Abuse Negl.* 1992;16(1):101-118

5. Kaplow JB, Widom CS. Age of onset of child maltreatment predicts long-term mental health outcomes. *J Abnorm Psychol.* 2007;116(1):176-187
6. Schreier HA, Libow JA. *Hurting for Love: Munchausen by Proxy Syndrome.* New York, NY: The Guilford Press; 1993
7. Parnell TF, Day DO, eds. *Munchausen by Proxy Syndrome.* Thousand Oaks, CA: Sage; 1998
8. American Psychiatric Association. *Diagnostic and Statistical Manual of Mental Disorders, Fourth Edition.* Washington, DC: American Psychiatric Association; 1994
9. Bools CN, Neale BA, Meadow SR. Co-morbidity associated with fabricated illness (Munchausen syndrome by proxy). *Arch Dis Child.* 1992;67(1):77-79
10. Gavin LA, Roesler TA. Posttraumatic distress in children and families after intubation. *Pediatr Emerg Care.* 1997;13(3):222-224
11. Roesler TA, Savin D, Grosz C. Family therapy of extrafamilial sexual abuse. *J Am Acad Child Adolesc Psychiatry.* 1993;32(5):967-970
12. Ayoub CC, Deutsch RM, Kinscherff R. Psychosocial management issues in Munchausen by proxy. In: Reece RM, ed. *Treatment of Child Abuse: Common Ground for Mental Health, Medical, Legal Practitioners.* Baltimore, MD: The Johns Hopkins University Press; 2000:226-235
13. Gregory J. *Sickened: The Memoir of a Munchausen by Proxy Childhood.* New York, NY: Bantam; 2003
14. Sanders MJ. Symptom coaching: factitious disorder by proxy with older children. *Clin Psychol Rev.* 1995;15:423-442
15. Libow JA. Beyond collusion: active illness falsification. *Child Abuse Negl.* 2002;26(5):525-536
16. Meadow SR. Munchausen syndrome by proxy. *Med Leg J.* 1995;63(Pt 3):89-104
17. Ayoub CC, Deutsch RM, Kinscherff R. Psychosocial management issues in Munchausen by proxy. In: Reece RM, ed. *Treatment of Child Abuse; Common Ground for Mental Health, Medical, Legal Practitioners.* Baltimore, MD: The Johns Hopkins University Press; 2000:226-235
18. Berg B, Jones DP. Outcome of psychiatric intervention in factitious illness by proxy (Munchausen's syndrome by proxy). *Arch Dis Child.* 1999;81(6):465-472

Chapter 14

Physicians as Part of the Problem

Munchausen syndrome by proxy therefore evolves as a product of the relationship between a parent who has both the capacity for abuse and the potential to be gratified by the medical system and a medical system that is specialized, investigation-oriented, fascinated by rare conditions, often ignorant of abusive behaviors, and too accepting of reported histories. —Donald and Jureidini, 1996[1]

Introduction

As much as we would like to pretend it isn't true, without doctors there would be no medical child abuse. Without doctors children could not be subjected to pointless medical care. Denny et al[2] wrote that the single biggest risk factor for Munchausen syndrome by proxy (MSBP) was exposure to the medical profession. However, we have seen that doctors can be conscious of their role and incorporate strategies into their medical practice to avoid hurting children with medical tests and procedures that are not needed. To do this physicians must be aware. They have to develop an ongoing observing ego that monitors the quality of their relationships with the parents of their patients, and to frequently make random checks for authentic information.

Physicians do not mean to hurt children in their care. In fact, when they find out they have been "professional participants"[3] they often feel guilty, betrayed, and angry about their involvement in the abuse. They have a fundamentally different reaction to the discovery of medical abuse than to all other forms of child maltreatment. After all, in other forms of child abuse physicians have a benevolent role, one consistent with their status as members of a helping profession. When they encounter other forms of maltreatment, they might have a tendency to deny that adults would hurt their children, because this is a not uncommon reaction by many in our society. But they know they were not involved in harming the children themselves. When other types of abuse are encountered, there is little ambivalence, no requirement to justify their previous behavior, and no reason to postpone advocating for the child.

In medical abuse the doctor's responsibility to a child is corrupted by the actions of the child's caretakers. The parent is not honoring the implied contract that dictates an appropriate doctor-patient relationship and sometimes it takes a long time before the physician realizes this to be the case. Certainly, physicians have been lied to before. Although most patients might be guilty of straying from the whole truth at one time or another, there are much more dramatic examples of people lying to their physician for various reasons.

For example, people go to doctors seeking prescription medicines they intend to take recreationally. They tell elaborate, convincing stories about why they need Valium, OxyContin, or Percocet. People also ask their physicians to diagnose disabilities so they can be paid without going to work. While many people making disability claims have medical conditions that justify declaring them disabled, others have minor physical ailments that should not keep them from participating in gainful employment. And others are simply malingering. Physicians are required to use their best medical judgment to sort out these different types of untruths.

Doctors have also come to terms with the need to recognize and treat adult patients with factitious illness. With or without an ulterior motive, adults sometimes inflict injuries on themselves, fabricate symptoms, or otherwise seek medical care they do not need. It is not the lying that makes medical child abuse special, nor is it the caretaker seeking a specific type of reaction from the medical care system. It is the fact that doctors have been placed in the position of "inadvertent collusion"[4] with people who are harming children in their care.

In this chapter we focus on the role of physicians in allowing medical child abuse to take place. In doing so we are only calling attention to something well recognized for decades. Here is Meadow[5] writing 25 years ago:

"Doctors behave in stereotyped ways—a symptom or sign is matched by an investigation or treatment. We still behave as if missing a core organic cause for a complaint is the greatest sin. It is not. It is far worse to batter a child to near death with investigations and treatment when the problem is the mother's behavior. We should develop broader shoulders on which to bear the knowledge that we might miss some organic diagnoses, learn to tolerate uncertainty and unresolved problems, and remember the vista of behavioural variation. This need is as great if not greater, for child psychiatrists as it is for paediatricians."

If Not Malpractice, What Is It?

Although they sometimes think so and occasionally are regarded as such by their patients, doctors are not perfect. They do make mistakes. They sometimes miss salient features of an illness. Occasionally they misread a diagnostic test. A physician might make the wrong diagnosis, or prescribe the wrong treatment for the correct diagnosis. Patients can develop symptoms as a result of medications or treatments administered for another infirmity. Sometimes, while receiving good medical care, patients do not improve and occasionally the treatment makes the illness worse. One study indicated that as many as 36% of the patients on a general hospital medical floor had an iatrogenic illness, one that was caused by the medical treatments given.[6]

Doctors try to minimize their mistakes. Their patients are usually tolerant of an occasional error. Making a mistake is not the same thing as committing malpractice. Malpractice is medical care that does not conform to generally accepted community standards and results in significant injury to the patient. Although all physicians have, at one time or another, been guilty of an oversight, many physicians practice their entire careers without ever being accused of malpractice.

We have said that the harm done to children in medical child abuse is not malpractice. Why not? If a doctor performs an unnecessary surgery, should he or she not be held accountable? To make a determination of malpractice we need to find that most physicians, given the same general circumstances, would not have given the same treatment. If most doctors, using the same false information, came to a similar treatment decision they could be mistaken but it would not be malpractice.

Unnecessary medical care given to a child based on false information supplied by a parent is best characterized as an honest mistake on the part of the physician. If 9 out of 10 doctors, listening to a child's heart, failed to detect a subtle murmur that had real clinical significance, it would not be malpractice, but it would be a mistake. It would be an honest, understandable mistake but a mistake just the same. In the case of medical abuse, even though 90% of physicians given the same false information might administer the same treatment, if it was not needed and harmful or potentially harmful, it has to be considered a mistake. And the reasonable response to finding out that one has made a mistake is to acknowledge it and try to correct it. This is the first thing a doctor should do when experiencing the "Oh, No!" reaction. He should look for a way to stop the abuse and resist the temptation to point fingers away from himself.

Why It's Important for Doctors to Get It Right

Medical abuse is completely preventable. Medical abuse begins with the caretaker's actions but continues with the inadvertent collusion of physicians and other medical care providers. While we do not agree with those who say that doctors are the biggest problem,[7] we assert that doctors should play a major role in *solving* the problem. To participate in stopping medical abuse and reversing its consequences, physicians need to consider that it might be happening. But as we have seen, having a doctor or other medical person call attention to the possibility of medical abuse may not be enough. Medical care is not delivered to one person from one person. This may have been the case long ago, but today medical decisions are made in complex networks of patients and providers. Someone seeking medical care for their child might become involved with literally dozens of medical care personnel. The more people involved, the more chance there is that someone might notice something is awry. But, at the same time, multiple providers make it more difficult to stop the abuse.

In describing our treatment of children with medical abuse and medical/psychiatric difficulties in the Hasbro Children's Partial Hospital Program (HCPHP), we emphasized how important it is to make all major treatment decisions by consensus. We made it plain that we assume there will be differences of opinion. It is the job of the treatment team to acknowledge the differences, to explore the reasons behind them, and to move forward to establish a unitary plan with which everyone can agree. This is consistent with the accepted practice of medicine. In many complicated cases, multiple medical providers gather the pertinent medical information, supplement it with further observations and medical tests, and then decide together on the best course of treatment. If the treatment is not successful, the response to that effort provides data that are used to decide on a new treatment. Treatment decisions flow from available information but are dictated by a process of medical personnel digesting that information and coming to an agreed-on treatment plan.

What happens if the treatment team cannot agree? If the data are interpreted in widely different ways, suggesting diametrically opposed treatment options, then at least one of the possible treatments is likely to be wrong. If the data obtained are incorrect, no treatment option is likely to work. Having doctors disagree is not uncommon. In cases of medical abuse, disagreement is frequent. However, it is often not just that well-meaning clinicians are coming to different conclusions based on the same information. The same caretaker might give different providers different information. Or, if the parent does not like the opinion offered by one doctor, she may approach another, either with new information or a different slant on what someone else has said.

The psychiatric term describing this process is *splitting*. A prototypical example is the child who asks his mother if he can have ice cream before dinner. If she says no he might go ask his father. If his father says, "Sure," the child can choose which answer he likes best. The parents are split with one saying one thing and the other the opposite. In this situation the judgment about what is best for the boy defaults to the child. Obviously, if the parents want to retain their authority with respect to their son it would be best for them to support one another and to coordinate their message. Hence, the answer all fathers need to learn in such a situation is, "What did your mother say?"

Once again, having disagreements about treatment is normal. Well-meaning physicians can and do advocate for children by suggesting a particular illness be addressed in contradictory ways. At times the differences can be trivial. For example, a pediatrician might suggest treating with an antibiotic before getting a positive test for streptococcal pharyngitis. Another physician might advocate holding off prescribing the antibiotic until the result of the microbiological test is known. This is not what we are talking about. In the struggle to identify medical child abuse, admitting the mistake and trying to rectify it, physicians can become irreconcilably split. While this can happen among groups of physicians who work well together, there are certain types of doctors who routinely offer more problems.

The Doctor Who Practices Nontraditional Medicine

A few doctors hold beliefs about medical practice that are far outside the mainstream. Certain parents who also have nontraditional beliefs about medical care gravitate toward them. The Internet provides an efficient way for them to find each other. In our experience doctors who practice nontraditional medicine offer some of the greatest opportunities for splitting. Generally, they have strong opinions and have long ago decided they are right and the rest of the medical community is wrong. These doctors seldom have an interest in forming a consensus with anyone else. As a result, they are a boon for parents who would expose their children to unnecessary or harmful medical care.

For example, there are physicians who believe that many nonspecific medical and psychological symptoms can be manifestations of chronic Lyme disease. Many, if not most, people who live on the East Coast of the United States test positive for antibodies to Lyme disease. This is an indication they have received a tick bite, been exposed to the infectious agent, and have mounted an antibody response. The Infectious Diseases Society of America has published recommendations for evaluation and treatment of Lyme disease.[8] Likewise, the American Academy of Neurology has also published guidelines for the treatment of central nervous system Lyme disease.[9] While Lyme disease can be a serious infectious process with major long-term consequences, it can also be a benign clinical entity where people become infected and never notice any significant symptoms.

We have treated several children whose parents took them to Lyme disease specialists with a reputation for diagnosing Lyme disease and treating it much more aggressively than indicated in accepted guidelines. One child with a documented history of sexual abuse in early childhood and psychological symptoms entirely consistent with her early trauma had received 1½ years of intravenous antibiotics prescribed to treat her chronic low level of depression and irritability. She came to us with her central line still in place. Her mother was appreciative of the help we offered but was adamant about continuing the intravenous antibiotic treatment for the entire 2 years prescribed by the specialist. Several months prior to coming to us the girl had a painful bout of cholecystitis requiring the removal of her gallbladder. This was a side effect of the antibiotic she was receiving. We felt the antibiotic treatment was unnecessary and the gallbladder surgery could have been avoided, and that the indwelling intravenous line was an invitation to potential life-threatening sepsis.

Although we attempted to engage the consultant in considering an alternative hypothesis for the girl's psychological difficulties, we were completely unsuccessful. The girl continued to receive unnecessary and harmful medical care prescribed by a licensed physician who believed he was practicing reasonable medicine. We consulted the local child protection agency but were told that because the family was following prescribed care, there were minimal grounds to support a protection order.

We had better success with a second case. In this instance the child was a young boy who had temper tantrums. During one of his angry outbursts he threatened his mother with a knife. At about the same time he received a tick bite, developed the typical rash, and was prescribed a standard course of antibiotics by his local physician. After completing the treatment he had another rage episode. His mother took him to a Lyme disease specialist who, predictably, diagnosed chronic Lyme disease and prescribed a year of intravenous antibiotics. The boy and his family were referred to us for a second opinion about whether Lyme disease could cause a child to be angry. In our day treatment program we were able to confirm that he had been appropriately treated for Lyme disease. We also determined that he had good reasons to be angry but needed to learn better ways of behaving. The family did not return to the Lyme disease specialist. Several years later the boy and his family are doing well.

Going to Mecca to Get Medical Care

Another group of doctors with whom we occasionally have difficulty collaborating are those who work at highly esteemed medical centers around the country. These are the super-specialists, the doctors who do research on rare conditions. People fly from all over the country to see them because of their special expertise. They have the latest diagnostic tests at their disposal. They are accustomed to making diagnoses that nobody else can make.

Terri was a 12-year-old girl who came to us with a diagnosis of chronic fatigue syndrome. She had not been attending school for more than a year. Her parents were divorced. She lived with her mother who worked at home so she was able to be with her daughter. Terri was intelligent and easily kept up with her schoolwork by studying an hour or two a day. She complained of being tired all the time. We enrolled her in the day treatment program and invited her to take part in all normal activities. We quickly noted a pattern in her behavior. If there was something that she really did not want to do, she complained of being tired. However, because most of the activities were interesting to her, she usually showed no evidence whatsoever of fatigue. We engaged her in a program of vigorous exercise and she thrived. We told her mother that after conducting a standard diagnostic workup and observing her for almost a month, we saw no evidence for chronic fatigue syndrome. Her mother acknowledged the progress she had made with us but said that Terri still complained of being tired at home.

Two days before she was discharged from the program, Terri's mother told us that she had scheduled a visit to a famous medical clinic in the Midwest. Terri left our program a healthy, happy 12-year-old and flew off for a 5-day schedule of medical tests. We sent the experts a detailed description of the 4 weeks Terri stayed with us, including the medical testing we conducted and our observations regarding her symptoms. They repeated many of our tests, had similar findings, and did many more. The doctors wrote a 10-page report saying that Terri didn't actually meet criteria for chronic fatigue syndrome but that she might have a minor variant of the condition. Terri's mother brought us the report and said, in effect, "See, I told you so."

In the HCPHP we sometimes treat what is now referred to as *complex regional pain syndrome*. The symptoms wax and wane, and the parents' description of symptoms is an essential piece in the diagnostic puzzle. We treated a teenager referred with this disease who responded very well to our therapeutic environment and showed no symptoms for several weeks. We reviewed her past medical records and noted that there had only been one time in the previous 3 years when a medical provider had observed what might be a confirmatory sign of the illness. Our conclusion was that if she had the disease at all, it was a very mild form and she should be encouraged to lead a normal life.

Her mother told us she wanted to seek a second opinion and took her to a well-respected expert in another city. After hearing the mother's account of the illness, including her version of all of the unsuccessful treatments the child had received, the expert recommended that the teen travel to Germany to get an experimental treatment that involved undergoing a drug-induced coma for 3 days.

Before taking this rather drastic step the family returned to us. We reiterated our treatment plan based on what we had learned previously about the child, and called the expert to confer. We explained to the expert that she had had no significant symptoms in the previous 3 years and had participated in 3 different sports at school. He expressed surprise to get this version of the child's medical history. His impression, based on his conversation with the mother, was that this was one of the worst cases of complex regional pain syndrome he had ever seen.

After we spoke with him, but before we put our treatment plan into effect, the mother e-mailed the expert to ask his opinion of what we proposed. The next day she brought us his e-mail response in which he advised her that she should follow the treatment as outlined by our program and assured her that she was "in good hands." In this case, the doctor who might have opened a big crack in the treatment team came back to heal the split.

Working With Specialist Colleagues

Among our regular colleagues and friends are some very good physicians who are particularly aggressive in making a diagnosis or starting a new treatment. They revel in the diagnostic dilemma presented by some of our more challenging patients. These doctors take great pride in their work. They really want to help patients get better. They practice mainstream medicine but sometimes do not seem to appreciate when to stop.

This aggressive approach to medical practice takes 2 general forms. The first type involves trying a series of new treatments, one after another, with the hope that one will eventually result in a cure. The second type is similar but with a twist. Some thoughtful physicians cannot stop looking for the cause of the illness. The first kind of physician is more likely to prescribe unnecessary medications and perform unneeded procedures, while the second will continue to do ever more obscure diagnostic tests.

Doctors are generally interested in curing illness. They see themselves as agents charged with eradicating pain and suffering. Some of our specialist colleagues are particularly dedicated. We spend a great deal of time with these doctors discussing how much treatment is enough. In his description of the treatment of several families with MSBP, Griffith[10] commented that his most difficult task was convincing doctors to stop giving medical care.

In Chapter 7 we introduced Richard. For 6 months prior to coming to our program, his mother would wake him up each morning in time to go to school. He would tell her, "I can't lift my legs, my feet won't move." She left him home in bed and went to work. At about 11:00 am he would get up and get some breakfast. He told us that his legs slowly got better during the day. At about the time school got out he would jump on his motocross bicycle and go out and practice with his friends, zooming around the track they had constructed in the woods. Motocross competitions involve jumping over tall mounds of dirt, spinning around sharp corners, and taking many a tumble. Richard was really good at this.

The first 2 days he attended the HCPHP he came in at about 11:00 am. After that he began showing up at the normal time between 8 and 8:30. We did a neurologic examination first thing each morning for the next 2 weeks, looking for weakness or loss of sensation in his legs. There were never any positive findings. We told Richard and his mother that we had no explanation for his previous difficulty but that he seemed to be fine now and recommended that he return to school.

Before starting the day program Richard had been scheduled to see a highly respected surgeon as part of the search for the answer to his mysterious neurologic condition. The surgeon ordered x-rays of Richard's spine. We told the surgeon about the boy's experience with us, including his many normal examinations. He responded that the story as related by Richard and his mother reminded him of children with a tethered spinal cord. He said in such cases the symptoms were always worse first thing in the morning. He felt the radiographs of the spine confirmed his diagnosis and scheduled Richard for surgery.

Surgery for a tethered cord consists of making an incision at the bottom of the back, opening the spine, and severing a piece of tissue. This tissue is attached to the spinal cord and keeps it from pulling back up into the spinal canal where it belongs. Richard had the surgery. It made no difference in his symptoms.

Practicing good, evidence-based medicine does not only mean knowing when to stop ordering more diagnostic tests. It also means knowing when one more test will make the difference in understanding why the child is sick. An adolescent was referred to us because of uncontrollable vomiting.

He was admitted to the hospital after several days of not being able to keep any food in his stomach. He was dehydrated and distraught. Specialists in gastroenterology, endocrinology, neurology, and infectious diseases, looking for an explanation for his illness, examined him. Two weeks went by and no one could find an answer. During that time, however, the young man's father had threatened to remove him from the hospital, gotten into major arguments with attending physicians, and interfered with the medical staff's treatment of his son. The hospital's child protection team was consulted to determine if the child needed to be protected from his father. They helped negotiate an appropriate relationship between the treatment team and the boy's father and enlisted him in cooperating with treatment for his son.

The boy was discharged from the hospital to the day treatment unit for ongoing monitoring. By this time he was living on nasogastric feeds dripped slowly into his stomach 24 hours a day. Any time he received any quantity of food he would vomit. We had no explanation for his medical condition. We considered a possible diagnosis of psychogenic vomiting but had no clear evidence that there was a psychological etiology for his symptoms. We called together all of the subspecialists for a conference and the decision was made to make one more attempt to find a neurologic cause for his illness. This time, on a specialized scan, a rare inflammatory process was discovered in a particular part of his brain that explained his medical difficulty.

The aggressive specialists are sometimes right. Sometimes we really do need to do one more procedure, or schedule one more diagnostic test. The key to practicing good medicine is to keep an open mind and follow the data. Sometimes the facts lead to a rare brain disease, and other times they dictate stopping unnecessary treatment.

Conclusion

We began this chapter by recognizing that without doctors there would be no medical child abuse. It is just as axiomatic that without doctors there could be no solution to the problem of medical child abuse. Physicians are best able to determine when medical care is not necessary. They are the appropriate source for initiating modifications in the treatment regimen. They are responsible for maintaining the doctor-patient contract and monitoring that it is functioning on behalf of the child. Doctors are responsible for looking at the evidence and applying it appropriately.

If we were to highlight 2 principles that can help doctors undo medical child abuse, the first would be to recognize the importance of directly observing perplexing symptoms reported by parents of children who are receiving unusual amounts of medical care. The second would be to appreciate the value of collaboration and communication with colleagues. In the HCPHP we have the luxury of observing a child 8 hours a day, 5 days a week. We can take any symptom described by a parent and subject it to direct scrutiny by a team of trained observers. If a parent claims that her child is "coughing all the time," we can count the number of times per hour the child coughs. This is not always possible in a busy medical practice. But there is no substitute for actually confirming the claims made by parents. Most of the time we can expect what parents say about their children will turn out to be consistent with what we observe. But some of our most effective medical judgments will occur when we discover discrepancy between parent claims and what we see ourselves.

We can extend the notion that it is important to directly observe children by recognizing the benefit to be gained by bringing in multiple points of view. Close collaboration with our colleagues is essential. The practice of medicine has become, more and more, a group endeavor. Gathering together providers from different disciplines allows us to see things from multiple points of view. Having the opportunity to apply many different perspectives to the same set of facts helps us avoid getting off on blind paths. Time and again we have found the answer to tough clinical problems by gathering a team of providers together to bring clarity to a confusing case. Finding consensus among colleagues is not a guarantee of practicing mistake-free medicine, but it is a very good place to start.

References

1. Donald T, Jureidini J. Munchausen syndrome by proxy. Child abuse in the medical system. *Arch Pediatr Adolesc Med.* 1996;150(7):753-758
2. Denny SJ, Grant CC, Pinnock R. Epidemiology of Munchausen syndrome by proxy in New Zealand. *J Paediatr Child Health.* 2001;37(3):240-243
3. Zitelli BJ, Seltman MF, Shannon RM. Munchausen's syndrome by proxy and its professional participants. *Am J Dis Child.* 1987;141(10):1099-1102
4. Hyman PE. Chronic intestinal pseudo-obstruction in childhood: progress in diagnosis and treatment. *Scand J Gastroenterol Suppl.* 1995;213:39-46
5. Meadow R. Munchausen syndrome by proxy. *Arch Dis Child.* 1982;57(2):92-98

6. Franks P, Clancy CM. Gatekeeping revisited-protecting patients from overtreatment. *N Engl J Med.* 1992;327:424-420
7. von Hahn L, Harper G, McDaniel SH, Siegel DM, Feldman MD, Libow JA. A case of factitious disorder by proxy: the role of the health-care system, diagnostic dilemmas, and family dynamics. *Harv Rev Psychiatry.* 2001;9(3):124-135
8. Wormser GP, Dattwyler RJ, Shapiro ED, Halperin JJ, Steere AC, Klempner MS. The clinical assessment, treatment, and prevention of Lyme disease, human granulocytic anaplasmosis, and babesiosis: clinical practice guidelines by the Infectious Diseases Society of America. *Clin Infect Dis.* 2006;43(9):1089-1134
9. Halperin JJ, Shapiro ED, Logigian E, Belmon AL, Dotevall L, Wormser GP. Practice parameter: treatment of nervous system Lyme disease (an evidence-based review): report of the Quality Standards Subcommittee of the American Academy of Neurology. *Neurology.* 2007;69(1):91-102
10. Griffith JL. The family systems of Munchausen syndrome by proxy. *Fam Process.* 1988;27(4):423-437

Chapter 15

Lawyers as Part of the Solution

"Abused child" means a child…whose parent or other person legally responsible for his care…creates or allows to be created a substantial risk of physical injury to such child by other than accidental means which would be likely to cause death or serious or protracted disfigurement, or protracted impairment of physical or emotional health.… —New York Family Court Act, Section 1012

Introduction

Doctors and lawyers think differently. Doctors use Aristotelian logic. They gather as many facts as they can, sift them into different categories, and come to conclusions based on how the facts fit together. A diagnostic and treatment plan follows from this reasoned interpretation of the available evidence. Lawyers use Platonic thinking. They start with a general premise and muster evidence to support or refute that premise.

Inductive logic is the foundation of evidence-based medicine. First start with the evidence and then come to an understanding of what organizes the evidence in the best way. Deductive logic is the foundation of legal advocacy. One starts with a general principle, guilt or innocence for example. The person using deductive logic then gathers whatever pieces of evidence give credence to the general principle while discarding the rest. Physicians live in a world of probability. They are comfortable considering what might be the "best possible solution." Lawyers live in a world of absolutes, and spend their efforts looking for Truth and Justice.

Once a physician determines that the medical contract is irreparably broken and that a child may be harmed by ongoing inappropriate medical care, he or she begins the process of moving between the worlds of medicine and law. Traditionally, this has not always been an easy transition. Doctors tend to believe that their kind of thinking is best. The same can be said for lawyers.

We have emphasized that medical care functions best when care providers collaborate with one another and work to achieve consensus. The legal system begins with the assumption that something is either black or white rather than some shade of gray. When a child is being mistreated there comes a time when someone has to decide if the treatment is right or wrong.

The legal system is by definition adversarial. It is based on the notion that to come to a fair judgment one must examine the best arguments from both sides. A neutral party, the judge or jury, then decides who has the best arguments. The system is designed so that for every question, someone argues for one side while someone else argues for the other.

By recognizing that the central issue in medical child abuse is whether the child needs protection, physicians are compelled to cooperate with the legal system. If medical child abuse were solely a disease that doctors could treat, the medical profession would feel much more comfortable. In a way, calling medical abuse an illness, namely Munchausen syndrome by proxy (MSBP), was an attempt by the medical profession to keep this type of child abuse within its own problem-solving context. But it is not an illness. It is a bad thing that happens to children, and doctors may not be able to stop it on their own.

As physicians begin to function in the legal world they most likely encounter a lawyer who will defend their point of view, their interpretation of the facts. But another lawyer will dispute that interpretation. Lawyers assume that someone will take the opposite point of view. Physicians, on the other hand, think that because they have put so much effort into evaluating all the facts, and they have come to agreement with knowledgeable peers, arguing with the other side should not be necessary. From the doctor's point of view, if all of the facts are presented and confirmed by their peers, there really should not be another side to the question.

We were provided recently with an excellent example of the discrepancy between how doctors and lawyers think in the case of Alice, who was discussed in Chapter 10. Several months after Alice's father filed for divorce, he remained the sole custodian of his children. Alice and her siblings were doing well. Their mother then requested unsupervised visitation. She came to the court hearing with a new attorney. The argument the attorney made on her behalf was that she was being barred from caring for the children because of her diagnosis of depression. The mother had spent several weeks in the hospital receiving treatment for depression and suicidal ideation. The lawyer for the children argued that over a number of years, Alice's mother had exposed her children to medical harm. The mother's attorney argued that she should have unsupervised visitation and, indeed, joint custody of the children because no one should be discriminated against because of mental illness. He argued that her right not to be discriminated against was more important than the right of the children to be safe. Fortunately, the arguments of the children's attorney prevailed.

Child Abuse Pediatrics

The legal community exists to interpret rules for society. The legal system cannot enforce the laws without help. For example, it needs police to catch lawbreakers and prisons to segregate lawbreakers from the rest of society. As a society we have decided that some children need protection from harm inflicted by caretakers. We have laws against harming children. In many cases of child abuse, the legal system also needs doctors to help enforce the laws by providing medical opinions in courts. We have described the natural antagonism that exists between legal and medical thinking and the discomfort many doctors feel when compelled to function in a legal environment. As the body of knowledge surrounding child abuse in all its forms has grown, it has become increasingly more difficult for the generalist physician to keep fully informed. In response to this need for professionals with this special knowledge, a new pediatric subspecialty has come into being.[1]

There are more than 500 pediatricians who belong to the child abuse interest group of the American Academy of Pediatrics. In November 2009, approximately 200 pediatricians will take a board examination in a new subspecialty approved by the American Board of Pediatrics called *child abuse pediatrics*. The availability of a new cadre of specialized pediatricians makes it possible for doctors of all kinds to consult with medical colleagues about concerns regarding suspected child maltreatment. These professional child abuse doctors are trained to communicate with the civil authorities, to testify in trials, and to use their pediatric knowledge of child abuse to advocate for children.

After the original "grandfathering" of physicians currently functioning as child abuse pediatricians, all new subspecialists will be trained as general pediatricians before starting a subspecialty fellowship program.[2] They will learn how to evaluate and identify child maltreatment in all its forms. They will study research methodology so they can conduct original research leading to a better understanding of child abuse and neglect. And they will learn how to function within the legal system as advisers to the court and as expert witnesses. On a day-to-day basis they will do what most physicians would rather avoid. They will provide a buffer between the general medical community and the child protection system.

While not all communities have one, child abuse specialists are becoming more available all the time. Their presence makes it easier for physicians seeing children who they suspect are victims of medical abuse to make the transition from being the vector of the abuse to being part of the solution. And conversely, the presence of child abuse pediatricians provides a necessary element for the legal system to advocate for children. Without medical professionals who function within the child protection system, the system would be missing critical information it needs to make the right decisions.

Child abuse pediatricians advocate for children but retain their medical identity. They are not required to be investigators, prosecutors, or judges. They use their special expertise as expert witnesses to state their opinions about the health issues pertaining to a child. The civil authority can use this information to decide whether the child needs protection. In practice this means that a doctor can look at a specific injury, a particular burn pattern for example, and render a medical judgment that the injury is not likely to be accidental. A child forced by an adult to stand in a tub filled with water at 180° F for a few seconds will develop a distinct red stocking-like burn pattern with a clear demarcation between burned flesh and normal skin. The child who accidentally sticks his leg in very hot tub water will jump out and have a totally different burn pattern, complete with splash marks. Once this observation is made, based on medical evidence, the decision about whether to report possible abuse is taken from the doctor's hands. A legally mandated report is made and the appropriate people investigate whether the child was burned intentionally, whether criminal charges need to be filed, or whether the child can return home safely.

Child abuse pediatricians are especially valuable for investigating suspected medical child abuse. A doctor who thinks medical abuse is occurring can consult the local child protection team in his or her jurisdiction and get an opinion from a child abuse specialist. As part of the medical community, a child abuse pediatrician can interpret the need for protection from unnecessary medical care to the appropriate civil authorities. This makes for a significantly easier transition between the medical context and the legal system.

Mandatory Reporting Laws and Malpractice

Doctors are not only uncomfortable dealing with medical child abuse; they often shy away from getting involved in any type of child maltreatment issues. In fact, before children could be adequately protected in this country, laws had to be passed mandating that physicians and others report suspected abuse to civil authorities. The choice whether to become involved was taken away from them. Mandatory reporting laws apply not only to the medical profession but also to other professionals, such as teachers, directly involved in helping children.

Mandatory reporting laws did 2 things. First, by taking away the choice of whether to report child maltreatment, they greatly improved the chances that the professional community would identify children being harmed in their home environment. Second, the laws provided immunity from litigation for professionals reporting suspected abuse or neglect. In this country, if you suspect child abuse, not only are you mandated to report, but, in theory, you cannot be sued for reporting the maltreatment "in good faith." Without mandatory reporting laws children would be much more vulnerable. Most physicians have come to appreciate the benefits of having these laws on the books.

This does not mean that doctors cannot face legal challenges. One report documents the case of a child with nodules covering her body that her pediatrician felt might be caused by injecting a foreign substance under the skin.[3] The pediatrician made a report to social services for suspected abuse. The child was removed from her family for 1 month and treated in a hospital, where she was eventually diagnosed with dermatomyositis. An important part of the diagnosis was the development of new nodules while not under the care of her parents. The parents filed a malpractice suit against the reporting physician. The parents lost at the pretrial summary judgment phase. The authors of this report conclude by saying, "Practitioners should also recognize that, regardless of the state statutes mandating reports, FDP [factitious disorder by proxy] is a form of 'medical' child abuse that carries with it invariable short-term morbidity, a high risk of long-term morbidity, and an estimated death rate of 9%. With this knowledge, physicians and others should never allow themselves to be dissuaded from reporting their suspicions to the appropriate authorities."

Rather than stating that FDP is a form of medical child abuse, we maintain that it *is* medical child abuse. (The death rate estimate of 9% in the above quotation refers to the number from the article, "Web of Deceit"[4] that has not been validated.) However, the message remains that the suspicion of illness induction by a caretaker represents child abuse and constitutes behavior protected under mandatory reporting statutes. In this case, a physician reported possible medical child abuse that was not confirmed. Yet he was still protected by the legal system.

The fact that mandatory reporters are protected from litigation also helped a prominent child abuse pediatrician in Seattle. Five different families sued him after he made reports of suspected child abuse by MSBP.[5] He was also reported to the local medical board by a physician hired by the families as an expert witness. The suits and complaints to the medical board were dismissed. Perman[6] reviews several recent court decisions that confirm protection for physicians who make reports of abuse in suspected MSBP. His review also notes court decisions that protect physicians from suits claiming malpractice by negligently diagnosing a parent with MSBP. We expect this will occur more and more frequently until awareness grows and standards emerge about what constitutes medically abusive behavior that requires protection of the child by public agencies.

When considering medical child abuse, physicians face another type of threat from the legal system. They are hesitant to stop searching for a medical answer in a perplexing case because they are afraid of being accused of malpractice if a diagnosis is missed. We mentioned earlier that many physicians practice an entire career without having a suit filed against them. But it happens frequently enough, and it is unpleasant enough, to produce a phenomenon referred to as *defensive medicine*. Defensive medicine is the practice of ordering extra diagnostic tests to make sure that one has not missed an important clinical finding. In fact, whenever we speak about medical child abuse to groups of physicians and advocate limiting the number of possibly unwarranted invasive medical tests on children, invariably a physician will express concern about being sued for malpractice. This motivation for excessive medical care has been cited often.[7]

Our response to this observation is to agree that doctors should, in the course of practicing good medicine, consider reasonable alternatives and take whatever medical steps are necessary to make an appropriate diagnosis. However, this does not extend to ordering tests or performing procedures when one suspects that the information on which the test is based might be inaccurate. It is incumbent on the physician to at least consider that the information might not be correct and to pursue alternative sources of history that could alleviate or confirm that suspicion.

The real danger for physicians in the legal environment may come from an unusual direction. It is entirely possible that, as people become more alert to the presence of medical abuse, doctors will be expected to recognize it much more readily than they do now. This could result in a new community standard of care that holds doctors responsible for *not* considering the possibility of false information entering the medical care setting resulting in harm to children from excessive medical care. Failure to report other forms of abuse has led physicians to run afoul of mandatory reporting laws.

There is one well-cited example of an adult suing her doctors for malpractice, and negotiating a judgment against them for failing to recognize that she was fabricating illness in herself.[8] The woman who brought suit had attended medical school but had not graduated. Instead, she was admitted many times to a hospital to treat a nonexistent cancer in her stomach. She brought suit against 35 doctors asking for $14 million based on their failure to diagnose that she was fabricating symptoms. She eventually settled for $315,000.

The Growing Awareness of Medical Child Abuse in the Legal System

Correctly designating medical child abuse as a form of child maltreatment paves the way for the medical profession to interact successfully with the legal process. Child abuse is already established as the purview of social service agencies and courts of law. Lawyers cannot cure diseases, but they can help determine whether a child deserves protection from maltreatment. By giving up their claim that a child (or a parent) is suffering from an illness, the medical community cedes jurisdiction regarding protection while retaining the ability to treat any of the consequences of the abuse.

Even if the medical profession has been slow to acknowledge that medical child abuse is behavior that has to be judged by social services and the legal system, the courts are making that determination. Schreier[9] describes the legal outcome of the Kathy Bush case:

> It took three years to bring the mother to trial for child abuse and fraud. Neither MBP nor any other testimony as to her motivation was permitted in the trial. The jurors all believed that Mrs. Bush loved her daughter, despite the overwhelming, but circumstantial evidence of her eight years of abuse of this child.
>
> Testimony at her trial as to the possible motives for the mother's actions was strickly [sic] excluded by the judge. Though he agreed that there was such a thing as MBP, he relied on the statement of one expert that it was a diagnosis of the child, and therefore the motivation of the mother was seen as irrelevant. All the jurors agreed that this verdict to convict was a difficult one, as all felt that Mrs. Bush loved her daughter. On January 28, a judge sentenced Mrs. Bush to five years in prison, but as in another high profile case, he took the unusual step of allowing her to return home rather than start her term while she filed an appeal.

When all was said and done, this parent was found guilty of child abuse. She was held accountable for what she did to her child. It did not matter to the jury why she subjected her child to such harm. It did not matter if she had a diagnosis of MSBP, or if her child had a diagnosis of MSBP. What did matter was that a child was harmed and needed protection from her mother's behavior.

The Queensland Decision

Further evidence that thinking in the legal system has progressed beyond that of the medical community is found in a landmark appellate decision from Australia.[10] In the Kathy Bush case the judge did not allow expert testimony explaining MSBP. In the Queensland decision the Court of Appeal determined that a woman was entitled to a new trial because the judge *did allow* expert testimony regarding MSBP.

The case involved a mother medically abusing all 4 of her children. She gave them laxatives in the form of magnesium sulfate (Epsom salts), which resulted in diarrhea, severe anemia, and failure to thrive. The children required indwelling lines to treat their malnutrition and dehydration, and subsequently experienced episodes of polymicrobial sepsis. They underwent bone biopsy, biopsies of the gut, numerous diagnostic procedures, and feeding by total parenteral nutrition. The abuse went on for years. Finally, the treating physician concluded the children were being abused and received consultation from experts in child abuse and MSBP. He admitted the youngest child to a special hospital unit where he could be observed and videotaped. The mother was given specific instructions not to feed the child anything but a special formula. She was observed breastfeeding the boy, giving him apple juice, pouring the formula into the sink, diluting the remaining formula with water, putting magnesium sulfate into his feeding tube via a syringe, and diluting the stool in his "nappy," making it look like diarrhea.

At trial the jury members were shown hours of videotape to determine whether this woman had harmed her child. The prosecution had a psychiatrist testify about MSBP. The expert, as recounted in the appeal decision, gave an excellent description of what is commonly referred to as MSBP or FDP. "There are no agreed sets of symptoms and signs which enabled the behavior to be classified into a recognized, psychiatric diagnostic system. It is a behaviour that occurs occasionally within the community but it is not necessarily within the expertise of a psychiatrist to comment on such behaviour because it is not a disorder. It is akin to recognizing that there is a thing such as laughing. It is merely a name for a type of behavior, comparable to the expressions 'malingering' or 'engaged in criminal conduct.'" He went on to summarize in considerable detail what is known about FDP. The prosecution also had 3 physicians testify that the behaviors engaged in by the mother were consistent with FDP.

The jury found the mother guilty and she was sentenced to 7 years in prison. The jury agreed with the prosecution's characterization that the mother had subjected the children to torture. The defendant appealed on several grounds. Her attorneys argued that the evidence about FDP was wrongly admitted. In addition they maintained that allowing the experts to testify had been unfair for their client.

The 3-judge panel of the Court of Appeal agreed. It wrote:

> The issues for the jury's determination of trial were whether the prosecution established that the appellant committed acts causing symptoms in and, or alternatively, falsely reported or fabricated symptoms of B, C and D [the children] with the intention that medical professionals would perform otherwise unnecessary procedures on them. It is purely a matter for the jury to decide the question of the appellant's past intentions.[10]

In other words there was no need for medical experts to testify about the motivation of the perpetrator. The jury was perfectly competent to decide whether the mother had hurt the children. In his decision the president of the Court of Appeal gave examples of other behaviors that people might find puzzling but that juries are often asked to take into consideration. "Who would think a wealthy, successful woman would steal small items of no apparent use to her? Who would think a dedicated, hard-working schoolteacher would sexually abuse some of his vulnerable young pupils whilst being greatly respected and valued by other students?"

In supporting the position of the mother with regard to the testimony of the 3 experts, the judges maintained that allowing the psychiatrist and others to testify about MSBP might have given the prosecution an advantage by making it seem as if there was a special explanation the jury might not be able to understand without expert help. The chief judge went on to say, "Ordinary people are capable of understanding that some mothers may harm their children through deceitfully manipulating unnecessary medical treatment."

As another example of the court system getting it right, a ruling from the Supreme Court of New York recently confirmed a lower court's finding on appeal that a parent subjecting a child to harmful medical care constituted child abuse.[11] Prior to this ruling MSBP was considered to be a form of neglect and as such was adjudicated as a misdemeanor.

The child in question was a 14-month-old girl. Her mother claimed she had a seizure disorder. The child had been taken to several different hospitals for evaluation and treatment. Dr Debra Esernio-Jenssen, a child abuse expert, explained during the original fact-finding hearing that the child had been subjected to many unnecessary tests and potentially harmful treatments, including the administration of anticonvulsant medications. The doctor testified that when she explained to the child's mother that the girl was perfectly healthy, the mother became angry and tried to take her to another hospital. The doctor testified that the "…pediatric community is changing the child victim's diagnosis from MSP to medical child abuse in order to shift the emphasis away from the perpetrator and place it on the abused child, disregarding the psychological motivation or emotional state of the parent."[11]

The defense in this case introduced evidence from a psychologist who argued that the defendant did not have MSBP. Later the defense argued that the mother's intellectual limitations explained why she made inaccuracies when reporting her child's symptoms. This explanation extended to numerous other false statements made by the mother as well. The defense went on to say that at worst, the mother should be found guilty of neglect because she only fabricated, not caused, illness in her child.

The trial judge, in offering her original opinion, referred to the New York state legal definitions of child abuse that includes the statement that child abuse exists when a person "…creates or allows to be created a substantial risk of physical injury to such child by other than accidental means which could be likely to cause death or serious or protracted disfigurement, or protracted impairment of physical or emotional health or protracted loss of impairment of the function of any bodily organ…." The judge found that the "…mother's affirmative and intentional acts of repeatedly bringing her infant and then toddler to multiple hospitals and doctors, repeatedly claiming that Anesia suffered from repeated and severe seizures for more than a year, created and allowed to be created by the medical community, a substantial risk of physical injury leading to serious physical injury to Anesia."[11] The judge ruled that the mother's actions constituted physical child abuse. She dismissed the argument that the mother's behavior was accidental or could be explained by her mental disabilities saying, "No specific intent to injure or specific motive is necessary for a finding of abuse."

The case was appealed to the Supreme Court of New York and upheld by a unanimous decision.[12]

Rewriting Abuse and Neglect Statutes

In our own jurisdiction we were recently asked to help rewrite the definitions of child abuse used by our state child protection agency. The previous departmental guidelines gave definitions for physical abuse, sexual abuse, emotional abuse, and various forms of neglect. Cases involving children harmed in the medical environment were treated under definitions for "physical neglect" and "other neglect."

In collaboration with the Rhode Island Department of Children, Youth and Families, we agreed that a definition be inserted in the guidelines that reads

> **Medical Abuse**
>
> *Definition:* Acts by a caretaker resulting in unnecessary and harmful or potentially harmful medical care to a child. The unnecessary medical care can be the result of either a pattern of persistent misinformation provided by the caretaker to medical care provider(s), or by falsification of symptoms, or by actual induction of illness in the child by the caretaker.
>
> *Usage:* The abuse must be attributable to a pattern of behavior by the caretaker. Direct harm to a child resulting from the induction of illness, such as non-accidental poisoning or suffocation, shall be considered assault.
>
> *Caveat:* The harmful or potentially harmful medical care cannot be solely the result of medical provider error.

With this language in place children in the state of Rhode Island can be protected from medical abuse just as they are from other forms of child abuse. On a case-by-case basis concerns can be raised and a report can be filed with the state. This results in an investigation to determine if the allegations can be substantiated and whether a child requires protection. The process is no different for this type of abuse than for any other.

Conclusion

As difficult as it may be to acknowledge, our colleagues in the legal profession may be in the process of saving physicians from themselves. In the cases cited here we see legal decisions that bypass the notion of motivation and essentially absolve physicians of the need to ascertain what that motivation might be. The legal system is not only giving us permission but is offering the medical community specific directions to follow the medical evidence and look at the medical care children have received in order to determine if they have been harmed.

As mentioned earlier, in legal proceedings there are 2 sides to every argument. Judges in 3 different jurisdictions agreed that motivation of the perpetrator was unnecessary to reach judgment. In 2 cases, Queensland and Florida (Kathy Bush), lawyers representing doctors were arguing that evidence for MSBP should be admitted and lawyers for the defense were arguing against this position. In the New York case, Dr Esernio-Jenssen and lawyers for the state maintained that there was no need to invoke MSBP. In all 3 situations evidence for MSBP was disregarded.

This leaves attorneys defending mothers accused of medical abuse in a curious position. They have been able to argue that their clients were not guilty because they did not suffer from MSBP. And if this did not work they could advocate that MSBP does not exist and therefore no crime was committed and the child was not harmed. In the New York case, even though no accusation of MSBP was made by the attorneys attempting to protect the child, the mother's defense team called a psychologist who testified that the defendant did not have it. The testimony was later ruled as irrelevant. Despite this, newspaper articles regarding this case and another similar case from the same institution, focused on "…a controversial, rare diagnosis."[13] The child abuse team at Schneider Children's Hospital made no allegations of MSBP but newspaper accounts gave it front-page coverage. In the article parents found guilty of medically abusing their children argued that they did not suffer from MSBP.

A high-profile case in Texas recently played out in a similar fashion. A mother of 3 children was found guilty of having one of her children receive 2 surgeries, a gastric feeding tube, and implantation of a nerve stimulation device to treat nonexistent diseases. She raised about $150,000 from community resources purportedly to help with their care. Dr Reena Isaac and the child protection team at Texas Children's Hospital in Houston investigated the case and recommended to state authorities they use *medical child abuse* instead of *MSBP* (R. Isaac, personal communication, 2008). Nevertheless, attorneys for the defense introduced witnesses who testified that the mother who perpetrated the abuse did not suffer from MSBP. In spite of her defense, the jury convicted her of 2 counts of injury to a child and sentenced her to 15 years in prison.[14]

Mike Trent, the assistant district attorney who tried the case, wrote an account of the trial that reads like a primer for authorities wanting to hold parents accountable for the medical abuse of their children.[15] Earlier we described a situation where a mother poisoned her daughter with ipecac in our hospital bathroom. Two weeks later we received a telephone call from a juvenile court judge. She was calling from the bench in the middle of a hearing regarding this child. She asked if we knew any experts on MSBP who would be willing to evaluate the mother. The mother's attorney was specifically asking the court for permission to spend $20,000 to retain an MSBP expert as part of his client's defense. The judge felt that might be a little expensive and wanted to know if we were aware of any more reasonably priced experts. Once we sorted out exactly what the judge was requesting we explained that finding an expert was not necessary. No one would be accusing the mother of having an illness called MSBP. The basis for the child protection case was simply that the mother had poisoned her daughter and got caught. The judge said, "Oh, I get it!" She told the defense attorney that the state would not be calling any experts on MSBP so he did not need to be looking for one either.

References

1. Block RW, Palusci VJ. Child abuse pediatrics: a new pediatric subspecialty. *J Pediatr.* 2006;148(6):711-712
2. Starling SP, Sirotnak AP, Jenny C. Child abuse and forensic pediatric medicine fellowship curriculum statement. *Child Maltreat.* 2000;5(1):58-62
3. Feldman MD, Allen DB. "False-positive" factitious disorder by proxy. *South Med J.* 1996;89(4):452-453
4. Rosenberg DA. Web of deceit: a literature review of Munchausen syndrome by proxy. *Child Abuse Negl.* 1987;11(4):547-563
5. Smith C. Persecuted parents or protected children? Allegations cost their reputations, their money and nearly their kids. *Seattle Post-Intelligencer.* August 7, 2002
6. Perman CM. The suspicious physician—legal protections and ramifications for the medical community in identifying and treating Munchausen syndrome by proxy. *Health Care Law Mon.* 2008;2008(1):2-7
7. Kessler DP, Summerton N, Graham JR. Effects of the medical liability system in Australia, the UK, and the USA. *Lancet.* 2006;368(9531):240-246
8. Lipsett DR. The factitious patient who sues. *Am J Psychiatry.* 1986;143(11):1482
9. Schreier HA. Proposed definitional guidelines for Munchausen by proxy: a cautionary note. *AACAP News.* 2000;March/April:77-78
10. R v LM. Vol QCA 192: Supreme Court of Queensland; 2004

11. In the Matter of Anesia E. A Child under Eighteen Years of Age Alleged to be Abused by Antoinette W., Respondent. Sangenito I, Whittig T, Fee L, trans: Family Court of New York; 2004
12. In the Matter of Anesia E. (Anonymous). Administration for Children's services, respondent; and Antoinetta W. (Anonymous), appellant: Supreme Court of New York, Appellate Division, Second Department; 2005
13. Lefkowitz M. Did they hurt their own kids? Two Long Island mothers deny they have a disorder that causes them to fake illnesses in their children. *Newsday*. November 26, 2006
14. Lezon D. Spring mom gets 15 years for son's unneeded surgeries. *Houston Chronicle*. April 30, 2008
15. Trent M. A horrific casue of 'medical child abuse.' *The Prosecutor*. 2008;38

Chapter 16

Where Do We Go From Here?

Many mothers exaggerate the details of their children's illness to ensure more prompt or better medical help. Is Munchausen syndrome by proxy one end of that spectrum? It may be so, for some of the actions described in this paper share similarities with the many less striking and more common cases one encounters: mothers who seem reluctant to let their children grow up and be independent, who keep them away from school for long periods because of colds, headaches, or some minor symptom, or who continually remind their children of symptoms which if left unmentioned would soon be forgotten. —Meadow, 1982[1]

Introduction

In the introduction to this book we advocated that it is time to adopt a new paradigm to explain child abuse that occurs in the medical setting. We explained the shortcomings of the old paradigm *Munchausen syndrome by proxy (MSBP)*. We introduced the definition of *medical child abuse* and described how it shares many features with other forms of child maltreatment. It does have one significant individual characteristic. Specifically, medical abuse is a particular kind of child abuse that includes "… the active engagement with the medical profession in the production of morbidity."[2]

We explained that the motivation of the perpetrator of medical abuse is just as important as it is for any other kind of abuse, but no more necessary to invoke than for other forms of child maltreatment. We also explained that the reason the term *MSBP* and all of its synonyms has not been discarded previously has to do with the psychology of the medical profession. More than anything else we presented in the first half of this book, this point is the most important. For if we ever are to get beyond MSBP, the medical profession must come to terms with its involvement in the abuse. It must get beyond feeling ashamed and guilty, sad or angry, and admit that sometimes, thankfully not very often, people manage to have their children be harmed with inappropriate medical care.

We said earlier that we feel the rest of the child protection community has been waiting for us to do the difficult work and come to terms with the central fact of this type of abuse. As described in the last chapter, judges have begun to do the work for us by declaring irrelevant whatever it is we might have to say about MSBP. We think the medical community involved in the treatment of children can make this shift, that the time is finally right. We also think that it is time for professionals in our community to begin taking the lead in protecting children from medical abuse.

So what do we have to do? We have to try on a new way of thinking and, realizing it may take some time to get used to it, allow this new thinking to inform our medical treatment. In the *International Classification of Diseases, Ninth Revision (ICD-9)* system there is an external injury code for "motor vehicle traffic accident involving collision with pedestrian injuring pedestrian" (E814.7). If a child shows up in the hospital emergency department and this code gets written on the chart, it does not specify what kind of motor vehicle, or the state of mind of the driver, or even what kind of injury the person sustained. But it does convey the idea that something important has taken place. We have a similar diagnostic code for medical child abuse. It already exists, albeit lacking a fifth digit describing the type of abuse. The *ICD-9* code for child maltreatment (995.5) works quite well. Essentially, it indicates that something bad has happened in the life of the child. The salient feature is that a child is harmed.

Donald and Jureidini[2] have commented about how difficult it might be to get rid of the term *MSBP*. They wrote, "...it is unlikely that the term MSBP will be dispensed with now that it is the subject of hundreds of published articles." We hope they are wrong and that the term can fade into the recesses of medical history as many others have done before. Some remember when tuberculosis (along with a mixture of other pulmonary diseases) was referred to as *consumption*. But who would know that mumps was once called *branks*? As recently as 30 years ago *pseudoneurotic schizophrenia* was a common psychiatric diagnosis. This clumsy term was replaced with the name of a particular kind of personality disorder. More to the point, the diagnostic expression that began the field of child abuse, *battered child syndrome*, has long since given way to more descriptive terms. No one would write in a medical chart or appear in court today and testify that a child suffered from battered child syndrome.[3] Instead, the injuries the child received would be carefully described and not as non-accidental trauma.

Chapter 16
Where Do We Go From Here?

In our opinion, we could all do away with the term *MSBP* and be the better for it. In the introduction to this book we described a conversation with a prosecuting attorney that took place 15 years ago. He was very eager to hear the story about MSBP. We had a different set of priorities. We wanted him to know that a mother had almost killed our patient and we wanted his help in protecting the child. At that particular time we had no need to get into a discussion about the psychological makeup of the potential perpetrator. We just wanted to allow this little boy to grow up healthy.

The sooner we can get on with this change in our thinking the better. We owe it to the children and we owe it to ourselves. We think a good way to start is to agree with Mothers Against Munchausen's Syndrome by Proxy Allegations (MAMA) that MSBP is a failed concept and needs to be abandoned.

What MAMA Says

The following is taken directly from the home page of MAMA. (the emphasis is in the original):

> **M.A.M.A.** was begun in response to the fast-growing numbers of false allegations of **Munchausen syndrome by proxy (MSBP)**. Parents are being accused of making their own children ill. Increasingly, families across America, Britain, Australia, Canada and New Zealand are being destroyed by doctors and other professionals who make false and even **malicious** allegations against desperate mothers of chronically/critically ill children.
>
> The inventor of this label/diagnosis, Sir Roy Meadow, has now been completely discredited in the UK courts and there is a tremendous public outcry for review of all cases in which he has been involved.... We believe there should be a review of all cases worldwide in which MSP label has been used.
>
> The motives of the accusers can be multi-faceted. Often, allegations are used by a doctor or institution to evade medical malpractice lawsuits, or to simply rid themselves of a troublesome mom when frustrated and unable to diagnose a child's condition. Increasingly, this label is being deliberately misused

by opposing parents in child custody suits. Many nurses and even doctors have been accused. **SIDS deaths** are the new frontier of prosecution.

EVERY PARENT who is seriously advocating for their child is in imminent danger of this cruel and ridiculous allegation! Mothers are emotionally raped, publicly slandered, criminally charged and jailed. Even if their child is returned, they will suffer a lifetime from the trauma and maybe tens or hundreds of thousands of dollars in debt from the legal fees!

The word syndrome is usually used when there is a collection of abnormal symptoms or characteristics to diagnose many different genetic illnesses. The word "syndrome" in the diagnosis of Munchausen syndrome by proxy, is a collection of normal **personality characteristics** (sometimes called warning signs) of the caregiver. Never should a pediatrician engage in evaluating a parent's motives for the suspected abuse. A pediatrician must deal with science, not innuendo or personal bias. Even the most seasoned psychologists would avoid evaluating someone during a life crisis, yet this diagnosis relies on the unqualified evaluation of the parent's emotions during just such a time. It is serious misconduct to refer to a parent's demeanor as a basis for suspecting abuse.

The madness continues as the "experts" debate over this controversial diagnosis. Some say it is rare, while others claim it is common. The evolution of this diagnosis continues as even the name is debated...Factitious Disorder by Proxy, Meadows Syndrome, Pediatric Falsification, etc. All while vying to be the top expert in this field, some claim it is a psychiatric condition, while others state it is a medical diagnosis, or a pattern of behavior. Yet they all involve identifying the psychological motivation of the parent. Munchausen by Proxy is not recognized by the American Medical Association or the American Psychiatric Association. Any physician who diagnoses this 'disorder' rather than identifying actual abuse by medical evidence, should be reported to the Ethics board.

Innocent Mothers Are Profiled and removed from their medically fragile child **without any evidence that a crime has even occurred**. Often, on the basis of a single phone call from a doctor, CPS will rush in and confiscate a child without even interviewing the parents, **leaving the "investigation" to the accusing physician!** Mom and dad will be instantly treated as criminals, *guilty until proven innocent*, and may lose the rest of their children as well. In reality, the accusers, medical caregivers and **Child Protective Service (CPS)** workers often perpetrate the real abuse.

The child is held up like a carrot, causing the mother to dance to their tune and agree to "MSBP counseling". Much of the purpose of this is to extract a false "confession," while assuring the mother that cooperation will enable a quicker reunification. Financially and emotionally drained from their child's long illness, many moms are manipulated and then trapped in this "web of deceit" because of their inability to fight.

The false MSBP diagnosis can be gravely detrimental; adding deep emotional stress to an ill child from *maternal deprivation*. Aggressive treatment may be stopped with the assumption that just "removing the mother" will get results, risking serious consequences to the child's well-being. Also, the child's health is further jeopardized because the mother's watchful eye is replaced with rotating nurses who have little or no experience with the child and his/her intricacies….

If the MSBP diagnosis is eventually proven to be erroneous and negligent, causing real harm or **even death** to the child, both the physician and CPS workers hide behind the guise of **Good Faith Immunity Laws**. The physician will proclaim that he had a legal responsibility to report even the slightest *suspicion of abuse, even if he hadn't followed standard medical guidelines for researching all possible conditions which would produce the same symptoms*. CPS, in turn, will cry that they were only responding to the expert opinion.

> *Special note*: We acknowledge that occurrences of child abuse are very real in our society and if the physician has **real evidence** to suspect child abuse, regardless of the motive of the perpetrator, it must be investigated and the perpetrators brought to swift and effective justice!
>
> In contrast, often the agenda behind Munchausen Syndrome by Proxy is to be able to make an accusation **without evidence**, but by the Munchausen Syndrome by Proxy profile. If it is in fact a crime has been committed [sic], call it by its real name…suffocation, poisoning, tampering with urine sample, etc…offer evidence! You don't need fancy labels or self-proclaimed experts to line their pockets pretending to be the only ones who know how to diagnose a crime.

We quote this long passage from the MAMA Web site not because it represents the most articulate criticism of MSBP. There are lawyers who defend mothers in court, and psychologists who testify that MSBP does not exist who present the arguments more elegantly.[4] Physicians with concerns regarding ethics in medicine weigh in thoughtfully about covert video surveillance. But MAMA purports to be the voice of the mothers being wronged by the child protection system. For this reason if no other, it is useful to note their concerns.

In the introductory statement for their Web site the authors for MAMA succinctly summarize the difficulties of the MSBP concept. They state that the professional community cannot decide what to call it. They say that we don't know how frequently it occurs. They point out that MSBP does not meet the criteria of a syndrome. They complain that it is unfair to take a collection of personality characteristics, call it a profile, and use it to identify potential child abusers. They maintain that guessing or otherwise determining the psychological motivation of the parent is no way to make a medical diagnosis. They call attention to the confusion caused in the legal community with the use of *MSBP* and cite efforts in various countries to review all cases where MSBP was involved. They call attention to the plight of Meadow, saying he has been "completely discredited in the UK courts." They even pick up the unfortunate term *web of deceit* and turn it back on the professional community, suggesting that doctors are deceiving poor unfortunate mothers.

We agree with many of these concerns. There is no clear definition. Profiles are ineffective. Munchausen syndrome by proxy is not really a medical diagnosis. We disagree that Meadow has been discredited and that cases where children were abused should be reopened. But we do find common ground with the writers of this statement, that a physician with real evidence to suspect child abuse must report it and help society bring the perpetrators to justice. We find particular irony in the statement, "You don't need fancy labels or self-proclaimed experts to line their pockets pretending to be the only ones who know how to diagnose a crime." This sounds eerily like the judge in the Queensland decision saying that juries don't need experts to tell them if excessive health care precipitated by a parent is harmful to a child.

In contradiction to the statement by MAMA, there are numerous examples of children who have been terribly injured in the medical care environment because of the actions of their mothers. There are many examples of parents who *do* cause their children to be ill. Others fabricate symptoms or give false information that doctors rely on when giving harmful medical treatments. We advocate that a person who has caused his or her child to be harmed in the medical environment should receive the same treatment as someone who has harmed her child in another way, and that this treatment could also include prosecution if indicated.

Is There a Downside to the New Paradigm?

What is the risk of declaring an end to an old paradigm and embracing a new one? The introduction of anything new has the potential to generate anxiety. The old way of looking at things is often more comfortable than applying a novel perspective. But even a pair of comfortable old shoes eventually gets worn out and must be thrown away. In this case it seems we have much to gain by giving up the old concept.

Still, we may have problems with the new paradigm. Munchausen syndrome by proxy has often been described as rare. A defense attorney commenting on a physician who diagnosed MSBP said, "Even if he were seeing a million patients a year, he couldn't diagnose that many."[5] The prevailing wisdom is that MSBP is something the ordinary physician sees only a few times in a lifetime of practice. Frequently after lecturing about medical child abuse we have someone approach us and say, "I saw a case on the wards a few years ago…."

On the other hand, medical child abuse has the potential to be commonplace. If we conceptualize it as a failure in the doctor-patient relationship caused by a parent's actions that result in a child being harmed in the medical environment, then most physicians can identify examples in everyday practice. When using the MSBP terminology people commonly assume that we are talking about something extremely unusual—the mother who puts ground glass in the formula, or the caretaker rubbing feces in open wounds. Medical child abuse, on the other hand, describes behavior found at the far end of a long continuum of parental actions, many of which will not reach the level of seriousness to be considered abusive. Parental behaviors that fall below or just above the threshold may be much more difficult to diagnose as medical child abuse.

As we adapt the new paradigm there is the prospect that everything will start looking like medical child abuse. For example, if an anxious mother frequently calls the doctor in the middle of the night about her basically healthy child, could or should someone begin to suspect abuse? As doctors begin to examine routinely the quality of information being received from caretakers, it is reasonable to assume they will find more and more instances where they feel the treatment contract has been violated or at least grossly distorted. A new set of criteria must emerge that defines what is abusive and what is not. The medical community will need help in this effort from members of the public to set standards about what constitutes abusive parenting.

There is precedent for this process of acquiring a new awareness, overreaction, and gradual development of reasonable standards. In the 1970s, awareness of sexual abuse of children, especially incest, changed dramatically. The professional community came to know that incest is fairly common and not an extremely rare, "one in a million" occurrence. There was a realization, for example, that people hospitalized in mental health facilities had a high probability of having been sexually abused by a family member or family friend. A simple study conducted by Briere and Zaidi[6] demonstrated the growth of the understanding of this phenomenon. They reviewed 50 random charts of nonpsychotic female patients seen in a psychiatric emergency department for evidence of sexual abuse experienced in childhood. They then instructed physicians to ask each of the next 50 female patients seen whether they were sexually abused as a child. The frequency of positive responses recorded in the medical record went from 6% to 70% just by making sure the question was asked.

This flood of new information presented difficulty for child psychiatrists, mental health professionals treating adults, and also pediatricians. Pediatricians performing medical examinations on children alleged to have been sexually abused frequently thought they were seeing physical evidence of abuse. As a noteworthy example, in response to an early paper,[7] dozens of pediatricians around the country began measuring the width of the hymenal opening in young female children. Evidence of a hymenal opening greater than 4 mm in diameter was used in court proceedings as evidence of penetration. Potential perpetrators were sent to jail based on this evidence. Subsequently, investigators learned that hymenal opening width has little relationship to penetration, and that the hymenal opening of a normal child can vary widely depending on examination techniques.[7]

Years went by as investigators gathered information and came to understand that the signs and symptoms of trauma seen on vaginal examinations were subtle in many cases. Only after comparison of colposcopic photographs could child abuse experts begin to agree on what constituted true evidence of trauma.[9] Studies of normal controls have resulted in diminishing the number of positive physical findings, even in children with a clear history of abuse.[10] In fact, we now have evidence that children assessed after a perpetrator confesses to digital or penile penetration only show abnormal physical findings in 61% of cases.[11] The point we are making is not that children don't get sexually abused, but that physicians investigating possible consequences of abuse took a number of years before finding reasonable standards that met criteria for medical certainty. We assume that a similar process will occur as suspicions of medical abuse become more widespread and we decide on methods of establishing what observations to accept as positive evidence.

A medical student who recently heard us speak about medical child abuse approached us with an apocryphal observation. She said, "I've just been working on the pediatric ward and I swear half the children I saw have been medically abused." One of the possible downside risks of adapting a new paradigm is that it might be severely overused. As we proceed we need to keep this in mind and follow the tenets of evidence-based medicine.

Unusual Manifestations of Battered Child Syndrome?

In Chapter 4 we documented how physicians have come to understand that certain illnesses are more likely to be associated with false information provided by caretakers. Rather than focusing on specific attributes of alleged perpetrators, these investigators looked at illnesses such as recurrent suffocation and noted that faulty information frequently was associated with the diagnosis. We called these *the unusual manifestations of battered child syndrome* and commented that C. Henry Kempe would be proud of these efforts.

Is this where the field should be focusing its attention? Should we be identifying specific illnesses with a high propensity for false information as part of the clinical presentation? A special issue of *Child Maltreatment* (May 2002) dedicated to MSBP included a series of papers that represent this approach. Feldman and colleagues[12] wrote about asthma and allergy presentations. Hyman and colleagues[13] gave a thoughtful review of chronic intestinal pseudo-obstruction and the possibilities for falsifying symptoms. Truman and Ayoub[14] added new information regarding recurrent suffocation. These are significant contributions to the literature.

It might be possible to conceptualize medical abuse as a collection of specific illnesses like these. A clear example is polymicrobial sepsis in an immunologically competent child. One could easily imagine how a child could get different types of bacteria growing in his or her blood if someone were contaminating a central venous line with saliva, feces, or dirt. And it is equally *difficult* to imagine how a child without an underlying compromised immune system and whose central line had been carefully handled could get infected any other way. Given current knowledge, physicians should be instructed to consider possible induction of illness in all cases of polymicrobial sepsis in children with competent immune systems. But polymicrobial sepsis without a clear medical explanation is rare. Equally rare is chronic unexplained vomiting associated with ipecac administration, or seizures caused by lack of oxygen following suffocation by a parent. McClure and colleagues[15] found that fatal poisoning and suffocation by parents had a low annual incidence in Great Britain (0.5 cases/100,000 children).

While it is important to keep these illnesses in mind, there is a potentially much larger group of children hurt in the medical environment because doctors take parents' histories as truth when, in fact, they may be providing inaccurate information. It will not be enough to teach doctors to think about parent involvement in a small number of dramatic illness presentations. In our sample, 87 children met our criteria for medical child abuse. Among them were examples of unproven medical illnesses treated in almost every organ system. While we did have examples of polymicrobial sepsis, recurrent suffocation, and non-accidental poisoning, more importantly, we saw parents able to induce physicians to treat a wide variety of nonexistent illnesses.

So, while continued research into specific disease entities is warranted, we feel physician efforts should be more broadly based. We advocate introducing a new awareness into the interview and examination process that takes into account the possibility of false information, particularly in cases that are confusing or extreme. Physicians should remember that not only is it possible but it occurs frequently enough to warrant special attention. What we are asking pediatricians to do is similar to the recent admonishment of emergency department personnel to recognize domestic violence. For many years women were assaulted in the home, went to the hospital, and gave a history of walking into a door. It took a major effort to change the mindset of physicians evaluating women presenting with trauma to think about things differently. Awareness of the high prevalence of domestic violence gave doctors specific permission to consider alternatives to implausible histories.

Awareness of medical child abuse requires a doctor to think that it might be occurring. For this to happen there has to be permission not to accept the parent's description of every event at face value. An extra step should be added to the history-gathering process. The mindset change required involves returning to an oft-neglected aspect of medical history-taking. That is, the process of commenting on the *quality* of the information obtained.

When a psychologist performs psychological testing and details the findings, he includes in the report a comment on the nature of the testing environment and the quality of the effort put into the test by the subject. This observation is a judgment made by the evaluator about whether the results should be considered a "best effort." Without this piece of control information, it would be difficult to assess the validity of the findings. In a comparable fashion, medical students have long been instructed to comment on the quality of the history they receive from the patient. In geriatric and psychiatric settings it is common to see in medical records comments about the person giving the history such as, "Patient appears to be a good (or poor) historian." But in pediatric treatment a parent giving a history about the patient is rarely questioned. Too often the parent can give information without the physician assessing its accuracy. It is assumed a parent is always benevolently concerned about the child. Fortunately, this is true most of the time. But sometimes this is not the case. We need to reinstitute the process by which physicians routinely reflect and comment on the information gained from parents.

As we reviewed medical records for the data presented in Chapter 7, we had frequent examples of this loss of medical objectivity. Although at times the record included comments such as, "Parent maintains that child vomited 13 times in last 24 hours," there were just as many examples reading, "Child vomited 13 times in last 24 hours." We can assume the physician was not present in the home to count the number of episodes. By taking the parent's claim at face value, however, and reporting it without any qualification, the doctor in the second case is leaving an ambiguous record. Vomiting 13 times in a 24-hour period is a significant piece of medical information. If it is true, severe dehydration is a possibility, and the medical workup will be considerably different than if the child vomited only 3 times. Reading the second notation in the medical record, one is unable to tell whether the physician actually believes the statement. It is written as if it is a fact. We understand that physicians' time is valuable and shortcuts in notation are necessary. Nevertheless, writing in the medical record in a way that indicates one is taking a parent's history at face value might also be an indication that the physician is indeed doing just that. If this is true, the doctor is vulnerable to becoming an unwitting accomplice to medical abuse.

It all comes back to practicing good medicine. Maintaining objectivity in taking a medical history is something all physicians are trained to do. They are also trained to be empathic, and to develop positive doctor-patient relationships. These 2 objectives are not mutually exclusive. Practicing good medicine includes feeling comfortable saying, "Did your child *really* vomit 13 times or did it just seem like that many?" Likewise, there is nothing lost, and much gained, by writing in the record, "Despite additional questioning parent maintained that child literally vomited 13 times." Taking this extra step, maintaining objectivity, thinking that parent history need not always be accurate is the sine qua non for identifying medical child abuse.

The change we are advocating is not so much introducing something new as returning to historical expectations for good medical practice. We are encouraging special attention to objectivity, to taking and recording a thorough medical history, and to corroborating the parent's history with physical examination findings, laboratory testing and, if necessary, secondary sources.

Developing Research Criteria

In constructing tools for assessing medical child abuse as described in Chapter 7, we followed research protocols developed for other forms of child maltreatment. Researchers studying physical or sexual abuse identify specific behaviors that can be described objectively and that most people would consider abusive. Research of child maltreatment, similar to other kinds of research, depends on defining variables and finding ways to measure them. For example, to study sexual abuse one begins with a general definition and then adds specific questions to characterize severity. The general question might be, "Have you ever experienced unwanted sexual contact prior to age 14 by someone at least 4 years older?" Following this would be a series of questions indicating the severity of abuse. The questions could include such things as, "Did this involve contact with your genitals through your clothing?" or "Did this involve digital or penile penetration?" By asking the questions regarding specific actions on a spectrum from least to most severe, one can construct a simple measure of severity. With physical abuse a general question might be, "In childhood did you ever experience something that most people would consider to be physically abusive?" Severity questions could include, "Have you ever been struck by a parent with a physical object such as a stick or a belt?" or "Have you ever been thrown against a wall?" or "Have you ever been threatened or assaulted by a parent with a lethal object such as a knife or gun?"

Questions we used to describe medical child abuse fell into 2 general categories. We wanted information about the severity of the abuse itself and also information regarding the contribution of the parent caretaker. To determine the nature of the medical abuse we asked ourselves, based on the review of medical records, the first general question, "Did this child receive unnecessary and harmful or potentially harmful medical care at the instigation of a caretaker?" We then went on to ask a series of questions that we felt indicated increasing levels of severity of abuse.

1. Did the child receive unnecessary medical or psychological examinations?
2. Did the child receive unnecessary but noninvasive medical testing (eg, urinalysis, throat cultures)?
3. Did the child receive unnecessary but minimally invasive medical testing (eg, blood tests, x-rays)?
4. Did the child receive unnecessary medicine as a result of actions of the caretaker?
5. Did the child receive invasive medical testing (eg, endoscopy, spinal taps)?
6. Did the child receive unnecessary surgery (eg, placement of pressure equalization tubes in the eardrums, Nissen fundoplication)?

An affirmative answer to any of these questions represents an example of possible medical child abuse. Obviously, receiving multiple medical examinations is less harmful to a child than having a central line placed or receiving a bowel transplant. Establishing research criteria to indicate possible severity of the condition is different from a legal definition and clearly distinct from how that legal definition might be interpreted in a particular situation. Developing research criteria is important in coming to understand medical abuse and informing us about its extent, variability of expression, and what child might be most vulnerable. These are different questions than whether a particular child should be protected from his mother.

While we used these questions to indicate severity of medical abuse in our sample, we expect other investigators might have other questions or interpret the severity continuum in a different way. For example, we ranked receiving any unnecessary prescribed medication as more serious than undergoing noninvasive testing but less serious than invasive testing. Our thinking involved the consideration that noninvasive testing might be necessary to rule out a potential diagnostic entity suggested by the parents' history. However, the same argument could be used for more invasive procedures. It seemed to us that invasive procedures involve violating the child's personhood in a way that prescribing unnecessary medications might not.

To examine the parent's behavior we followed commonly accepted descriptions of increasing involvement in causing medical treatment to occur. The questions we used included

1. Did the parent exhibit persistent anxiety that resulted in unnecessary medical care?

2. Did the parent persistently exaggerate existing symptoms resulting in unnecessary medical care?

3. Did the parent fabricate symptoms (in the absence of any symptom) or fabricate medical test results in a way that resulted in unnecessary medical care?

4. Did the parent induce symptoms in a child resulting in unnecessary medical care? (Doing something to a child to make them ill constitutes physical abuse. Medical treatment given based on a parent's deception regarding what he or she did to the child constitutes medical abuse.)

Intuitively one would expect morbidity in the child to increase with the severity of the medical abuse. The more invasive the medical treatment received, the more impact there should be on the child. Our preliminary results do not indicate a linear relationship between a parent's increasing level of involvement and severity of abuse of the child. It seems to us that a parent can cause a child to have just as high a level of medical abuse with exaggerating symptoms as with actually physically assaulting the child. Laura, for example, who received more abusive medical treatment than anyone else in our series had a mother who primarily exaggerated symptoms. We never found evidence that she induced any medical condition.

The Financial Cost of Medical Child Abuse

We suggest high priority be given to research regarding the cost of medical child abuse, both in financial terms and in the allocation of medical resources. We stated previously that we estimated more than $3 million was spent on unnecessary medical treatment for one of our patients, Laura. There were 6 other children in our sample who we estimate consumed at least $1 million in unnecessary care. These are startling numbers. It is difficult to imagine how one can spend $1 million for health care in the first few years of a child's life unless they are very critically ill.

Perhaps more important than the monetary cost is the significant waste of medical resources. For example, the child we evaluated who had been to his pediatrician's office an average of every 2½ days for the first 24 months of his life did not meet our million-dollar benchmark but did take away opportunity for treatment from other children with demonstrable illnesses who may have benefited from the services of that pediatric practice. Our index case, who predated our chart review study, would not meet the $1 million threshold either. But he did require several weeks in the intensive care unit (ICU) on a respirator that was therefore not available to treat another child. He was in the ICU because he was seriously ill but, had we discovered earlier that his mother was frequently inducing illness, he would not have required such expensive treatment.

Starfield and colleagues[16] pointed out 30 years ago that a small portion of pediatric patients can be identified as "high utilizers" of pediatric care. Some of these children are seriously ill with chronic debilitating disease. Others are not. At present, we do not know what portion of medical care resources is consumed by victims of medical child abuse. It is important to find out.

Finally, Some Thoughts About Hippocrates

It is commonly believed that somewhere in the Hippocratic oath is the statement, "First, do no harm." In researching this book we went back to our graduation ceremony from medical school to look at the oath we swore. We were surprised to find that, "First, do no harm" was not there. We did swear, "I will apply, for the benefit of the sick, all measures that are required, avoiding those twin traps of overtreatment and therapeutic nihilism." We did agree to admit when we didn't know what was wrong with the patient, to ask for help when needed, and to respect the patient's privacy. But we did not swear to "do no harm."

It turns out that the phrase for which Hippocrates is most famous probably did originate with him. In his book, *Epidemics* (Book I, Section XI), is the phrase that reads in translation, "Declare the past, diagnose a patient, foretell the future; practice these acts. As to diseases, make a habit of two things—to help, or least to do no harm."

It is in this spirit that we invite our medical colleagues and the families who help us treat their children to join together to "first, do no harm."

References

1. Meadow R. Munchausen syndrome by proxy. *Arch Dis Child.* 1982;57(2):92-98
2. Donald T, Jureidini J. Munchausen syndrome by proxy. Child abuse in the medical system. *Arch Pediatr Adolesc Med.* 1996;150(7):753-758
3. Boros SJ, Ophoven JP, Andersen R, Brubaker LC. Munchausen syndrome by proxy: a profile for medical child abuse. *Aust Fam Physician.* 1995;24(5):768-769, 772-763
4. Mart E. *Munchausen's Syndrome by Proxy Reconsidered.* Manchester, NH: Bally Vaughn Publishing; 2002
5. Smith C. Persecuted parents or protected children? Allegations cost their reputations, their money and nearly their kids. *Seattle Post-Intelligencer.* August 7, 2002
6. Briere J, Zaidi LY. Sexual abuse histories and sequelae in female psychiatric emergency room patients. *Am J Psychiatry.* 1989;146(12):1602-1606
7. Cantwell HB. Vaginal inspection as it relates to child sexual abuse in girls under thirteen. *Child Abuse Negl.* 1983;7(2):171-176
8. Berenson AB, Chacko MR, Wiemann CM, Mishaw CO, Friedrich WN, Grady JJ. Use of hymenal measurements in the diagnosis of previous penetration. *Pediatrics.* 2002;109(2):228-235
9. McCann J. The appearance of acute, healing, and healed anogenital trauma. *Child Abuse Negl.* 1998;22(6):605-615; discussion 617-622
10. Adams JA, Harper K, Knudson S, Revilla J. Examination findings in legally confirmed child sexual abuse: it's normal to be normal. *Pediatrics.* 1994; 94(3):310-317
11. Muram D. Child sexual abuse: relationship between sexual acts and genital findings. *Child Abuse Negl.* 1989;13(2):211-216
12. Feldman KW, Stout JW, Inglis AF Jr. Asthma, allergy, and sinopulmonary disease in pediatric condition falsification. *Child Maltreat.* 2002;7(2):125-131
13. Hyman PE, Bursch B, Beck D, DiLorenzo C, Zeltzer LK. Discriminating pediatric condition falsification from chronic intestinal pseudo-obstruction in toddlers. *Child Maltreat.* 2002;7(2):132-137
14. Truman TL, Ayoub CC. Considering suffocatory abuse and Munchausen by proxy in the evaluation of children experiencing apparent life-threatening events and sudden infant death syndrome. *Child Maltreat.* 2002;7(2):138-148
15. McClure RJ, Davis PM, Meadow SR, Sibert JR. Epidemiology of Munchausen syndrome by proxy, non-accidental poisoning, and non-accidental suffocation. *Arch Dis Child.* 1996;75(1):57-61
16. Starfield B, van den Berg BJ, Steinwachs DM, Katz HP, Horn SD. Variations in utilization of health services by children. *Pediatrics.* 1979;63(4):633-641

Index

A

Abdominal pain. *See* Gastrointestinal cases
Achievement by proxy, 25
"Acute Water Intoxication as Another Unusual Manifestation of Child Abuse," 65
Allergy cases, 51
    extreme aero-allergen avoidance, 70
    informing session, use of, 207–208
Alveolitis, type III, 79–80
Anecdotal information, use of, 14
Anemia, iron deficiency, 25–26, 64
Anorexia nervosa, 245–246
Anxiety
    parental anxiety, 183, 190–191
    PTSD-related, 13
Apnea, recurrent, 8, 103
APSAC Taskforce on Munchausen by Proxy, Definitions Working Group, 52–53
Aspiration pneumonia, 2
Asthma cases, 26–27, 51
    HCPHP/*ChildSafe* program cases, 135
    informing session, use of, 207–208
    MSBP prevalence rates, 31
Attachment difficulties, 262–263
Attachment theory, 116
Attorneys, 293–295. *See also* Legal system
    awareness of medical child abuse, 299–300
    as "guardians ad litem," 14
    how attorneys think, 293–295
    as part of the solution, 13–14, 293–306
Availability heuristic, 8

B

"Bacteriologically Battered Baby, The: Another Case of Munchausen by Proxy," 67
Barbiturate poisoning, 67
Battered child syndrome, 17
    unusual manifestations of, 7, 8, 63, 77–88, 318–321
"Battered Child Syndrome, The," 7
Briquet's syndrome, 123
Bleeding disorders, 71–72, 155–156
    detecting illness fabrication, 71–72
"Blended cases," 270
Bloody urine, 3
Bowel obstruction, 87–88, 103
Bulimia nervosa, 243
Burns on cheek, 26

C

Cardiac anomalies
    detecting abuse in cases involving, 170–171, 192
    HCPHP/*ChildSafe* program cases, 135
    recurrent cardiorespiratory arrest, 68–69
Case studies, 9–10
    1983–1987 case reports, 63–73
    HCPHP/*ChildSafe* program(s). *See* HCPHP/*ChildSafe* program(s)
Chart notes, 228

Chart review, 14
"Chemical abuse," 65, 66. *See also* Poisoning cases
"Chemically Abused Child, The," 65
Child abuse
  life-threatening, 83
  medical. *See* Medical child abuse
  Munchausen syndrome by proxy as, 1–2
  renaming MSBP as, 35
Child abuse specialists, 175–176, 177, 295–297
  evaluations by, 177–182
Child maltreatment
  and medical child abuse, 44, 45, 49–53
  treatment of, 160–161
  what is, 44–45
Child neglect, 20, 44
Child protection. *See* Protection of child
Child protection team (CPT), 11, 214–215, 217
ChildSafe program. *See* HCPHP/*ChildSafe* program(s)
Chlorpromazine poisoning, 65–66
Chronic fatigue syndrome, 137, 285–286
Chronic intestinal pseudo-obstruction, 87–88, 103
Clostridium difficile infection, 186
Cognitive distortions, 13
  treatment of, 268–271
Complex regional syndrome, 286–287
Constipation. *See* Gastrointestinal cases
Consulting specialists. *See* Specialty care physicians
Covert video surveillance, 194–196
  arguments against using, 194–195
  arguments in favor of using, 195–196
  as "entrapment," 195
  informed consent, 194
  Meadow's use in suffocation cases, 4
  privacy issues, 195
  suffocation cases, use in, 4, 81–83
CPT. *See* Child protection team (CPT)
Crohn's disease, 135
"Crossing the line," 50–51, 123
Cult diets, 66
CVS. *See* Covert video surveillance
Cystic fibrosis case, 72–73

D

"Dauphin of Munchausen: Factitious Passage of Renal Stones in a Child, The," 22
Defensive medicine, 298–299
Depression, 13
Diagnosis
  child focus, need for, 93–94
  emotionally deprived/disturbed perpetrator, 114, 115–116
  mental illness of perpetrator, 98–101, 105–106, 113
  Munchausen syndrome by proxy, 18–20
  preliminary interventions, use of, 190–193
  psychological explanations, 113, 114, 115–118
  psychoses of perpetrator, 113, 114
  video surveillance, use of. *See* Covert video surveillance
  of whom, 23–24, 56
Diagnostic and Statistical Manual of Mental Disorders, Fourth Edition (DSM-IV)
  APSAC Taskforce discussion of classifications, 53
  factitious disorder, not otherwise specified, 24–25

factitious disorder by proxy, 19, 20, 23, 144–145
somatization disorder, 123
Diarrhea cases, 134, 186. *See also* Gastrointestinal cases
Diets
cult diets, 66
food allergy, 80
Discharge summaries, 228
Disordered Mother or Disordered Diagnosis? 20
Doctor-patient relationship, 125–127, 167. *See also* Medical community
Doctor shopping, 22, 270

E

Ear infections, 203–204
Eating disorders, 243, 245–246
Electroencephalogram (EEG) evidence, 78
Emotional abuse, 45
Emotionally deprived/disturbed perpetrators, 114, 115–116
Emotional neglect, 44
Epilepsy
false, 78–79
seizures. *See* Seizure cases
Evidence-based medicine, 166
Exaggeration of illness, 10
detecting, 184, 185, 191–192
extreme illness exaggeration, 79–80

F

Fabricated illnesses, 52
Fabricated or induced illness in a child by a carer, 23, 93
Fabrication/falsification of illness, 10
as child abuse, 46
detecting, 184, 185, 189–190
reasons for, 119–122

Factitious disorder, not otherwise specified (NOS), 24–25
Factitious disorder by proxy (FDP), 1, 22, 23, 24, 98. *See also* Munchausen syndrome by proxy (MSBP)
APSAC Taskforce classification, 52–53
as caretaker focused, 93
DSM-IV criteria, 19, 20, 23, 144–145
HCPHP/*ChildSafe* program case studies, 144–145
Failure to thrive (FTT), 52, 64
from food allergy diets, 80
HCPHP/*ChildSafe* program cases, 137
False epilepsy, 78–79
Falsification of illness. *See* Fabrication/falsification of illness
Family cooperation/involvement
HCPHP/*ChildSafe* program(s), 242–247
after the informing session, 211–212
Family systems response, need for, 216–217
Family systems theory, 117
Family unit, 239–240
preservation of, 275–277
Fatality rates. *See* Mortality rates
Fatigue, 137, 285–286
Fever, exaggeration/fabrication of, 172
Financial costs, 323–324
Flashback phenomena, 264
Food allergy diets, 80
Foster care, medical, 233–234
Future directions, 309–324

G

Gasoline poisoning, 117
Gastrointestinal cases
   bleeding in the GI tract, 71–72
   HCPHP/*ChildSafe* program cases, 138–141, 248–255
   identifying the abuse, 173
   pseudo-obstruction, 87–88, 103
"Guardians ad litem," 14

H

Hasbro Children's Partial Hospital Program (HCPHP). *See* HCPHP/*ChildSafe* program(s)
HCPHP/*ChildSafe* program(s), 131–132, 241–248
   abused versus non-abused children in, 145–148
   case examples, 133–138, 243–246, 248–255
   case involvement, 138–141
   "factitious disorder by proxy" criteria, 144–145
   family involvement/partnership, 242–247
   identification of victims, 132–133
   illness presentations in abused group, 148–150
   interventions in abuse cases, 151–152
   "medical child abuse" criteria, 141–144
   patients in, 241
   philosophy of, 242
   specialist colleagues, working with, 285–289
   staff, 241
   starting at different places, 255–257
   treatment/treatment model, 151–152, 241–243, 244, 245, 282–283
   unnecessary medical care received, 143, 148

Head trauma, abusive, 17
Hematuria, 3
Hippocratic Oath, 324
Historical backdrop, 7–8, 61–62
   pre-1977 years, 62–66
   1977–1982 acceptance of MSBP, 66–68
   1983–1987 case reports, 68–73
   1987 "Web of Deceit . . ." report, 73–74
Hospital environment
   safety of child in, 230–232
   separation of child from parent, 190
Hurting for Love, 22, 24, 116
Hypoglycemia, 66, 102
Hysteria, 123

I

Identifying the abuse, 11, 165–169
   child abuse expert's evaluation, 177–182
   child abuse specialists, 175–176, 177, 295–297
   covert video surveillance. *See* Covert video surveillance
   HCPHP, children in, 132–133
   illness exaggeration and, 184, 185, 191–192
   illness fabrication and, 184, 185, 189–190
   illness induction and, 185, 190, 192–193
   medical record review, 177–182, 249–250
   parental anxiety and, 183, 190–191
   preliminary interventions, use of, 190–193
   in primary care practices, 169–173, 176–177
   in specialty care practices, 173–175, 177
Illness behavior, role of, 118–119

Illness exaggeration. *See* Exaggeration of illness
Illness fabrication. *See* Fabrication/falsification of illness
Illness induction. *See* Induction of illness
Illness induction syndrome, 22
Induction of illness, 10
  detecting, 185, 190, 192–193
Informing session, the, 11, 206–211
  family cooperation, 211–212
"Intentional Poisoning of Two Siblings by Prescription Drugs: An Unusual Form of Child Abuse," 67
Intergenerational patterns, 34–35
Intervention, 34
  HCPHP/*ChildSafe* case studies, 151–152
  minimum necessary, 221–227
  persuasive intervention, 223–226
  preliminary, for diagnostic purposes, 190–193
Intestinal conditions. *See* Gastrointestinal cases
Intravenous poisoning, 135
Ipecac-induced vomiting, 101–102
Iron deficiency anemia, 25–26, 64

K
Kaspar Hauser syndrome, 21

L
Lawyers. *See* Attorneys
Learning theory, 116–117
Legal system. *See also* Attorneys
  cooperation of, 156
  medical child abuse, growing awareness of, 299–300
  Queensland decision, 300–303
  reporting abuse. *See* Reporting abuse
  rewriting statutory law, 303–304
  stopping the abuse, 215–216
Leg paralysis, 137
Letters to other physicians, 228–229, 253–254
Long-term hospitalization. *See* Hospital environment
Long-term safety. *See* Ongoing safety
Lying about illness. *See* Fabrication/falsification of illness
Lyme disease, 284–285

M
"Malingering," 28
Malnutrition
  from cult diets, 66
  HCPHP/*ChildSafe* program cases, 137, 256–257
  starvation cases, 105
Malpractice
  and defensive medicine, 298–299
  medical child abuse, distinguished, 46, 56
  versus unnecessary medical care, 281–282
MAMA (Mothers Against Munchausen Syndrome by Proxy Allegations), 4, 106, 311–315
Meadow's syndrome, 22
  as caretaker focused, 93
"Medea complex, the," 115
Medical abuse, 45, 47, 54, 58
Medical child abuse, 43
  and child maltreatment, 44, 45, 49–53
  HCPHP/*ChildSafe* case studies, 141–148
  distinguished from other types of abuse, 54–55
  financial costs, 323–324
  future directions, 309–324
  growing acceptance of term, 46–48

Medical child abuse, *continued*
   historical developments. *See* Historical backdrop
   identifying. *See* Identifying the abuse
   malpractice, distinguished, 46, 56
   as a new paradigm, 6–7, 44, 315–317
   non-abused children, importance of distinguishing, 153–154
   putting the concept into practice, 55–58
   statutory law, 303–304
   treatment of. *See* Treatment
   what is, 1, 43–46
   when MSBP does not exist, 101–103
Medical community
   building consensus, 11, 199–205, 282–283
   child abuse specialists. *See* Child abuse specialists
   cooperation of, 156
   defensive medicine, 298–299
   doctor-patient relationship, 125–127, 167
   at esteemed medical centers, 285–287
   as FDP perpetrators, 25
   Hippocratic Oath, 324
   how doctors think, 293–295
   inadvertent role in abuse, 95–98, 167
   letters to members of, 228–229, 253–254
   malpractice. *See* Malpractice
   mental illness of mother rationalization, 98–101
   nontraditional practitioners, 284–285
   as part of the problem, 13, 279–290
   "practicing good medicine," 165–169
   primary care pediatricians, 169–173, 176–177
   roles and responsibilities, 93–108, 124–127, 279–281
   self-protective reaction, avoidance of, 104
   specialty care physicians. *See* Specialty care physicians
   "trust but verify" approach, 168
   what doctors *should* do, 103–104
Medical foster care, 233–234
"Medical game, the," 71, 168
Medical malpractice. *See* Malpractice
Medical neglect, 125
Medical records
   ongoing safety, use for promotion of, 227–229
   review to identify abuse, 177–182, 249–250
   sample chart used to review, 179
Medicinal abuse, 47. *See also* Poisoning cases
Mental illness diagnosis/explanation, 98–101, 105–106, 113
Minimum intervention necessary, use of, 221–227
Mortality rates, 30, 31, 32
   presumption about, 51
Motivation of perpetrator, 9, 111–112
   conscious awareness, 27–28
   difficulty in determining, 139–140
   DSM-IV criteria, 19
   emotional deprivation/disturbance explanation, 114, 115–116
   as inappropriate diagnostic focus, 93–94
   lying, reasons for, 119–122
   mental illness explanation, 98–101, 105–106, 113
   no conscious intent, 28

physician's roles and
    responsibilities, 124–127
psychological explanations, 113,
    114, 115–118
psychopathic explanation, 114
psychotic explanation, 113
relevancy of, 28–29, 44, 56, 93–94
sociological theories, 118–119
somatization disorder, 123–124
vulnerable child syndrome,
    122–123
"Munchausen Syndrome by Proxy:
    The Hinterland of Child Abuse,"
    3, 7–8, 61, 66
Munchausen syndrome by proxy
    abuse, 48, 84
Munchausen syndrome by proxy/
    fabricated and induced illness,
    23
Munchausen syndrome by proxy
    (MSBP)
    1977–1982 acceptance of, 66–68
    as caretaker focused, 93
    as child abuse, 1–2
    diagnostic criteria, 18–20
    DSM-IV criteria, 19, 20
    Hasbro Children's Partial Hospital
        Program (HCPHP). *See*
        HCPHP/*ChildSafe* program(s)
    historical developments. *See*
        Historical backdrop
    as an "interactional disorder," 220
    medical abuse as synonym for, 47
    motivation of perpetrator. *See*
        Motivation of perpetrator
    multiple uses of term, 24–27
    need for a new paradigm, 17–35
    nonexistent, abuse when, 101–103
    origin of term, 17, 21
    prevalence of, 30–32, 57
    profile of perpetrator, 32–33, 57
    psychoanalytic formulation for,
        115–116

renaming the term, 21–23
Rosenberg's criteria, 18, 20,
    142–144, 145
scope of concept, 24–27, 56
seriousness of, 32, 57
as a "syndrome," 18–20, 55
treatment of. *See* Treatment
use of term, 1, 5, 47–48, 94,
    310–311
who should be diagnosed, 23–24,
    56

N

"Nonaccidental Poisoning: An
    Extended Syndrome of Child
    Abuse," 65
Nontraditional medical practitioners,
    284–285

O

"Obstacles to the Treatment of
    Munchausen by Proxy
    Syndrome," 155
"Oh, No!" event, significance of, 95–98
Ongoing safety, 219–220
    defining, 235–236
    medical foster care, 233–234
    medical record, promotion of
        ongoing safety with, 227–229
    minimum intervention necessary,
        use of, 221–227
    out-of-home placements, 229–232
    parent education, 222–224
    persuasive intervention, 223–226
    removal of child from caretaker. *See*
        Removal of child from caretaker
    termination of parental rights, 221,
        234–235
Out-of-home placements, 229–232

P

Pancreatitis, 120
"Pansinusitis," 120, 184

Paradigms
  and scientific thought, 6
  shift in. *See* Paradigm shift
Paradigm shift
  concept of, 6
  medical child abuse as, 6–7, 44, 315–317
Paralysis, 137
Parental anxiety, 183, 190–191
Parental rights termination, 221, 234–235
Parent education, 222–224
Parent-perpetrators
  emotionally deprived/disturbed, 114, 115–116
  mental illness, 98–101, 105–106, 113
  motivation of. *See* Motivation of perpetrator
  non-perpetrator parents, treatment of, 271–273
  profiling, 32–33, 57
  psychiatric treatment of, 34, 161–162, 273–275
  psychological explanations, 113, 114, 115–118
  removal of child from. *See* Removal of child from caretaker
  termination of parental rights, 221, 234–235
  treatment approach to, 107
  "trust but verify," 168
  video surveillance of. *See* Covert video surveillance
Parent's belief system
  as determinant of child's health, 191
  educating parents to alter, 222–223
  and vulnerable child syndrome, 122
Parents–non-perpetrators, treatment of, 271–273
Pediatric condition falsification, 1, 23, 24. *See also* Munchausen syndrome by proxy (MSBP)

APSAC Taskforce classification, 53
  as caretaker focused, 93
Perpetrators. *See* Parent-perpetrators
Perphenazine poisoning, 63–64
Persistent parent, the, 22
Persuasive intervention, 223–226
Pets as FDP victims, 25
Phenobarbital therapy, 71
Physical abuse, 50, 52
  fatal, 45
  treatment approach, 106–107
Physical consequences, treatment of, 12
HCPHP. *See* HCPHP/*ChildSafe* program(s)
  without a partial hospital program, 257–258
Physical neglect, 44
Physicians and other medical personnel. *See* Medical community
Pigeon fancier's lung, 79–80
Placement of child
  long-term hospitalization. *See* Hospital environment
  medical foster care, 233–234
  out-of-home placements, 229–232
Pneumonia, aspiration, 2
"Poisoning: A Syndrome of Child Abuse," 66
Poisoning cases
  1983–1987 case reports, 69–70
  barbiturate poisoning, 67
  chlorpromazine poisoning, 65–66
  gasoline poisoning, 117
  intravenous poisoning, 135
  ipecac-induced vomiting, 101–102
  perphenazine poisoning, 63–64
  pre-1977, 63–66
  prescription drugs, use of, 68
  salt poisoning, 3, 66, 157
  warfarin poisoning, 67
Polle syndrome, 21, 67

Polymicrobial sepsis, 3, 8, 66, 67, 69, 85–87
  HCPHP/*ChildSafe* program cases, 136
Porphyria cases, 136
  persuasive intervention in, 224–225
Post-traumatic stress disorder (PTSD), 13, 261, 264–265
  treatment of, 265–268
"Practicing good medicine," 165–169
  Hippocratic Oath, 324
Preliminary interventions, diagnostic use of, 190–193
Prescription drugs, poisoning with, 68
Prevalence rates, 30–32, 57
Prevention of reoccurrence. *See* Protection of child
Primary care pediatricians, 169–173, 176–177
Profiling perpetrators, 32–33, 57
Protection of child
  identifying the abuse. *See* Identifying the abuse
  intervention. *See* Intervention
  ongoing protection. *See* Ongoing safety
  steps in, 10
  stopping the abuse. *See* Stopping the abuse
  through treatment. *See* Treatment
Protection orders, 215–216
Psychiatric treatment of child, 12–13, 259–262
  attachment difficulties, 263
  building consensus about, 282–283
  cognitive distortions, 268–271
  disagreements about, 283
  family integrity, maintenance of, 275–277
  nontraditional medical practitioners, 284–285
  post-traumatic stress disorder, 265–268

Psychiatric treatment of parents
  non-perpetrator parents, 271–273
  perpetrator parents, 34, 161–162, 273–275
Psychological abuse, 44, 54
Psychological diagnoses/explanations, 113, 114, 115–118
Psychological neglect, 44
Psychopathic diagnosis/explanation, 114
"Psychotherapy for Munchausen by Proxy Syndrome," 155
Psychotic diagnosis/explanation, 113

Q
Queensland decision, 300–303

R
Removal of child from caretaker, 220–221, 227
  medical foster care, 233–234
  out-of-home placements, 229–232
  therapeutic separation, 190
Reoccurrence, prevention of. *See* Protection of child
Reporting abuse, 193, 212–213
  mandatory reporting laws, 297–298
  warning parent to prevent abuse, 225–226
Research
  criteria, development of, 321–323
  methodology, 14

S
Safety of child. *See* Protection of child
"Salicylate Poisoning as a Manifestation of the Battered Child Syndrome," 63
Salt poisoning, 3, 66, 157
School absences, 248
  HCPHP/*ChildSafe* program cases, 134

Seizure cases
　identifying the abuse, 188–189
　Phenobarbital therapy, 71
Separation of child from caretaker. *See* Removal of child from caretaker
Sepsis cases
　HCPHP/*ChildSafe* program cases, 134
　identifying the abuse, 166–167
　polymicrobial. *See* Polymicrobial sepsis
　stopping the abuse, 204–205
Seriousness of MSBP, 32, 57
Sexual abuse, 45, 50, 51, 52, 54
"Sexual neglect," 44
Shaken baby syndrome, 17
"Sick role," 118–119
Skin lesions, 26
Smothered children, 81, 117–118. *See also* Suffocation cases
Social services involvement, 212–216
Sociological theories of motivation, 118–119
Somatization disorder, 123–124
　treatment of, 126
Specialty care physicians, 173–175, 177
　working with, 285–289
"Splitting," 283
Starvation cases, 105. *See also* Malnutrition
Statutory law
　mandatory reporting laws, 297–298
　rewriting abuse and neglect statutes, 303–304
Stopping the abuse, 11, 160, 161, 199. *See also* Ongoing safety
　building consensus, 199–205
　family cooperation, 211–212
　family systems response, need for, 216–217
　informing session, the, 11, 206–212
　leadership necessary, 201
　legal system, 215–216
　removal of child. *See* Removal of child from caretaker
　social services involvement, 212–216
Sudden infant death syndrome (SIDS), 80, 81, 84–85, 183
Suffocation cases
　acute water intoxication, 65
　covert video surveillance, use of, 4, 81–83
　HCPHP/*ChildSafe* program cases, 136
　psychological explanations, 117–118
　recurrent cardiorespiratory arrest and, 69
　recurrent suffocation, 66, 80–85
　throat obstruction, 103
"Symptom coaching," 270

T

Termination of parental rights, 221, 234–235
Treatment, 155–163
　child maltreatment cases, compared, 160–161
　ChildSafe/HCPHP program(s), children in, 151–152, 241–242, 244, 245, 282–283
　effectiveness of, 33–35, 57, 155–163
　framework necessary for, 125
　goals of, 220
　ideas important in, 158–159
　informing session, the. *See* Informing session, the
　model/program, 12, 13. *See also* HCPHP/*ChildSafe* program(s)
　options, 104–107
　of physical consequences. *See* Physical consequences, treatment of

of psychological consequences. *See* Psychiatric treatment of child; Psychiatric treatment of parents
somatization disorder, 126
steps important in, 160
therapeutic separation, 190

U

"Uncommon Manifestations of the Battered Child Syndrome," 7, 63
"Untreatable Family, The," 234–235
Urethra, stones in, 26
Urinary tract infections, recurrent, 3

V

Video surveillance. *See* Covert video surveillance
Virtual factitious disorder by proxy, 25
Vomiting cases
   bulimia nervosa, 243
   HCPHP/*ChildSafe* program cases, 136–137
   ipecac-induced vomiting, 101–102
   out-of-home placements, 229–230
   termination of parental rights, 234
von Munchausen, Baron, 21, 61
Vulnerable child syndrome, 122–123
   and parental anxiety, 183

W

Warfarin poisoning, 67
Water intoxication, 65, 66
"Web of Deceit: A Literature Review of Munchausen Syndrome by Proxy," 8, 30, 31, 62, 73–74
"Witch hunts," 201, 202